SEXUAL HEALTH
IN A DIVERSE WORLD

Consuelo A. Bonillas, Ph.D
Kean University

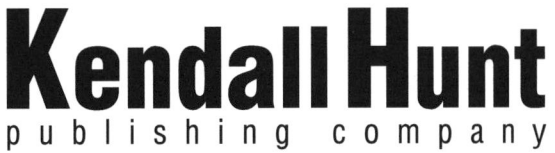

Cover image © Shutterstock, Inc.

Kendall Hunt
publishing company

www.kendallhunt.com
Send all inquiries to:
4050 Westmark Drive
Dubuque, IA 52004-1840

Copyright © 2012 by Consuelo A. Bonillas

ISBN 978-0-7575-9786-2

Kendall Hunt Publishing Company has the exclusive rights to reproduce this work,
to prepare derivative works from this work, to publicly distribute this work,
to publicly perform this work and to publicly display this work.

All rights reserved. No part of this publication may be reproduced,
stored in a retrieval system, or transmitted, in any form or by any
means, electronic, mechanical, photocopying, recording, or otherwise,
without the prior written permission of the copyright owner.

Printed in the United States of America
10 9 8 7 6 5 4 3 2 1

Table of Contents

ONE	Sexual Health in the United States	1
TWO	Social Media & Sexual Health	17
THREE	Theories That Promote Sexual Health	29
FOUR	Female Sexual/Reproductive Anatomy & Physiology	39
FIVE	Male Sexual/Reproductive Anatomy & Physiology	71
SIX	Female & Male Sexual Arousal & Response	93
SEVEN	Reproductive Tract Infections	117
EIGHT	Gender Issues	139
NINE	Sexual Orientations	159
TEN	Companionship & Marriage	173
ELEVEN	Conception, Pregnancy, & Outcomes	189
TWELVE	Contraception	225
THIRTEEN	Sex as a Business	247
FOURTEEN	Paraphilias	259

chapter one

SEXUAL HEALTH IN THE UNITED STATES

CHAPTER OBJECTIVES

On completion of this chapter, students will be able to:

- comprehend what broadly constitutes sexual health;
- describe past laws used to restrict the rights of others in sexual health;
- discuss laws enacted to expand the rights of others in sexual health.

ABBREVIATIONS AND ACRONYMS USED IN THIS CHAPTER

CDC	Centers for Disease Control and Prevention
IDU	injection drug use
IUD	intra-uterine device
MSM	men who have sex with men
SIECUS	Sexuality Information Education Council of the United States
STIs	Sexually Transmitted Infections

WHAT IS SEXUAL HEALTH?

How would you define *sexual health*? For example, would your definition of sexual health include living without a sexually transmitted infection (STI) or being able to prevent an unintended pregnancy? Does your sexual health depend on the sexual health of another? For example, how do you know that your sexual partner does not have an STI? Moreover, how do you know that *you* don't have an STI? Do you place your sexual health above all else, regardless of the well-being of others? For example, do you care if your sexual partner is sexually satisfied during your sexual interactions with each other or is it "all about you"? The scope of sexual health varies by gender, culture, and religion (to name a few influences). For example, a woman can visit a gynecologist in the United States to discuss her sexual health needs, but with whom does a man regularly visit to discuss his own sexual health needs?

> *The World Health Organization (2006) defines sexual health as a state of physical, emotional, mental, and social well-being related to sexuality. It is not merely the absence of disease, dysfunction or infirmity. Sexual health requires a positive and respectful approach to sexuality and sexual relationships, as well as the possibility of having pleasurable and safe sexual experiences, free of coercion, discrimination and violence. For sexual health to be attained and maintained, the sexual rights of all persons must be respected, protected and fulfilled.*

This definition of sexual health may be hard to achieve in countries where some members of society are not considered equal to others, for example, women, children, adolescents, individuals from a minority (or disempowered) religion, people from a minority (or disempowered) ethnic/racial background, and individuals with perceived disabilities (emotional, mental, physical, and/or visual). Many cultures also include a value system with their definition of sexual health. For example, some countries and religions only expect sexual health to exist within a heterosexual marriage and only for the primary reason of procreation. Other countries and religions broadly define sexual health and welcome the diversity that exists within humanity. As is discussed later in this chapter, throughout history legal restrictions (or punishment) have been enacted in this country and around the world to make societies conform to religious or cultural beliefs on contraception, sexual behavior, abortion, and marriage.

According to the Sexuality Information Education Council of the United States (SIECUS, 2004), the goal of sexuality education is to promote adult sexual health. Sexuality education can assist youth and young adults in developing a positive view of sexuality, provide them with medically accurate information they need to maintain their sexual health and help them acquire the necessary skills to make informed decisions. Sexuality education should not end in high school (if one even had it in high school). Just as one keeps informed about what physical activity and diet are appropriate as our bodies change with age, similarly, one should practice a lifelong process of obtaining sexual health information, and of shaping attitudes, beliefs, and values about such significant topics as identity, pregnancy, relationships, and intimacy (SIECUS, 2004). SIECUS developed a list of life behaviors of a sexually healthy adult to help individuals understand the factors that promote sexual health (review Table 1.1).

Table 1.1 SIECUS LIFE BEHAVIORS OF A SEXUALLY HEALTHY ADULT

- Appreciate one's own body
- Seek further information about reproduction as needed
- Affirm that human development includes sexual development, which may or may not include reproduction or sexual experience
- Interact with all genders in respectful and appropriate ways
- Affirm one's own sexual orientation and respect the sexual orientations of others
- Affirm one's own gender identities and respect the gender identities of others
- Express love and intimacy in appropriate ways
- Develop and maintain meaningful relationships
- Avoid exploitative or manipulative relationships
- Make informed choices about family options and relationships
- Exhibit skills that enhance personal relationships
- Identify and live according to one's own values
- Take responsibility for one's own behavior
- Practice effective decision making
- Develop critical thinking skills
- Communicate effectively with family, peers, and romantic partners
- Enjoy and express one's sexuality throughout life
- Express one's sexuality in ways that are congruent with one's values
- Enjoy sexual feelings without necessarily acting on them
- Discriminate between life-enhancing sexual behaviors and those that are harmful to self and/or others
- Express one's sexuality while respecting the rights of others
- Seek new information to enhance one's sexuality
- Engage in sexual relationships that are consensual, non-exploitative, honest, pleasurable, and protected
- Practice health-promoting behaviors, such as regular check-ups, breast and testicular self-exam, and early identification of potential problems
- Use contraception effectively to avoid unintended pregnancy
- Avoid contracting or transmitting a sexually transmitted disease, including HIV
- Act consistently with one's own values when dealing with an unintended pregnancy

Table 1.1	SIECUS LIFE BEHAVIORS OF A SEXUALLY HEALTHY ADULT (CONTINUED)

Seek early prenatal care

Help prevent sexual abuse

Demonstrate respect for people with different sexual values

Exercise democratic responsibility to influence legislation dealing with sexual issues

Assess the impact of family, cultural, media, and societal messages on one's thoughts, feelings, values, and behaviors related to sexuality

Critically examine the world around them for biases based on gender, sexual orientation, culture, ethnicity, and race

Promote the rights of all people to accurate sexuality information

Avoid behaviors that exhibit prejudice and bigotry

Reject stereotypes about the sexuality of different populations

Educate others about sexuality

Source: SIECUS. (2004). *Guidelines for comprehensive sexuality education: Kindergarten through 12th grade, 3rd ed.* Washington, DC: Author. Http://www.siecus.org/_data/global/images/guidelines.pdf
Copyright © 2004 by the Sexuality Information and Education Council of the United States. Reprinted by permission.

After reviewing the SIECUS list of life behaviors of a sexually healthy adult, which ones do you feel you need to work on in your own life? Which ones do you feel are not needed to determine if you are sexually healthy or not? About which ones do you need more information before you can make a conscious decision whether you practice them in your life?

The first formal government recognition of the importance of a sexual health framework to enhance population health in the United States was released in 2001 by the Surgeon General (U.S. Department of Health and Human Services, 2001). A decade since the publication, the rates of STIs, HIV infections, and unintended pregnancies in the United States unfortunately continue to increase, thereby creating a high health burden on our society. There are numerous, complex factors that influence the rates of any of these health issues in this country. The Centers for Disease Control and Prevention (CDC, 2010) outlined a more positive, health-based approach to address sexual behaviors across one's lifespan to serve as a potential framework for public health action to build on and advance the Surgeon General's *Call to Action*. However, there are a number of obstacles impeding the achievement of optimal sexual health, as well as a meaningful reduction of sexually related problems in the United States (CDC, 2010). We touch on some obstacles in the next section.

Sexually Transmitted Infections in the United States

Every year, there are at least 19 million new cases of STIs in the United States alone (Weinstock, Berman, & Cates, 2004). Although young adults (15–24 years old) represent only one-quarter of the sexually active population, they account

Table 1.2 STATISTICS ON STIs IN THE UNITED STATES	
STI	**Yearly Cases**
Human papillomavirus (HPV)	6,000,000
Chlamydia	2,000,000
Gonorrhea	700,000
Genital herpes	500,000
Human immunodeficiency virus (HIV)	56,000
Syphilis	36,000

Source: Centers for Disease Control and Prevention (CDC). (2008). *Trends in reportable sexually transmitted diseases in the United States, 2007: National surveillance data for Chlamydia, Gonorrhea, and Syphilis.* Atlanta, GA: Author.

for nearly half of all new STIs each year (Weinstock, Berman, & Cates, 2004). These numbers are worrisome, and the public goal to decrease the spread and negative health consequences of STIs has been a top priority for centuries for many countries globally. Table 1.2 includes a list of some of the STIs diagnosed in this country and their yearly estimated cases of occurrence (these STIs are discussed at length in chapter 7).

Why do America's youth experience such high rates of STIs compared to lower rates in other Western countries such as Sweden? What could be some possible obstacles to lowering these incidences of infection? Is it because America's youth are becoming sexually active before they understand the implications (positive and negative) to such behavior? Perhaps it is because they are not using condoms consistently (if at all) to reduce the risk of STIs. Or is it because they have multiple sexual partners whose STI status may be unknown?

Then again, youths could be too embarrassed to buy condoms or too uncomfortable to talk to their doctors, their parents, or another trusted adult about topics such as abstinence, STI prevention, and healthy sexual behaviors. Does poverty have a negative effect on the use of contraceptives? What role do some religions play in discouraging condom use, such as those religions that advocate natural family planning and frown on contraception—let alone non-marital sexual activity? Can the media play a role in the decisions youths

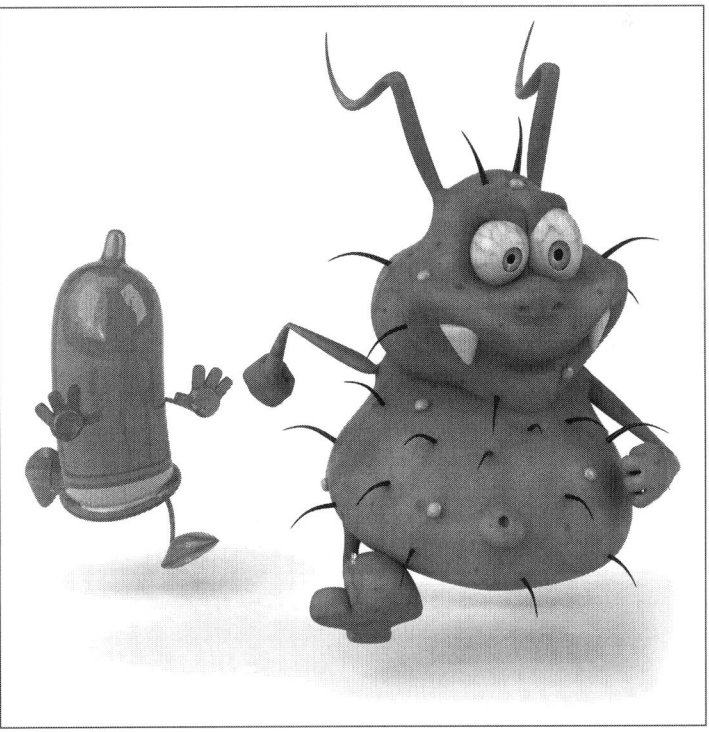

make about becoming sexually active and exhibiting healthy sexual behaviors? These are difficult questions to answer across such a broad population.

Countries like Sweden that have lower rates of STIs than the United States take a public health approach—not a moralistic one—to preventing STI exposure. Access to education, screening, and treatment is universal in Sweden, which helps promote healthy sexual behaviors to reduce exposure to STIs and HIV. Since the 1950s, Sweden has provided youth from kindergarten to the end of high school with comprehensive sexuality education and *free* access to sexual and reproductive health services, including contraception and STI screening and treatment (Francoeur & Noonan, 2004). Access to education, screening, and treatment in the United States varies not only by state, but by county and even municipality (The Alan Guttmacher Institute, 2011a). For example, states located on the East Coast are considered more liberal in their stance on providing comprehensive sexuality education in public schools than states located in the southern region of the U.S. Without a federal mandate, responsibility lies with state, county, and local governments to dictate the focus (e.g., comprehensive vs. abstinence-only) of sexuality education targeted at youth (if any is even provided).

Recent estimates of HIV incidence in the U.S. have revealed that approximately 50,000 infections occurred *annually* between 2006 and 2009 (Prejean et al., 2011). In 2009, men who have sex with men (MSM) accounted for 61 percent of new infections, heterosexual contact was 27 percent, injection drug use (IDU) was 9 percent, and MSM/IDU was 3 percent. There was an estimated 21 percent increase in HIV infection for people between the ages of 13–20 years old. According to the CDC, African Americans represent approximately 14 percent of the U.S. population, but accounted for 44 percent of all new HIV infections in 2009. Hispanics represent approximately 16 percent of the U.S. population, but accounted for 20 percent of all new HIV infections in 2009 (Prejean et al., 2011). Overall, in 2009, African American men had the highest rate of new HIV infections (103.9 new infections per 100,000 persons), followed by Hispanic men (39.9 per 100,000), and African American women (39.7 per 100,000). A more concerted effort is needed to reach individuals most at risk of acquiring an HIV infection. Stigma toward same-sex sexual contact, poverty, lack of access to medical and social services, racism, and sexism need to be addressed simultaneously to reduce the rate of HIV infection in the African American and Hispanic communities.

Pregnancy in the United States

In the U.S., an estimated 6 million women become pregnant annually (Martin et al., 2009). According to Ventura and her colleagues (2009), of the 6.4 million pregnancies in the U.S. in 2006, 4 million resulted in births, 1.3 million in abortions, and 1.1 million in miscarriages and stillbirths. The proportions of pregnancies that were intended (51 percent) and unintended (49 percent) were almost identical (pregnancy and its outcomes are discussed at length in chapter 11). Why do you think we have such a high rate of unintended pregnancies? How can the U.S. increase the rate of *intended* pregnancies? Do we provide enough focus on education about contraception, pregnancy spacing, or the importance of prenatal care? Do we concentrate our efforts mostly on women or should we reach out equally to men? Perhaps we need to educate primary care physicians and pediatricians to discuss family planning with their patients (of reproductive age) even if the patient doesn't initiate the conversation. Moreover, perhaps social media can be used to influence our understanding of the importance of family planning to decrease the rate of unintended pregnancies.

Exploring the Meaning of Sex

The meanings we place on sexual terms are socially constructed by the time period and various institutions (e.g., religion, government, etc.) that have a strong influence on a culture's perception of sexuality. "Sex" is a term many use loosely to refer to vaginal-penile intercourse. The medical term for vaginal-penile intercourse, though, is *coitus* (koi-t s) (Jones & Lopez, 2006). Thus, the word "sex" will not be ambiguously used to refer to vaginal-penile intercourse in this textbook. The word *sex* is also the clinical term used to identify us as a biological female or male.

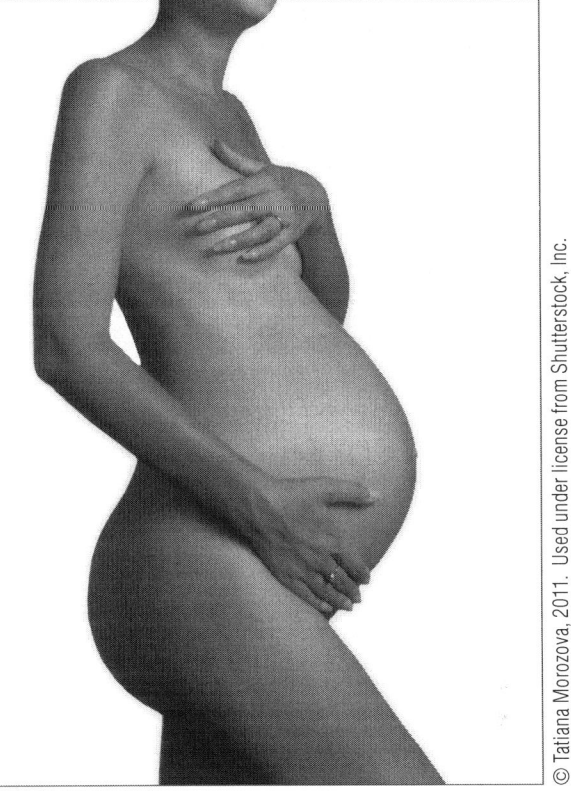

Many of us use the term *gender* to categorize someone as female or male, but "sex" and "gender" (i.e., a collection of attitudes and behaviors that are considered normal and appropriate in a specific culture for people of a particular sex) are two separate constructs to consider when identifying someone (or yourself) as a girl/boy, female/male, or woman/man. Moreover, even though the term "biological sex" is referred to as a dichotomous variable differentiating between females and males, it is recognized that not all individuals agree with what makes someone a female or what makes someone a male (these concepts are discussed at length in chapter 8).

Also, when comparing females and males, the term "other" is used instead of "opposite" to promote the numerous similarities instead of the differences between the sexes (Crooks & Baur, 2011). Thus, the term "sex" is either used to refer to a biological female, male, or intersexed individual, or as a broad term encompassing all forms of sexual activity, including oral sex, anal sex, masturbation, and vaginal-penile intercourse. Moreover, studies have shown that the term "sex" needs to be explicitly defined to help individuals correctly answer questions regarding sexual behavior (Brady & Halpern-Felsher, 2007).

By assigning the term sex to mean vaginal-penile intercourse, we place that behavior above all others, as well as devalue other forms of sexual behavior. No behavior between consenting adults should be depicted as more worthy or more satisfying than another (only you can determine that for yourself). That narrow definition of sex only limits our range of possibilities to experience sexual pleasure. Of course, one should never participate in or be forced to succumb to a sexual behavior that one is not comfortable with, or that one does not hold positive meaning to, including vaginal-penile intercourse.

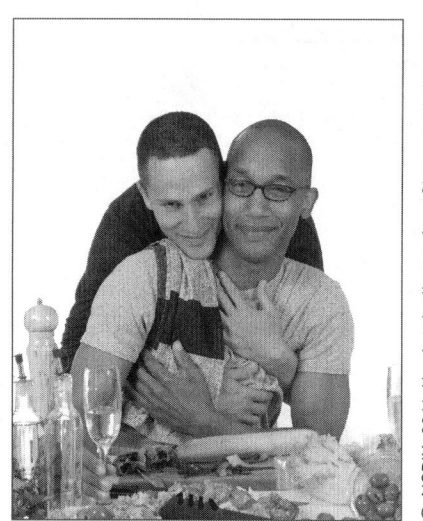 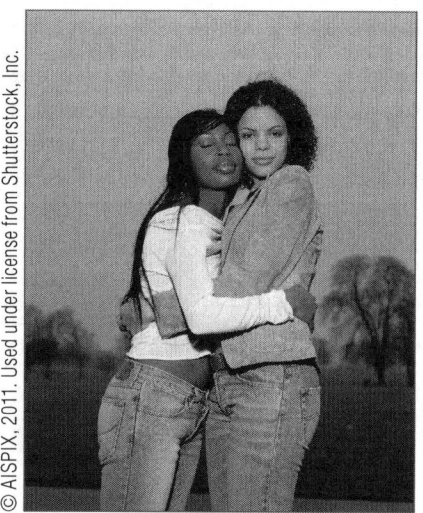 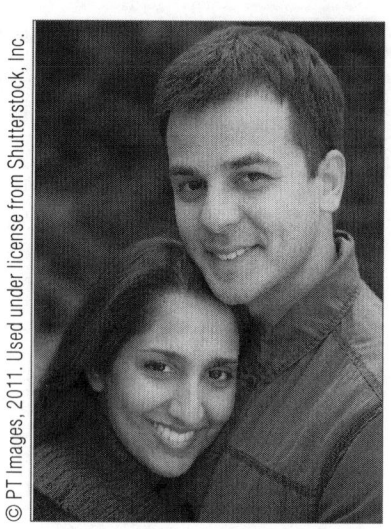

Similar to how vaginal-penile intercourse has been erroneously deemed as the "main" sexual behavior for humans, other sexuality-related terms also have been marginalized due to society's acceptance or disapproval of others. For example, even though it is not disputed that more people around the world identify as *heterosexual* (attracted to a member of the other sex), that should not demean other sexual orientations that exist. *Homosexuality* (attracted to a member of the same sex) and *bisexuality* (attracted to members of either sex) are seen by the medical community as normal and natural and need to be acknowledged as such (sexual orientations are discussed at length in chapter 9).

BIOLOGICAL SEX AND STEREOTYPED TRAITS

We live in a society that places a higher value on characteristics that have been defined as masculine. Being assertive, independent, unemotional, and competitive are just a few traits expected to be present in males more so than females. Caring, nurturing, cooperative, understanding, and emotional are a few qualities expected to be displayed in females more so than in males.

In the U.S., even though girls and women who exhibit masculine characteristics are not met with overt disapproval as much as in the past, boys and men who exhibit feminine characteristics can suffer alienation and verbal, physical, or emotional abuse. Girls and women can strive to better themselves by embracing masculine characteristics, yet it is not universally believed that boys and men adopting feminine characteristics are bettering themselves. Is it because we value males more than females? Is it because society has blurred the distinction between gender and sexual orientations, thus believing that males who exhibit feminine characteristics must be gay? All the characteristics mentioned above, though, are human traits that have been stereotyped by many societies to be present in one sex more than the other. We all have the ability to show emotion, be assertive, demonstrate compassion, etc. We owe it to ourselves to be the people we know we are on the inside, and not the people others expect us to be.

SEXUAL HEALTH AND THE LAW

People engage in sexual activity more for personal enjoyment and for physiological, emotional, and psychological satisfaction than for procreation (Philaretou, Phellas, & Karayianni, 2006). Yet, society has either ignored or denied this fact, depending on the culture, the particular time period's view of sexuality, and its place in an individual's life. Throughout our nation's history, each state has had a right to create any laws they saw fit for their residents, especially if it could be argued they were protecting the innocent (i.e., children or women) or restricting what was deemed unnatural or immoral at the time. Thus, limiting sexual expression (in public or in private) by criminalizing certain sexual behaviors was considered necessary for the greater good of the community. For example, at one time in this country, access to contraception was severely restricted, abortion was only allowed to save the mother's life, and a couple could be arrested if they were "caught" (even in the privacy of their own home) performing a sexual act that was considered "immoral" or "inappropriate" by societal standards.

Access to Contraception

The Comstock Act (17 Stat 598) was described as an act for the suppression of trade in and circulation of obscene literature and articles of immoral use. It was enacted in 1873 to prohibit the distribution of devices and information that could prevent conception (Heins, 2001). In 1932, Margaret Sanger, a strong proponent of family planning, sent a New York City doctor a box of diaphragms from Japan for his patients (see Figure below on what a diaphragm looks like and how it is used to prevent a pregnancy). This package was confiscated under the Comstock Act. Ms. Sanger sued and in 1936 a Second Circuit Federal Appeals Court ruled in *United States v. One Package of Japanese Pessaries* (86F.2d 737) that the federal government could not interfere with doctors providing contraception to their patients. Even so, women did not have the legal right to access and use contraception for almost 30 years (contraception is discussed at length in chapter 12).

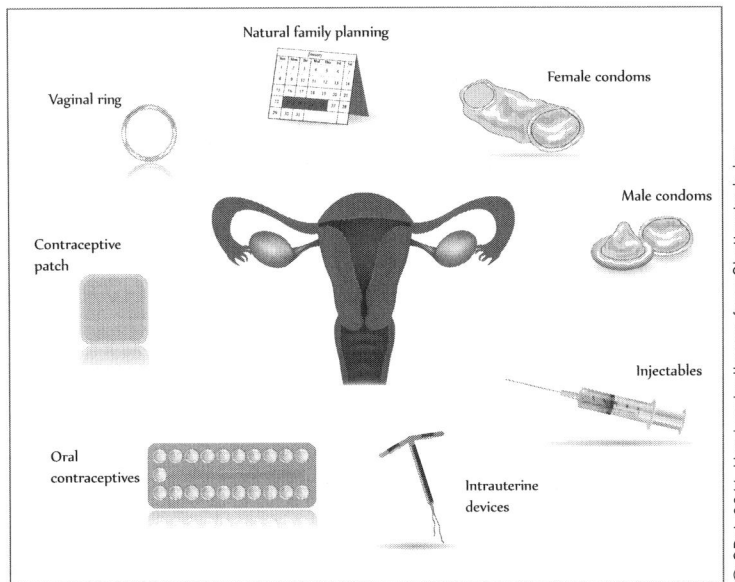

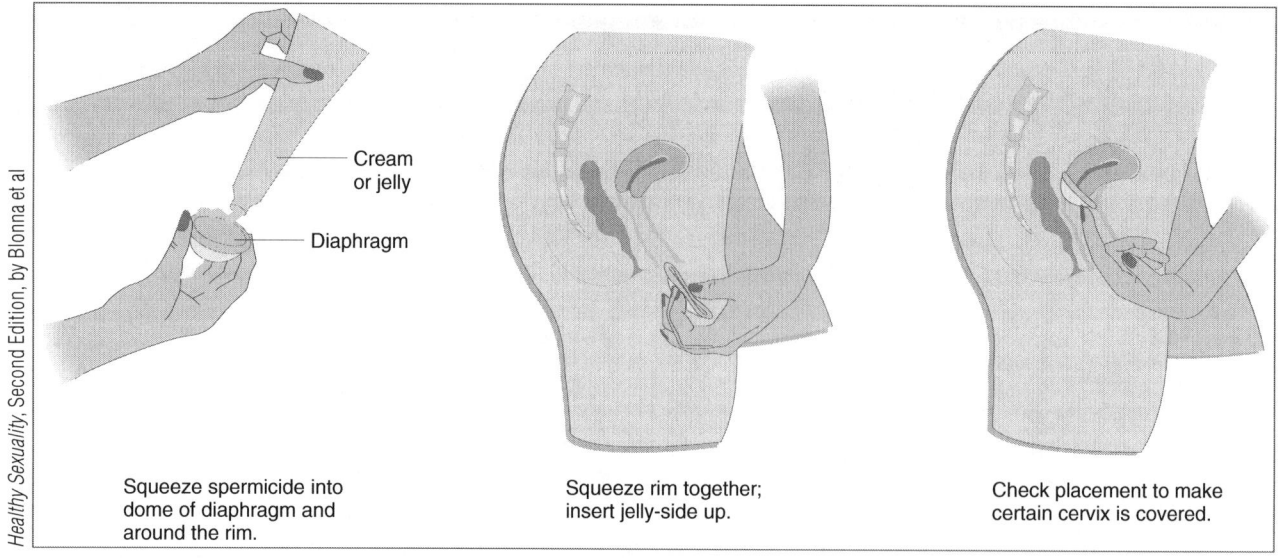

Squeeze spermicide into dome of diaphragm and around the rim.

Squeeze rim together; insert jelly-side up.

Check placement to make certain cervix is covered.

Even though oral contraceptives were developed in 1960, the majority of women who wanted to plan, space, or prevent future pregnancies could not obtain such a prescription from their doctors because the use of medication or devices to control one's fertility was against the law in most U.S. states. In 1965, that all changed—well, at least for married people! The U.S. Supreme Court ruling of *Griswold v. Connecticut* decriminalized every state law against married individuals using contraceptives, such as the pill (381 U.S. 479). It wasn't until 1972 that the Supreme Court extended the right of privacy to unmarried people by overruling every states' prohibition against single people using contraceptives in *Eisenstadt v. Baird* (405 U.S. 438).

Some religions or denominations, such as the Catholic church, condemn the use of a contraceptive method other than for natural family planning, which takes into account a woman's menstrual cycle to dictate when unprotected coitus (vaginal/penile intercourse) can be initiated without the fear of an unintended pregnancy (Crooks & Baur, 2011). Still, that doesn't seem to deter many religious women in the United States, though, from using a reliable method to prevent an unintended pregnancy or to plan a future pregnancy. For example, according to Jones and Dreweke (2011), among all women who have participated in coitus, it is believed that 99 percent of them have used a contraceptive method other than natural family planning. A similar number (98 percent) is believed to exist among sexually experienced Catholic women. Regardless of denomination, among sexually active women who do not want to become pregnant, 69 percent use a very effective method, such as an oral contraceptive or another hormonal method, sterilization, or the

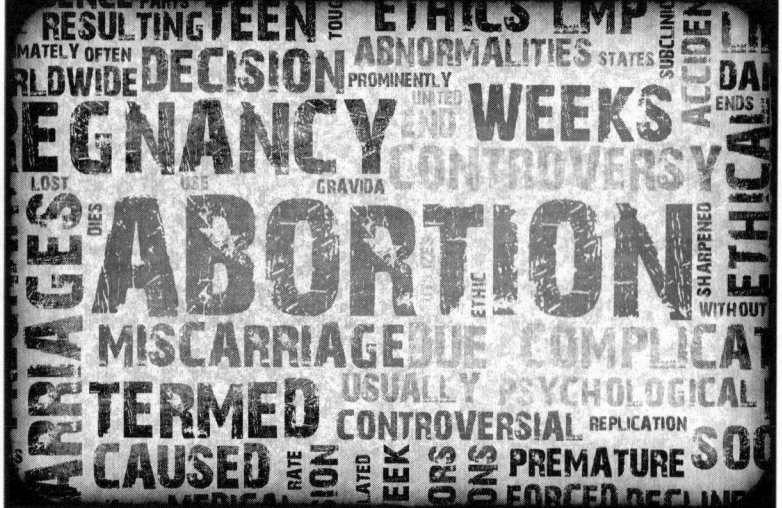

intra-uterine device (IUD). Among different denominations, 74 percent of Evangelical women, 73 percent of mainline Protestants, and 68 percent of Catholics use a highly effective method to prevent an unintended pregnancy. Only 2 percent of Catholic women supposedly rely on natural family planning as their approach to prevent an unintended pregnancy. Evangelicals (4 in 10) are more likely than other denominations to rely on female or male sterilization to prevent unintended pregnancies (Jones & Dreweke, 2011).

Access to Abortion

According to Crooks and Baur (2011), in the 13th century, St. Thomas Aquinas outlined the Catholic Church's stance on when human life begins. He stated that a fetus developed a soul (and thus life) after conception—90 days after conception if it was a female and 40 days after conception if it was a male. Thus, it can be assumed that abortion was allowed, or at least tolerated, depending on when the termination took place during this time period of the pregnancy. It wasn't until the 1860s that Pope Pius IX declared that human life begins at conception (Crooks & Baur, 2011). According to Haffner (2011), abortion is not mentioned in the Hebrew Bible or New Testament. Moreover, many religious traditions teach that the health and life of the woman must take precedence over the life of the fetus.

Early American law allowed the termination of a pregnancy until the woman felt fetal movements, which usually would be felt around the fourth gestational month (Crooks & Baur, 2011). In the late 1800s, abortion became illegal in the United States, except to save a woman's life. It wasn't until 1973 that women, in consultation with their physician, were given the right to choose to continue a pregnancy or not. Even before 1973, however, abortion existed illegally in the United States. The methods to terminate a pregnancy were usually dangerous for a woman, though. For example, in desperation women used wire coat hangers to try to expel the pregnancy themselves by puncturing their cervix in an effort to scrape the uterus. This usually led to internal bleeding and infection, and many times the women died (Crooks & Baur, 2011). Part of the reason why women (and men) fought to legalize abortion in this country was to stop the dangerous abortions that were taking place.

The U.S. Supreme Court case of *Roe v. Wade* established that a woman has a right to self-determination, including the right to abortion (410 U.S. 113). U.S. states were not allowed to intervene in barring a woman from seeking an abortion during her first trimester (i.e., the first three months of pregnancy), but could place restrictions during the second and third trimester—corresponding to the fetus' increasing viability (likelihood of survival outside the uterus). The U.S. Supreme Court cases *Webster v. Reproductive Rights* in 1989 (492 U.S. 490) and *Planned Parenthood v. Casey* in 1992 (505 U.S. 833) gave states the right to enact laws to restrict women's access to abortion (Crooks & Baur, 2011). Moreover, Congress has blocked the use of federal Medicaid funds to pay for abortions, except when the woman's life would be endangered by a full-term pregnancy or in cases of rape or incest (The Alan Guttmacher Institute, 2011b).

Abortion continues to be a contentious issue in the United States as well as in other parts of the world. Even though over 60 percent of Americans want *Roe v. Wade* to remain in place, younger generations seem to be less likely to support abortion rights than older generations (The Alan Guttmacher Institute, 2011c). During the past 40 years, many religious denominations have even passed policies in support of legalized abortion, including the Christian Church (the Disciples of Christ), the Episcopal Church (in the U.S.), the Evangelical Lutheran Church in America, the Jewish Reconstructionist Federation, the Presbyterian Church (in the U.S.), the Union for Reform Judaism, the Unitarian Universalist Association, the United Church of Christ, The United Methodist Church, and the United Synagogue of Conservative Judaism (Haffner, 2011).

Even so, the first half of 2011 saw a record number of provisions (162) enacted by U.S. states to restrict reproductive health and rights (Alan Guttmacher Institute, 2011b). Almost 50 percent were targeted attempts to limit abortion and, 80 out of the 162 provisions were enacted in only 19 states. Abortion stipulations included:

- mandatory counseling and waiting periods;
- gestational bans (i.e., unable to terminate a pregnancy after a certain week or month during pregnancy);
- banning abortion coverage in federal health insurance exchanges;
- making it obligatory to listen to the embryo or fetal heartbeat;
- setting restrictions on abortion by medication.

Sexual Behavior

Not only have laws been enacted to restrict access to contraception and abortion, but also to condemn sexual behaviors deemed "unnatural" or inappropriate, including oral sex, anal sex, and bestiality (i.e., sexual contact with animals). Enacted by states, *sodomy laws* (i.e., defined as anal and/or oral sex between adults of any sexual orientation) were often more focused on deterring sexual contact between consenting adults that would not lead to procreation (Crooks & Baur, 2011). For example, prior to 2002, a couple—even a married couple—could be imprisoned for participating in certain sexual activities considered "unnatural" (which could mean anything but coitus). These state laws were more likely to target men who participated in sexual activity with other men, as such laws were rarely enforced against heterosexual couples. By 2002, thirty-six states had repealed all sodomy laws or had them overturned. In 2003, the remaining laws were nullified by the landmark U.S. Supreme Court case

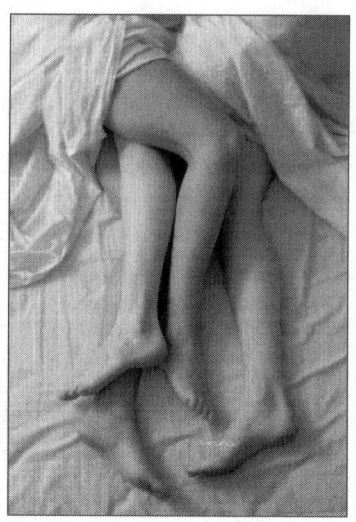

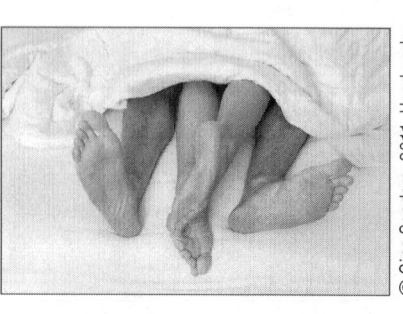
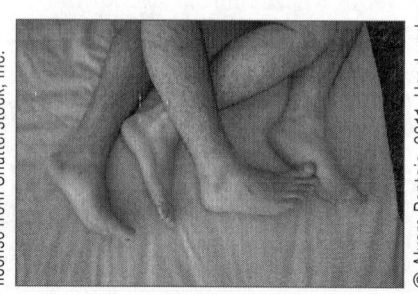

of *Lawrence v. Texas*, which struck down the sodomy law in Texas (539 U.S. 558), thus giving liberty and substantial protection to adult individuals in deciding how to conduct their private lives in matters pertaining to sexual behavior.

Other societies have laws against same-sex sexual contact with penalties such as life imprisonment (countries such as Barbados, Burma, Guyana, and Tanzania) or death (countries such as Mauritania, Saudi Arabia, and Yemen). Some countries, though, have not had laws against same-sex sexual activity for decades (i.e., Denmark, Norway, Sweden, and United Kingdom), if not centuries (i.e., Belgium, France, Luxembourg, Monaco, and The Netherlands).

Many societies, including the United States, have strict laws against adults having sexual contact with children, and against those forcing someone to engage in sexual activities. Even though many societies cannot agree on perceiving same-sex sexual activity as normal and natural, most countries do not tolerate sexual contact between a child and an adult. Depending on the time and the relation between the woman and the man, most societies condemn a woman being forced to participate in sexual activity against her will. Some cultures, though, have stricter laws if the alleged rapist was a stranger rather than if he was the husband or a current or prior sexual partner. Many countries, including the United States, vary on penalties against the rapist, depending on if a woman was raped by another woman, if a man was raped by a woman, or if a man was raped by another man.

Reflections

A more concerted effort is necessary to develop the strategies needed in the U.S. to significantly reduce STIs, HIV incidence, and unintended pregnancies that occur every year. Medically accurate education and access to reproductive and sexual health services (to name a few) can encourage healthy sexual behaviors throughout one's life. Encouragingly, the U.S. continues to redefine the meanings placed on a variety of issues related to sexual health. Even though many European countries have solidified their perspectives on granting the right to marriage equality to same-sex couples, when it comes to access to abortion and sexuality education, unfortunately, the U.S. remains divided in these matters. Education, politics, the judicial system, religion, the medical community, and even the business sector all play a role in how this country shapes its perspectives and whose will dominate our society.

Critical Thinking Questions

1. What factors prevent the U.S. from achieving optimal sexual health?
2. Why do you think there are some populations in this country that experience more negative sex-related health consequences than others?
3. How would restricted access to contraception affect your life today or in the future?
4. What laws do you think will be enacted in the near future that might restrict or broaden rights to others on sexual health?
5. How do you think past legal restrictions on sexual health affected your parents or grandparents?

How Much Do You Remember from the Chapter?

1. Prior to the 1965 U.S. Supreme Court ruling of _____, states could prohibit the use of contraception by married people.
   - a. Eisenstadt *v.* Baird
   - b. Brown *v.* the Board of Education
   - c. Griswold *v.* Connecticut
   - d. Roe *v.* Wade

2. In 1972, the U.S. Supreme Court case _____ extended the right of privacy to unmarried individuals by decriminalizing the use of contraception to single people.
   - a. Eisenstadt *v.* Baird
   - b. Brown *v.* the Board of Education
   - c. Griswold *v.* Connecticut
   - d. Roe *v.* Wade

(3–5) Match the term with its definition.

Coitus _____

Gender _____

Sex _____

a. biological female or male

b. vaginal-penile intercourse

c. collection of attitudes and behaviors that are considered normal and appropriate in a specific culture for people of a particular sex

Challenge Yourself!

Review the following laws online and try to find an argument that strengthens the case for the losing side or weakens the case for the winning side.

The Comstock Act (17 Stat 598)

United States *v.* One Package of Japanese Pessaries (86F.2d 737)

Griswold *v.* Connecticut (381 U.S. 479)

Eisenstadt *v.* Baird (405 U.S. 438)

Roe *v.* Wade (410 U.S. 113)

Webster *v.* Reproductive Rights (492 U.S. 490)

Planned Parenthood *v.* Casey (505 U.S. 833)

Lawrence *v.* Texas (539 U.S. 558)

Websites

www.cdc.gov/sexualhealth/
Centers for Disease Control and Prevention

www.guttmacher.org/
The Alan Guttmacher Institute

www.itsyoursexlife.com/
MTV - Its Your (Sex) Life

www.religiousinstitute.org
The Religious Institute

www.worldsexology.org
World Association for Sexual Health

References

The Alan Guttmacher Institute. (2011a). *Monthly state update: Major developments in 2011.* Retrieved from www.guttmacher.org/statecenter/updates/index.html

The Alan Guttmacher Institute. (2011b). *Facts on induced abortion in the United States.* Retrieved from www.guttmacher.org/pubs/fb_induced_abortion.pdf

The Alan Guttmacher Institute. (2011c). *States enact record number of abortion restrictions in first half of 2011.* Retrieved from www.guttmacher.org/media/inthenews/2011/07/13/index.html

Brady, S., & Halpern-Felsher, B. (2007). Adolescents' reported consequences of having oral sex versus vaginal sex. *Pediatrics, 119,* 229–236.

Centers for Disease Control and Prevention (CDC). (2008). *Trends in reportable sexually transmitted diseases in the United States, 2007: National surveillance data for Chlamydia, Gonorrhea, and Syphilis.* Atlanta, GA: Author.

Centers for Disease Control and Prevention (CDC). (2010). *A public health approach for advancing sexual health in the United States: Rationale and options for implementation, meeting report of an external consultation.* Atlanta, GA: Author.

Crooks, R., & Baur, K. (2011). *Our sexuality.* Belmont, CA: Wadsworth/Cengage.

Francoeur, R., & Noonan, R. (2004). *The continuum complete international encyclopedia of sexuality updated.* New York, NY: The Continuum International Publishing.

Haffner, D. (2011). *The religious reasons why abortion is a moral decision.* Retrieved from www.huffingtonpost.com/rev-debra-haffner/abortion-moral-decision_b_917160.html

Heins, M. (2001). *Not in front of the children: 'Indecency,' censorship and the innocence of youth.* New York, NY: Hill & Wang.

Jones, R., & Dreweke, J. (2011). *Countering conventional wisdom: New evidence on religion and contraceptive use.* New York, NY: The Alan Guttmacher Institute.

Jones, R., & Lopez, K. (2006). *Human reproductive biology* (3rd ed.). Burlington, MA: Elsevier.

Martin, J., Hamilton, B., Sutton, P., Ventura, S., Menacker, F., Kirmeyer, S. et al. (2009). Births: Final data for 2006. *National Vital Statistics Reports, 57*(7). Hyattsville, MD: National Center for Health Statistics.

Philaretou, A., Phellas, C., & Karayianni, S. (2006). *Sexual interactions: The social construction of atypical sexual behaviors.* Boca Raton, FL: Universal Publishers.

Prejean, J., Song, R., Hernandez, A., Ziebell, R., Green, T., Walker, F. et al. (2011). Estimated HIV incidence in the United States, 2006–2009. *PLoS ONE 6*(8), e17502. doi:10.1371/journal.pone.0017502

SIECUS. (2004). *Guidelines for comprehensive sexuality education: Kindergarten through 12th grade,* (3rd ed.). Washington, DC: Author.

U.S. Department of Health and Human Services. (2001). *The Surgeon General's call to action to promote sexual health and responsible sexual behavior.* Retrieved from http://www.surgeongeneral.gov/library/sexualhealth/call.htm

Ventura, S., Abma, J., Mosher, W., & Henshaw, S. (2009). Estimated pregnancy rates for the United States, 1990–2005: An update. *National Vital Statistics Reports, 58*(4). Hyattsville, MD: National Center for Health Statistics.

Weinstock, H., Berman, S., & Cates, W., Jr. (2004). Sexually transmitted diseases among American youth: Incidence and prevalence estimates, 2000. *Perspectives on Sexual & Reproductive Health, 36*(1), 6–10.

World Health Organization (WHO). (2006). *Defining sexual health: Report of a technical consultation on sexual health, 28–31 January 2002, Geneva.* Geneva, Switzerland: Author.

chapter two

SOCIAL MEDIA & SEXUAL HEALTH

CHAPTER OBJECTIVES

On completion of this chapter, students will be able to:

- understand how social media can affect sexual communication;
- describe means by which we can communicate with each other through social media.

ABBREVIATIONS AND ACRONYMS USED IN THIS CHAPTER

IM   instant messaging
LOL   laugh out loud

SOCIAL NETWORKS

Blogging, profile-based sites, instant messaging, and texting have all become part of daily life for millions of people around the world. By July 2011, Facebook had reached over 750 million users on its social networking site (Facebook, 2011). Yet, email remains the most popular form of communication online for adults over the age of 34 (Jones & Fox, 2009). Texting is the most frequently used method of communication for younger adults (Lenhart, Ling, Campbell, & Purcell, 2010).

Moreover, young people dominate the online community. In 2008, 93 percent of youths between the ages of 12–17 and 89 percent of young adults between the ages of 18–24 were Internet users in the United States, and similar rates were found in other developed countries (Jones & Fox, 2009). Women are just as likely as men to be online on a daily basis (Lenhart, 2009a).

In the United States, a majority of adolescents have grown up with Internet-based communication as part of their daily social interactions. Marston and King (2006) assert that social factors help mold our sexual identity. How do you think the Internet has shaped individuals' ideas about gender, sexuality, and relationships? How has this attractive communication medium helped construct a person's view of sexuality? Online environments are ideal for providing instant communication. It has been proposed that this may encourage the expression of repressed desires, such as sharing intimate information about oneself or seeking sexual partners online (Ross, 2005). Moreover, sexual boundaries can become skewed online. For example, can a person cheat on their sexual partner online even if they never touch another person? Can a couple experience sexual pleasure with one another online? Is it becoming acceptable to end a relationship via a text or email instead of face-to-face offline? Moreover, these instant online interactions can also encourage a false heightened sense of trust and familiarity (Ross, 2005). For instance, what if we had been communicating with someone online who we believed was a 22-year-old woman from England and found out it was a 43-year-old man living three blocks from our neighborhood? Also, what is "said" online stays

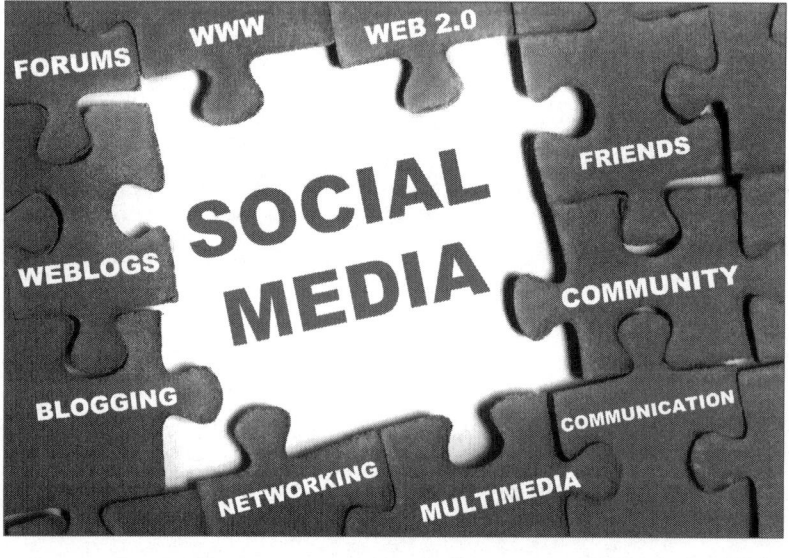

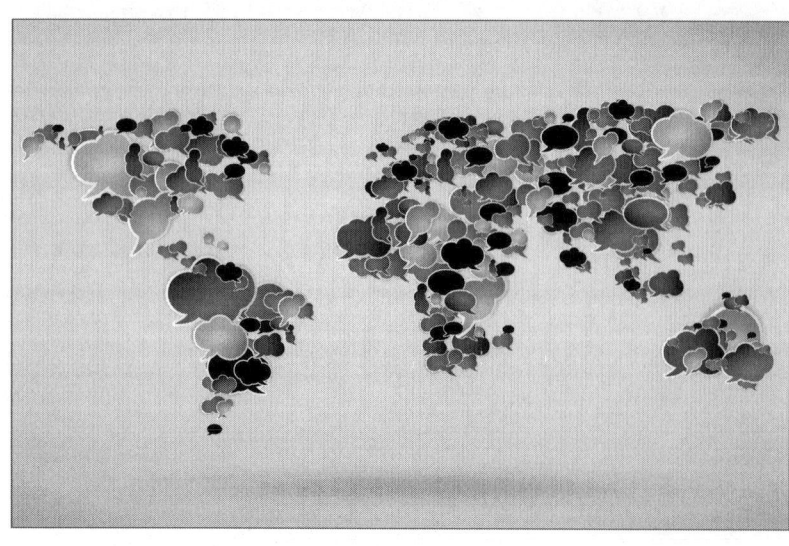

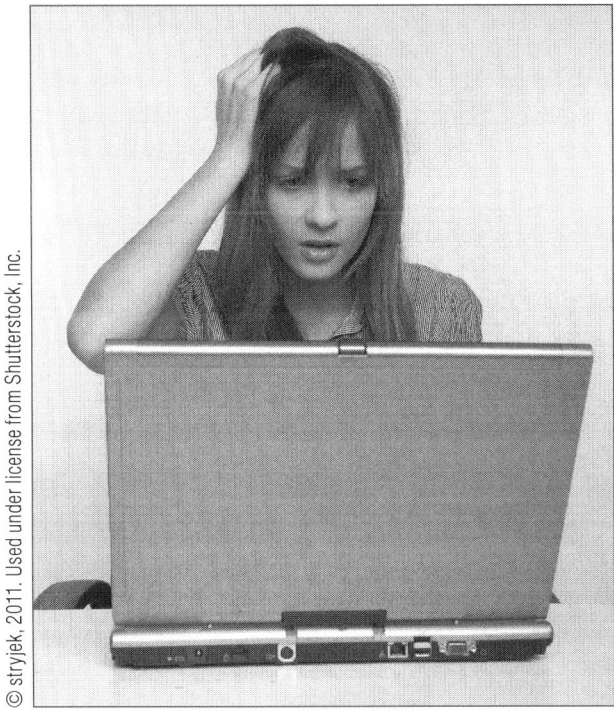
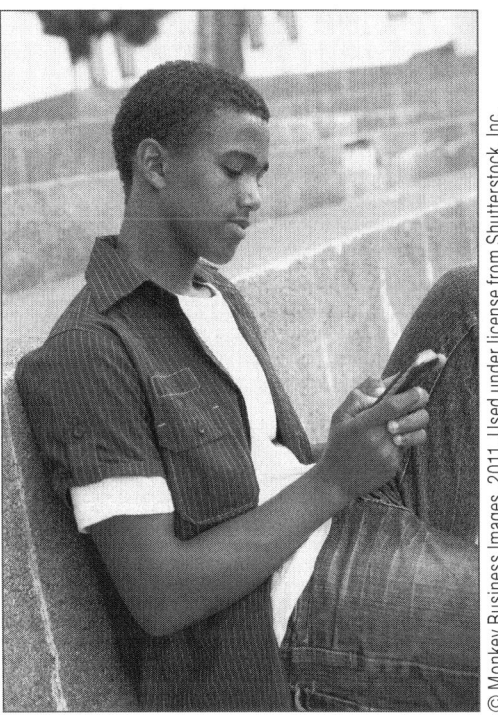

online! Keep in mind that certain social media, such as Facebook, IM (instant messaging), texting, and Twitter, allow messages to live online long after the conversation is over.

A relatively new concept in using social networking sites is in providing education or interventions in sexual health (Bennett & Glasgow, 2009). Governments and organizations have been creative in developing online strategies to influence specific behaviors to improve sexual health (Gold et al., 2011). For example, online interventions have focused on decreasing HIV exposure in youth (Bull, Pratte, Whitesell, Rietmeijer, & McFarlane, 2009), and decreasing exposure to syphilis or HIV among men who participate in sexual activity with other men (Klausner, Levine, & Kent, 2004; Rhodes et al., 2010) by providing education or available services on sites such as Facebook, MySpace, Twitter, or chat rooms. The Internet has been used to help individuals obtain anonymous sexual health advice (Lee et al., 2009), as well as to notify sexual partners of clinic patients of possible exposure to a sexually transmitted infection (Levine, Woodruff, Mocello, Lebrija, & Klausner, 2008). As online technology evolves, so will the methods, topics, and targeted populations for sexual health promotion.

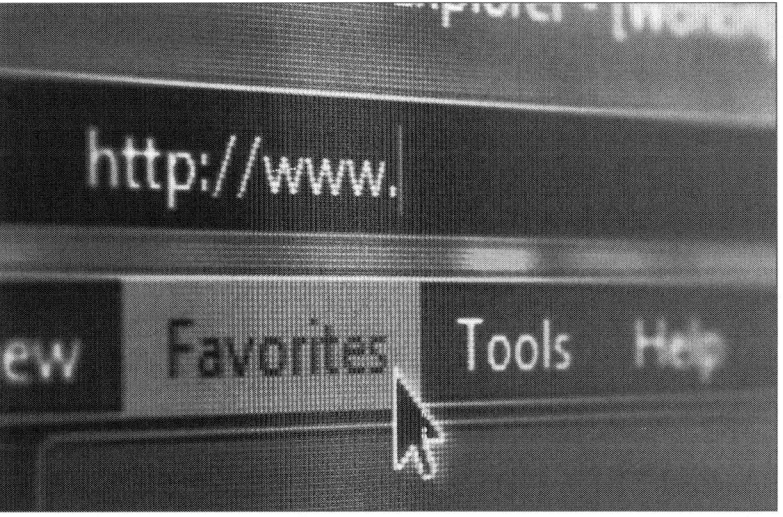

Profile-Based Sites

The first multimedia online identity formats were typically personal homepages (Marwick & boyd, 2010), which can be developed on websites such as Facebook, MySpace, and LinkedIn. These homepages are highly self-managed about how we want others to "see" us, and are limited (to some extent) in how others can change the content (Papacharissi, 2002). These sites have the capacity to facilitate private and public messaging, enable live updates, and allow photo, video, and other content sharing (Gold et al., 2011). In 2008, 75 percent of Internet users in the United States between the ages of 18–24 had a profile on a social networking site, compared to 57 percent of online adults between the ages of 25–34 (Lenhart, 2009a). Over half of all social network users had two or more online profiles, usually to separate their personal and professional lives.

What do profile-based sites have to do with sexual health? Some people use these sites to communicate to others about their relationship status—new relationship, married, divorced, single-and-looking, dissolving a relationship, etc. Ending a relationship is hard enough, but publicly sharing the reasons for the breakup or feeling the need to reveal unflattering information about the other person online should be strongly discouraged. Furthermore, disclosing personal information about others ironically divulges more about the person you are and how you treat others. Discretion is the best policy to follow. You cannot easily take back what you write or images of yourself or others that you display online!

Many people use profile-based sites to stay connected to family, friends, and colleagues. Individuals may also use these sites to seek casual sexual relationships or to find a partner for a more long-term relationship (Bauermeister, Leslie-Santana, Johns, Pingel, & Eisenberg, 2011; Dedobbeleer, Morissette, & Rojas-Viger, 2005). Even so, caution is warranted about the possibility of experiencing illusory feelings of closeness and mutual familiarity when seeking potential sexual partners online (Sevcikova & Daneback, 2011). Influenced by their own desires, some may erroneously read more into the intent of an online flirtation.

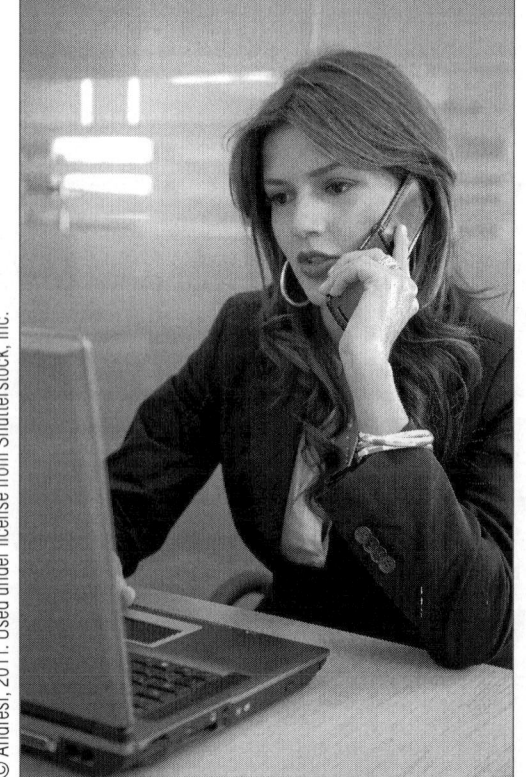
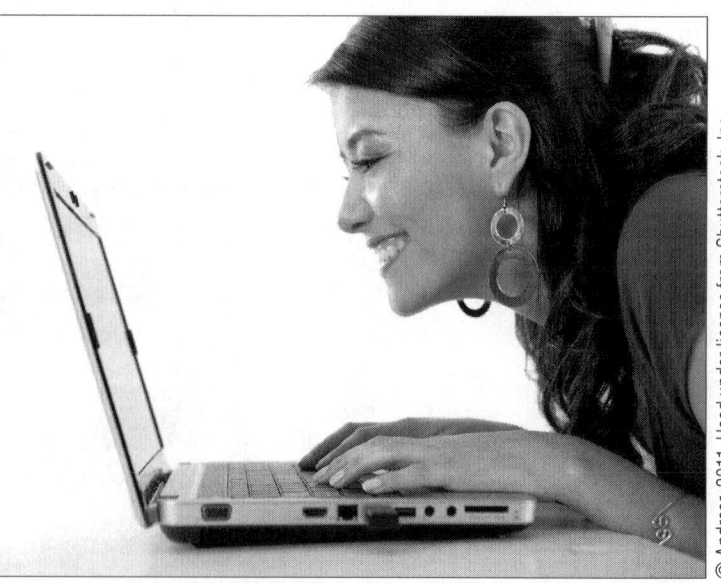

Others use these sites to promote particular views on social issues—for or against abortion, marriage equality for same sex couples, reproductive-assisted technology, contraceptive use, etc. These sites have also helped numerous groups mobilize hundreds of thousands of people to attend rallies, sign petitions, and increase awareness of specific social issues affecting their neighbors as well as strangers a thousand miles away (Liang, Commins, & Duffy, 2010).

Search Engines

Bing, Google, and Yahoo! are search engines that allow the online user to search the Internet for practically anything of interest. Cyberspace is a vast information system that can be used to search for sensitive information anonymously, depending on the country (China has strict Internet-use laws) and topic (most countries have restrictions on accessing child pornography or other material considered inappropriate for their citizens). Have you ever googled information on your sexual health to learn about symptoms related to sexually transmitted infections, premature ejaculation, "normal" sexual desire, or where to purchase a vibrator? For many individuals, accessing the Internet is quick and discreet, allowing them to gain information about their health or a particular topic of interest. But are all sites containing sexual health information medically accurate? How do you know you visited a site that contained accurate information?

The Medical Net Top 20 provides a list of the most popular and highest-rated sites for medical information on the Internet in 2011. Only the top 10 are included in Table 2.1. To review the whole list, visit www.medical.nettop20.com/.

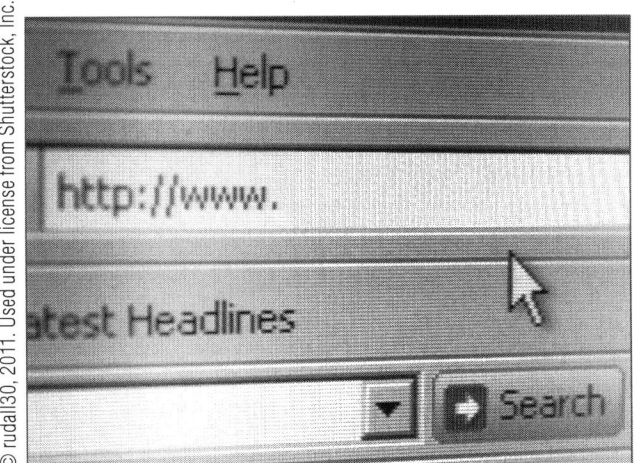
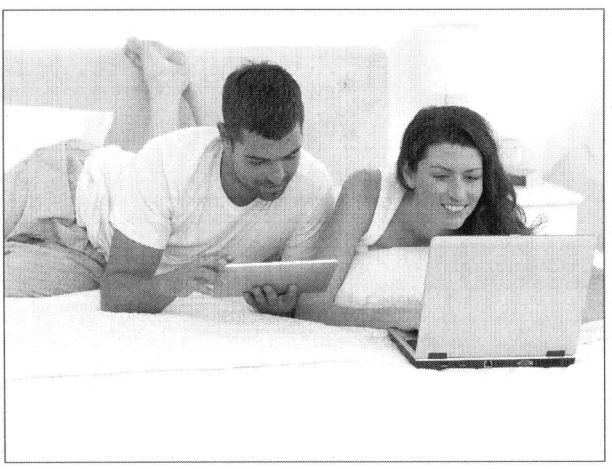

Table 2.1 TOP 10 INTERNET SITES FOR MEDICAL INFORMATION*

1. WebMD	4. Health A to Z
2. Health Central	5. CDC Health Topics A to Z
3. Wrong Diagnosis	6. Dr.Koop.com

Table 2.1	TOP 10 INTERNET SITES FOR MEDICAL INFORMATION* *(CONTINUED)*
7. The Merck Manual	9. MayoClinic.com
8. Medicine Online	10. Yahoo! Health

www.medical.nettop20.com, 8/11/11

Blogs

A blog is another way to communicate via the Internet. *Merriam-Webster's Collegiate Dictionary* (2008) defines a *blog* as a website that contains an online personal journal with reflections, comments, and often hyperlinks provided by the writer. Blog hosting services such as Blogger, LiveJournal, TypePad, and Xanga help individuals create Web space in which finite thoughts and ideas can be shared with the world (boyd, 2006). These thoughts and ideas can be broad and disconnected to the writer or very passionate and personal to the blogger. Many times bloggers write for a targeted audience, such as people empathic to a specific social cause, yet this imagined group of readers may not actually read the blog (boyd, 2006).

What does blogging have to do with sexual health? People write or read blogs for various reasons. For example, individuals may be compelled to write a blog on transitioning from a male to a female. One reason for revealing this private process online (thus sharing it globally) is to help others realize the struggle, as well as to normalize the people experiencing it. Access to news and information through blogging has been found to be a new medium to share and receive news updates, as well as a means to promote a specific angle on a social issue (Hargittai, 2008).

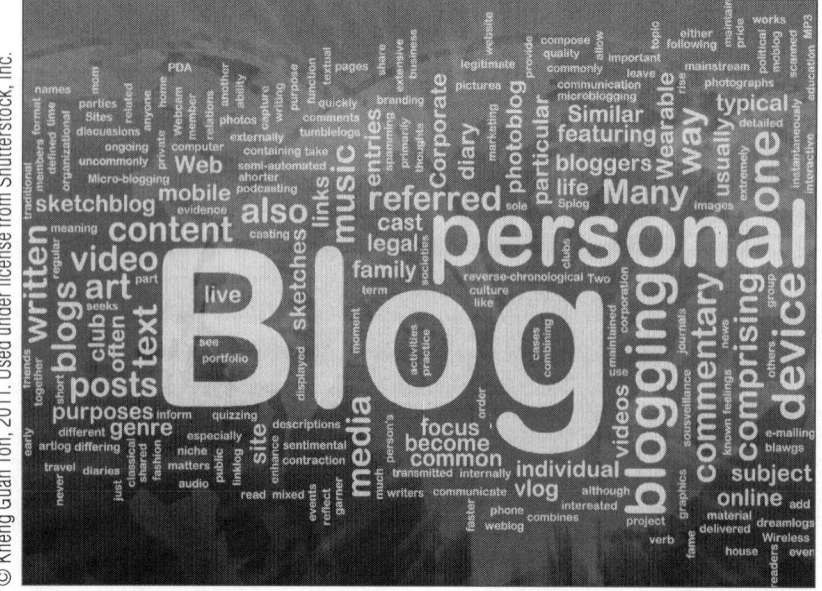

© Kheng Guan Toh, 2011. Used under license from Shutterstock, Inc.

Twitter

Originally created for mobile phones, Twitter was developed to let individuals post short, 140-character text updates or *tweets* to a network of others (Marwick & boyd, 2010). This microblogging site prompts users to answer the question, What are you doing? This creates a timeline that can be constantly updated and the stream of short messages can range from humor, to reflections on life, to links, to breaking news stories. Tweets can burst with an astonishing frequency and intensity. People choose what Twitter accounts to follow on their stream and they in turn can have their own group of followers (Marwick & boyd, 2010). Moreover, users can repost tweets (their own or others) to Facebook, MySpace, and blogs or forward via email to broaden their content to new audiences (boyd, Golder, & Lotan, 2010).

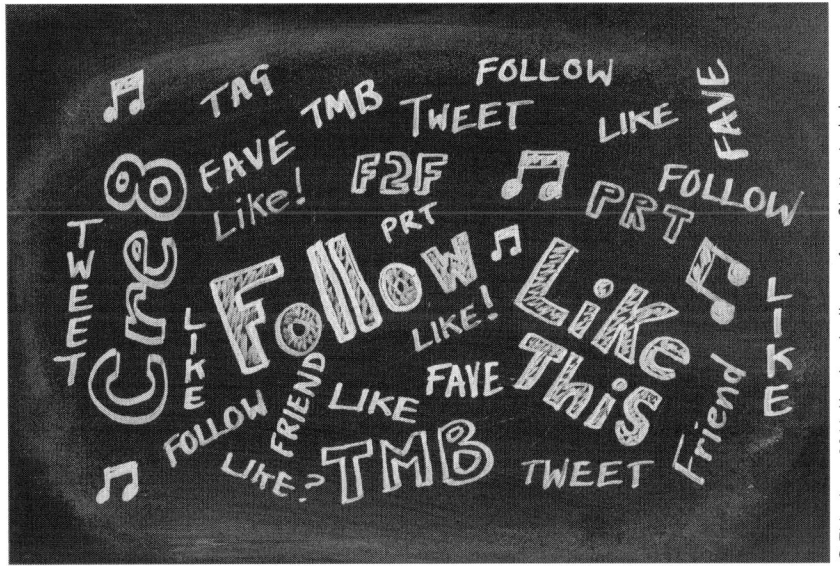

People can restrict access to who sees what content sent on Twitter, yet as a public domain, most tweets can be viewed by anyone or the respondent can forward the tweet to others. Thus, if a friend wants to share something personal with another friend, then tweeting the information should be strongly discouraged. According to Twitaholic.com, the top five most followed Twitter accounts in 2011 were: (1) Lady Gaga (with over 12 million followers); (2) Justin Bieber; (3) President Barack Obama; (4) Brittany Spears; and (5) Katy Perry.

What does Twitter have to do with sexual health? People can tweet to announce a new relationship, an end to one, or that one is in search of a new partner. Even though it is not common knowledge how tweeting sensitive information (i.e., containing sexual content) affects the majority of society, some politicians, celebrities, and influential businesspeople have all regretted a tweet or two!

Texting

In 2009, over half of all American young adults texted on a daily basis (Lenhart et al., 2010). A cell phone is no longer used just for talking to someone over the phone, but also to text, access the Internet, and take or share photos and videos. Sometimes individuals may share sexually suggestive images or texts to sexual partners, potential sexual partners, or friends (Lenhart, 2009b). The thought that these private images will be forwarded to an unintended audience in the future is not a salient concern to many individuals (Lenhart, 2009b). The sender is no longer in control of any material (sexually explicit or otherwise) sent to others. Thus, their own words or images can be forwarded to countless individuals, even months after it was sent! Moreover, because of the concern of abuse and reaching children, laws throughout the United States and in other countries have been enacted to restrict the use of sharing sexually suggestive images and sexting to minors. Depending on the U.S. state, an individual sending sexually explicit material (the definition for sexually explicit varies from state to state) of themselves or someone else, may end up being charged with child pornography and/or convicted as a sex offender.

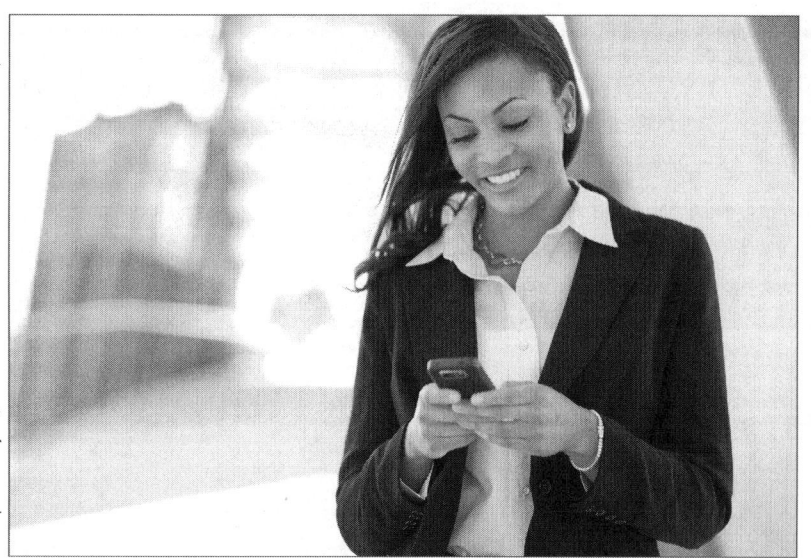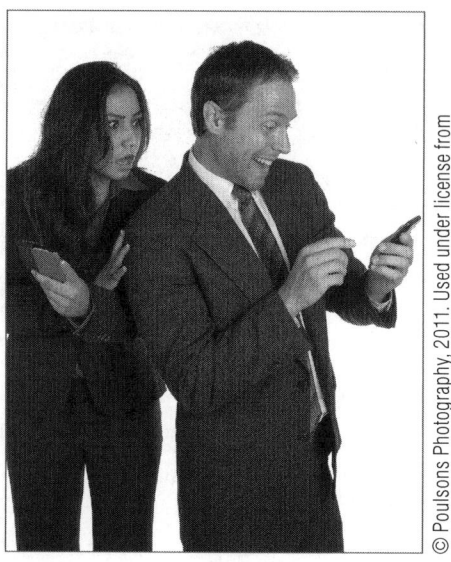

Has it become part of the social norm to ask someone out on a date through texting? Ever broken up with someone through texting? What if she/he says they never got your text (LOL—laugh out loud)? The lingo created for this form of communication has allowed individuals or groups of individuals to correspond with each other frequently and efficiently. Texting has allowed us to communicate with each other any time of the day or night, regardless of where we are and with minimal distraction to others (even though you may find it difficult to concentrate on the task at hand).

What does texting have to do with sexual health? Sexual communication has changed considerably given the advances in technology. We can express our love or hate through a text without ever having to be in front of the person. Yet, what we text can be easily misinterpreted, either because it was perceived as lacking in emotion or overflowing with it! Our body language and tone of voice are helpful in getting our message across, but neither form of communication is available through a text, thus, we may misread what another's intent was. Moreover, texting allows someone to avoid experiencing an uncomfortable situation face-to-face offline. At the same time, though, this form of communication may be the only way some individuals can easily express themselves to others.

Accessing Sexually Explicit Material Online

There are numerous websites that are sex oriented and intended to provide the viewers with sexually explicit material that can induce solitary arousal that may

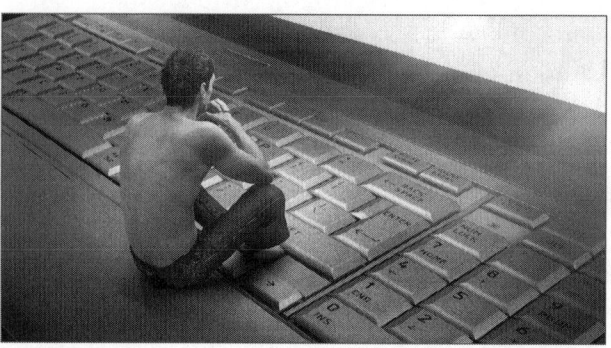

lead to masturbation, or partnered arousal that may lead to sexual activity with another person (Sevcikova & Daneback, 2011). Each of us needs to decide what we find comfortable when viewing sexually explicit images and what we don't. We need to realize how erotic material can enhance our sexual gratification. It can help us realize what arouses us and what doesn't. But it can also provide a false sense of reality in what is sexually pleasing to women and/or to men.

Soliciting Sexual Partners Online

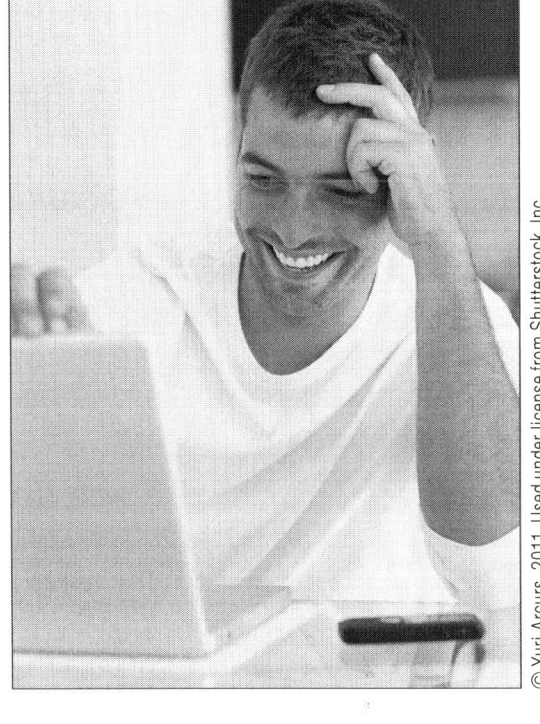

Would you find it easy to approach a total stranger and initiate a conversation regarding the possibility of becoming sexually intimate with one another? Would you find it easier if it was done online instead of face-to-face offline? Even though some individuals have no inhibitions in propositioning a total stranger, most of us do—shying away from fear of rejection, or worse, enduring a public spectacle. Most of us, at this time, would not approach a stranger regardless if it was on- or offline. Some people who wish to engage in less traditional sexual activity or have few opportunities to approach a person face-to-face offline take advantage of what the online world has to offer (Ross, 2005).

Men tend to look for sexual partners online more often than women. Men are more likely to visit Web contact sites and respond to sex ads (Shaughnessy, Byers, & Walsh, 2010). Yet women are more likely than men to meet an online sexual partner offline (Bolding, Davis, Hart, Sherr, & Elford, 2006). Pursuing or being pursued as a potential sexual partner online may precede meeting them face-to-face (Daneback, Mansson, & Ross, 2007). For example, studies have shown males who are interested in participating in sexual activity with other males go online to learn about their sexuality and to meet potential sexual partners (Franssens, Hospers, & Kok, 2010).

Finding "Love" Online

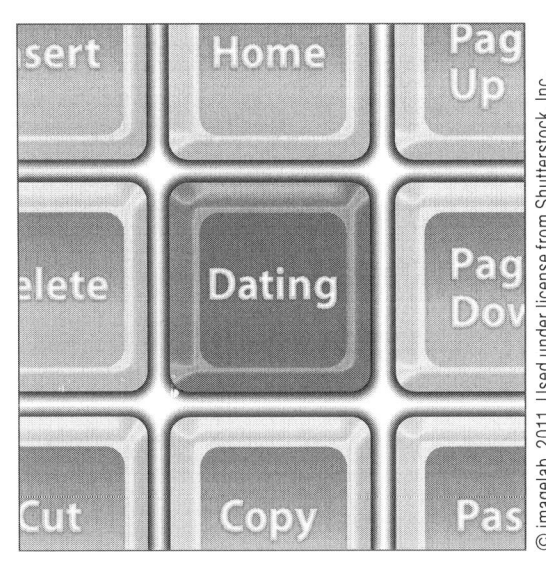

Online dating sites like Match.com, Chemistry.com, and eHarmony.com help individuals find potential partners for platonic or sexual relationships (Couch & Liamputtong, 2008). The user is able to control how they are perceived by others on the site and whom they choose to reach out to (Whitty, 2008). Online dating is not for everyone, but for individuals who do not have time or do not want to make time to find a partner offline, online dating sites may be an area to explore.

Reflections

Depending on where you live, you may be surrounded by the use of technology for personal use. We have computers, laptops, cell phones, texting mobile devices, and a variety of tablets or pads to communicate with others on cyberspace. The wealth of information on the Internet continues to expand at an astounding rate, with no end in sight. For example, we don't need to physically go to a doctor or visit a library to receive information on a variety of sexual health topics. Moreover, with Internet access, we can retrieve this information anonymously from the privacy of our own home or mobile device. Even so, medical misinformation is abundant on the Internet and the user needs to search for answers with caution. Moreover, a real visit to a doctor should never been seen as a last resort, and you can always use the Internet to find a reputable doctor or clinic nearest you!

Social media can be used to help us to find new ways to sexually express ourselves with others, as well. This field of study is in its infancy but the more generations take advantage of these innovative forms of communication, the more society will want to understand how individuals integrate them into their lives. Whatever the medium of expression, we need to realize the possible negative and positive outcomes of what we write or images we send online.

Critical Thinking Questions

1. How have relationships changed because of social media?
2. Does social media make it more challenging to maintain our individuality, by promoting adoption of behaviors from others in our network?
3. How does social media enhance sexual communication and how can it negatively affect it?
4. Has social media sacrificed the quality of our interpersonal relationships by broadening our circle of friends?
5. How do you think social media will change in the next 10 years?

Websites

www.aasect.org/
American Association of Sexuality Educators, Counselors and Therapists

www.answer.rutgers.edu/
ANSWER, Sex Ed Honestly

www.sexscience.org/
Society for the Scientific Study of Sexuality

References

Bauermeister, J., Leslie-Santana, M., Johns, M., Pingel, E., & Eisenberg, A. (2011). Mr. Right and Mr. Right now: Romantic and casual partner-seeking online among young men who have sex with men. *AIDS & Behavior, 15,* 261–272.

Bennett, G., & Glasgow, R. (2009). The delivery of public health interventions via the Internet: Actualizing their potential. *Annual Review of Public Health, 30,* 273–292.

Bolding, G., Davis, M., Hart, G., Sherr, L., & Elford, J. (2006). Heterosexual men and women who seek sex through the Internet. *International Journal of STD & AIDS, 17,* 530–534.

boyd, d. (2006). A blogger's blog: Exploring the definition of a medium. *Reconstruction, 6*(4). Retrieved from www.reconstruction.eserver.org/064/Boyd.shtml

boyd, d., Golder, S., & Lotan, G. (2010). Tweet, tweet, retweet: Conversational aspects of retweeting on Twitter. *Proceedings of the Forty-Third Hawaii International Conference on System Sciences* (HICSS-43). Kauai, HI: IEEE Press.

Bull, S., Pratte, K., Whitesell, N., Rietmeijer, C., & McFarlane, M. (2009). Effects of an Internet-based intervention for HIV prevention: The Youthnet trials. *AIDS & Behavior, 13*(3), 474–487.

Couch, D., & Liamputtong, P. (2008). Online dating and mating: The use of the Internet to meet sexual partners. *Qualitative Health Research, 18,* 268–279.

Daneback, K., Mansson, S., & Ross, M. (2007). Using the Internet to find offline sex partners. *CyberPsychology & Behavior, 10,* 100–107.

Dedobbeleer, N., Morissette, P., & Rojas-Viger, C. (2005). Social network normative influence and sexual risk-taking among women seeking a new partner. *Women & Health, 41*(3), 63–82.

Facebook. (2011). *Facebook statistics.* Retrieved from www.facebook.com/press/info.php?statistics

Franssens, D., Hospers, H., & Kok, G. (2010). First same-sex partner and the Internet. *AIDS & Behavior, 14*(6): 1384–1386.

Gold, J., Pedrana, A., Sacks-Davis, R., Hellard, M., Chang, S., Howard, S. et al. (2011). A systematic examination of the use of online social networking sites for sexual health promotion. *BioMed Central Public Health, 11,* 583–605.

Hargittai, E. (2008). The digital reproduction of inequality. In D. Grusky (Ed.), *Social stratification* (pp. 936–944). Boulder, CO: Westview Press.

Jones, S., & Fox, S. (2009). *Generations online in 2009.* Pew Internet & American Life Project. Retrieved from www.pewinternet.org/~/media//Files/Reports/2009/PIP_Generations_2009.pdf

Klausner, J., Levine, D., & Kent, C. (2004). Internet-based site-specific interventions for syphilis prevention among gay and bisexual men. *AIDS Care, 16*(8), 964–970.

Lee, D., Fairley, C., Sze, J., Kuo, T., Cummings, R., Bilardi, J. et al. (2009). Access to sexual health advice using an automated, Internet-based risk assessment service. *Sexual Health, 6*(1), 63–66.

Lenhart, A. (2009a). *Adults and social network websites.* Retrieved from www.pewinternet.org/~/media//Files/Reports/2009/PIP_Adult_social_networking_data_memo_FINAL.pdf

Lenhart, A. (2009b). *Teens and sexting*. Retrieved from pewinternet.org/~/media//Files/Reports/2009/PIP_Teens_and_Sexting.pdf

Lenhart, A., Ling, R., Campbell, S., & Purcell, K. (2010). *Teens and mobile phones*. Retrieved from www.pewinternet.org/~/media//Files/Reports/2010/PIP-Teens-and-Mobile-2010-with-topline.pdf

Levine, D., Woodruff, A., Mocello, A., Lebrija, J., & Klausner, J. (2008). inSPOT: The first online STD partner notification system using electronic postcards. *Public Library of Science Medicine, 5*(10), e213.

Liang, B., Commins, M., & Duffy, N. (2010). Using social media to engage youth: Education, social justice, & humanitarianism. *The Prevention Researcher, 17*, 13–16.

Marston, C., & King, E. (2006). Factors that shape young people's sexual behavior: A systematic review. *Lancet, 368*, 1581–1586.

Marwick, A., & boyd, d. (2010). I tweet honestly, I tweet passionately: Twitter users, context collapse, and the imagined audience. *New Media & Society, 13*(1), 114–133.

Merriam-Webster. (2008). *Merriam-Webster's Collegiate Dictionary* (11th ed.). Springfield, MA: Merriam-Webster.

Papacharissi, Z. (2002). The presentation of self in virtual life: Characteristics of personal home pages. *Journalism & Mass Communication Quarterly, 79*(3), 643–660.

Rhodes, S., Hergenrather, K., Duncan, J., Vissman, A., Miller, C., Wilkin, A. et al. (2010). A pilot intervention utilizing Internet chat rooms to prevent HIV risk behaviors among men who have sex with men. *Public Health Reports, 125*, 29–37.

Ross, M. (2005). Typing, doing, and being: Sexuality and the Internet. *Journal of Sex Research, 42*(4), 342–532.

Sevcikova, A., & Daneback, K. (2011): Anyone who wants sex? Seeking sex partners on sex-oriented contact websites. *Sexual & Relationship Therapy, 26*(2), 170–181.

Shaughnessy, K., Byers, E. S., & Walsh, L. (2011). Online sexual activity experience of heterosexual students: Gender similarities and differences. *Archives of Sexual Behavior, 40*(2), 419–427.

Whitty, M. (2008). Revealing the 'real' me, searching for the 'actual' you: Presentations of self on an Internet dating site. *Computers in Human Behavior, 24*, 1707–1723.

chapter three

THEORIES THAT PROMOTE SEXUAL HEALTH

CHAPTER OBJECTIVES
On completion of this chapter, students will be able to:
- understand why theoretical frameworks are needed to promote sexual health;
- compare the differences in theoretical underpinnings among the four models.

ABBREVIATIONS AND ACRONYMS USED IN THIS CHAPTER
HBM	Health Belief Model
STIs	Sexually transmitted infections
TPB	Theory of Planned Behavior
TTM	Transtheoretical Model

PROMOTING SEXUAL HEALTH?

If we want to decrease the rate of unintended pregnancies in the U.S., what do we need to know about the people experiencing unplanned pregnancies? Would it help to know how knowledgeable they are of the various methods of contraception and the likelihood of getting pregnant from participating in unprotected coitus (vaginal-penile intercourse)? Do we need to ascertain their attitudes on getting pregnant, on using contraception, and on obtaining contraception? Do we need to examine the societal influences that facilitate or hinder an individual's ability to protect against experiencing an unintended pregnancy?

Public health policy has increased emphasis on the importance of both individual responsibility and choice in participating in sexual behaviors that may potentially increase one's risk of negative health outcomes. Consequently, there is a need to improve our understanding of individual motivations that affect one's choice to participate in sexual health-related behaviors (Ogden, 1996).

Even though the focus of many theories is the individual, social norms and values related to sexuality in a specific culture need to be taken into consideration. Different societies govern what women and men do and how they behave sexually. Biologically, women and men experience different levels of susceptibility to, for example, sexually transmitted infections (STIs). Gender inequality within a culture (as well as age, racial/ethnic background, socioeconomic status, and sexual orientation), though, can magnify vulnerability to health risks through:

- specific actions that are socially acceptable or not (such as expecting women, but not men, to limit the number of lifetime sexual partners);
- through access to essential resources—or lack thereof (such as ability to obtain condoms or screening and treatment services), or the perceptions or treatment of women and men at health-related institutions (such as not providing men with sexual health services);
- through policies that may encourage gender inequities, or not protect one sex or the other against injustices (Cottingham & Ravindran, 2008).

Researchers have developed numerous theories to investigate the most efficient and effective approach to understand actions and encourage healthy behaviors that promote optimal sexual health. These theories differ in how each focuses on specific mental processes believed to influence the causes and mechanisms of human motivation and behavior. This chapter discusses four theoretical frameworks (Health Belief Model, Social Cognition Theory, Theory of Planned Behavior, and Transtheoretical Model) used to guide sexual health education and promotion, as well as offer a structured approach to understanding and meeting the sexual health needs of a population.

The Health Belief Model

The Health Belief Model (HBM) is a value-expectancy model for predicting health behavior and changes in health behavior (Rosenstock, 1974). According to the model, for an individual to take action to avoid a negative health outcome (e.g., STIs or an unintended pregnancy) that person is guided by four kinds of considerations:

1. *perceived susceptibility*—she or he is susceptible to that negative health consequence ("I am currently participating in a sexual activity with another person so it is possible that I might come into contact with an STI.");
2. *perceived severity*—the negative health outcome could have at least a moderately severe impact on some aspect of her or his life ("If I become infected with an STI, I might not be able to have children in the future.");
3. *perceived benefits*—certain behaviors could be beneficial in reducing his or her perceived susceptibility or severity in the event of experiencing an undesirable health outcome ("If I abstain from sexual contact with others, I cannot be exposed to an STI.");
4. *perceived barriers*—these behaviors could be hindered by factors such as cost, pain, and embarrassment ("I don't want to jeopardize my relationship with my partner by ending sexual relations with him/her.").

To prevent negative health outcomes using the HBM, individuals must expect that the protective actions suggested for avoiding an undesirable health consequence will actually prevent the unwanted effect (Strecher, Champion, & Rosenstock, 1997). The HBM posits that self-protective behavior will occur when individuals feel at risk to an undesirable health outcome, believe that the negative health effect would be severe, believe that the benefits of the protective actions outweigh the barriers to perform it, and feel that they are capable of acting on the protective behavior. The HBM has been used in research to study commercial sex workers' participation in condom use to prevent HIV transmission (Ragsdale, Anders, & Philippakos, 2007), the frequency of at-risk sexual behaviors in older adults (Maes & Louis, 2003), and different racial/ethnic backgrounds and the incidence of multiple sexual partners (Neff, Crawford, & MacMaster, 2002).

Social Cognitive Theory

Social Cognitive Theory (also known as Social Learning Theory) focuses on individual motivation and action based on three types of expectancy (Bandura, 1977). In this model, actions, cognition and other personal dynamics, and environmental factors interact to give shape and direction to behavior (Bandura, 1989). According to Bandura (2004), there are four constructs that guide behavior:

1. *knowledge* of health risks and benefits of healthy practices (i.e., "Wearing a condom during anal sex will protect me and my partner from HIV.");
2. *self-efficacy*, or confidence in one's ability to influence one's actions (i.e., "I can wear a condom every time I have anal sex.");
3. *outcome expectations* about the perceived costs and benefits for different behaviors (i.e., "My partner will be not want to have anal sex with me if I wear a condom.");
4. *perceived facilitators* and *impediments* or obstacles (i.e., "I don't have money to buy condoms.").

Knowledge and self-efficacy are needed for any behavior change. Outcome expectations include physical outcomes (i.e., "I will reduce my risk of HIV infection if I use condoms during anal sex."), social outcomes of approval or disapproval (i.e., "My partner wants me to use condoms when we have anal sex."), and positive and negative self-evaluative reactions (i.e., "I feel good about myself that I am wearing a condom when I have anal sex because I am protecting myself and my partner from HIV."). Perceived facilitators and impediments pertain to personal/situational factors and to those of the healthcare system (Bandura, 2004).

Thus, the lower a person's knowledge base and low self-efficacy (along with expecting negative health outcomes, and believing one's behavior is not under her or his control), the more interventions this individual needs in order to motivate healthy behaviors to promote sexual health. Social Cognitive Theory has been used in research to study healthy and unhealthy sexual behaviors in women and men (Colodro, Godoy-Izquierdo, & Godoy, 2010), sexual risk-taking among pregnant adolescents (King Jones, 2010), and healthy sexual behaviors among homeless youth (Taylor-Seehafer et al., 2007).

Theory of Planned Behavior

The Theory of Planned Behavior (TPB) was developed by Icek Ajzen in the 1980s. The TPB is a theoretical framework that can be used to strengthen intentions to participate in healthy behaviors during sexual activity. The TPB focuses on specific mental processes to encourage healthy sexual behaviors to prevent or reduce STIs, unintended pregnancies, and other undesirable outcomes in order to promote sexual health.

The TPB has been used in past studies (Aaro et al., 2006; Askelson et al., 2010), and has been shown to aid in the understanding and prediction of behavior, to direct the creation of instruments to measure the variables that determine behavior, and to guide the development of belief-based intervention techniques. According to the TPB (Ajzen, 1991, 2002; Francis et al., 2004), intention and perceived control over a specific behavior are guided by three kinds of considerations:

1. *behavioral beliefs*—beliefs about the likely outcomes of that behavior and the evaluations of these outcomes (i.e., "Using a condom each time I participate in sexual activity will reduce my risk of acquiring an STI and that is perceived as a positive outcome.");
2. *normative beliefs*—beliefs about the perceived expectations of others and motivation to comply with these expectations (i.e., "Important people in my life believe I should use a condom each time I participate in sexual activity and I want to follow their advice.");
3. *control beliefs*—beliefs about the presence of factors that may facilitate or impede performance of that behavior and the perceived power of these factors (i.e., "I believe it will be easy for me to find and purchase condoms.").

The theory states that behavioral beliefs will generate a favorable or unfavorable *attitude* toward the behavior; normative beliefs will result in perceived social pressure or *subjective norm*; and control beliefs will produce *perceived behavioral control*. In combination, attitude toward the behavior, subjective norm, and perception of behavioral control lead to the formation of a behavioral intention (Ajzen, 2002). Thus, the more favorable the attitude and subjective norm, and the greater the perceived control, the stronger should be the person's *intention* to perform the behavior of interest. Intention is an indication of a person's readiness to perform a given behavior. Researchers use the TBP to develop strategies that would improve these three constructs to strengthen an individual's intentions to take part in the behavior of interest (i.e., consistent condom use), and hopefully change future behavior to influence healthier lifestyles. This theory has been used in research to study adolescents' attitudes and intentions to remain sexually abstinent or not (Masters, Beadnell, Morrison, Hoppe, & Gillmore, 2008), the effects of alcohol on intentions to participate in unprotected sexual activity (Conner, Sutherland, Kennedy, Grearly, & Berry, 2008), and safer sex intentions among methamphetamine users (Mausbacha, Semplea, Strathdeeb, & Patterson, 2009).

Transtheoretical Model

The Transtheoretical Model (TTM) is based on a developmental sequence that motivates an individual to improve intention to participate in healthy behaviors (Prochaska, Redding, Harlow, Rossi, & Velicer, 1994). The model suggests that adopting healthy behaviors, or eliminating unhealthy ones, more likely occurs through a series of stages of change over time. This theory describes a series of five stages of behavior change that can result in long-term maintenance of a behavior (Prochaska et al., 1994):

1. *precontemplation stage*, individuals do not have a desire to change their behavior in question (i.e., "I will not get on the pill to prevent an unintended pregnancy.");
2. *contemplation stage*, individuals intend to change their behavior within the next six months but have no specific plans (i.e., "I intend to go on the pill to prevent an unintended pregnancy, but I haven't made an appointment to see my doctor.")
3. *preparation stage*, individuals have made plans to take specific actions to change their behavior in the immediate future (i.e., "I have made an appointment to see my doctor to start taking the pill.");
4. *action stage*, individuals have changed their behavior in the last six months (i.e., "I am taking the pill every day to prevent an unintended pregnancy."); and
5. *maintenance stage*, individuals have maintained the new behavior for at least six months and it has become a habit (i.e., "I have been taking the pill every day over the past six months to prevent an unintended pregnancy.").

TTM is guided by the principle that specific processes of change are used at different times to progress individuals to later stages of change to adopt healthy sexual behaviors. These processes can be translated into strategies to assist a targeted group to adopt healthy sexual behaviors or reduce the frequency of high-risk sexual behaviors (Horowitz, 2003). This theory has been used in research to study condom use in HIV-positive youth (Naar-King et al., 2006), pregnancy, and STI prevention (Horowitz, 2003), and the impact of readiness to change in couple therapy (Tambling & Johnson, 2008).

Reflections

Society continues to grapple with the negative health consequences of STIs, unintended pregnancies, and other sexually-related health problems. Researchers and community organizations continue to strive to find that theoretical "magic bullet" that could be successfully implemented in practice, in the form of community programs and services that will have an impressive impact on decreasing unhealthy sexual behaviors and promoting healthy ones. In the meantime, each of us should review these theoretical frameworks and ascertain which one works best for us in influencing healthy behaviors for ourselves and our sexual partners, and perhaps for those who are more ambitious, in spreading the word to others.

Critical Thinking Questions

1. If you were a health worker commissioned to evaluate and implement one of the theories discussed above to lower a particular large U.S. city's high incidence of STIs, which theory seems like it would be the most effective in practice? Would you expect the theory you chose to be prohibitively expensive to put into practice?

2. Would your choice be different if the city was experiencing a high rate of unintended pregnancies?

3. Which of the theories seems the least expensive to implement in real life, even if you expect that theory would not be as effective as your other choices above?

4. Which theory, if any, would be most challenging to implement if that city consisted of a high number of diverse religions and cultures?

How Much Do You Remember from the Chapter?

1. Which theory includes *perceived behavior control* as one of its constructs that guides behavior?
    a. Social Cognitive Theory
    b. Health Belief Model
    c. Transtheoretical Model
    d. Theory of Planned Behavior

2. Which theory includes a timeframe to determine if an individual has progressed to the next level of behavioral change?
   a. Social Cognitive Theory
   b. Health Belief Model
   c. Transtheoretical Model
   d. Theory of Planned Behavior

3. Which theory is the oldest?
   a. Social Cognitive Theory
   b. Health Belief Model
   c. Transtheoretical Model
   d. Theory of Planned Behavior

4. Which theory uses the most constructs to ascertain how behavior can be changed?
   a. Social Cognitive Theory
   b. Health Belief Model
   c. Transtheoretical Model
   d. Theory of Planned Behavior

5. Which theory was used in studying the frequency of at-risk sexual behaviors in older adults?
   a. Social Cognitive Theory
   b. Health Belief Model
   c. Transtheoretical Model
   d. Theory of Planned Behavior

Challenge Yourself!

Which individual developed which theory?

1. Albert Bandura _____
2. Irwin Rosenstock _____
3. Icek Ajzen _____
4. James Prochaska _____

a. Health Belief Model
b. Social Cognitive Theory
c. Theory of Planned Behavior
d. Transtheoretical Model

5. Find an example of an actual community program to reduce the occurrence of unwanted pregnancies, and compare its method of implementation to the theories in this chapter. Which one does it most closely resemble?

Websites

www.cdc.gov/hiv/topics/prev_prog/acdp/intervention/behavior.htm
Centers for Disease Control and Prevention–Determinants of Behavior Change

www.commonfund.nih.gov/behaviorchange/
National Institutes of Health–Science of Behavior Change

References

Aaro, L., Flisher, A., Kaaya, S., Onya, H., Fuglesang, M., Klepp, K. et al. (2006). Promoting sexual and reproductive health in early adolescence in South Africa and Tanzania: Development of a theory- and evidence-based intervention programme. *Scandinavian Journal of Public Health, 34*, 150–158.

Ajzen, I. (1991). The theory of planned behavior. *Organizational Behavior & Human Decision Processes, 50*, 179–211.

Ajzen, I. (2002). Perceived behavioral control, self-efficacy, locus of control and the Theory of Planned Behavior. *Journal of Applied Social Psychology, 32*, 665–683.

Askelson, N., Campo, S., Lowe, J., Smith, S., Dennis, L., & Andsager, J. (2010). Using the theory of planned behavior to predict mothers' intentions to vaccinate their daughters against HPV. *The Journal of School Nursing, 26*(3), 194–202.

Bandura, A. (1977). Self-efficacy: Toward a unifying theory of behavioral change. *Psychological Review, 84*, 191–215.

Bandura, A. (1989). Social cognitive theory. In R. Vasta (Ed.), *Annals of child development, Vol. 6. Six theories of child development* (pp. 1–60). Greenwich, CT: JAI Press.

Bandura, A. (2004). Health promotion by social cognitive means. *Health Education & Behavior, 31*, 143–164.

Colodro, H., Godoy-Izquierdo, D., & Godoy, J. (2010). Coping self-efficacy in a community-based sample of women and men from the United Kingdom: The impact of sex and health status. *Behavioral Medicine, 36*, 12–23.

Conner, M., Sutherland, E., Kennedy, F., Grearly, C., & Berry, C. (2008). Impact of alcohol on sexual decision making: Intentions to have unprotected sex. *Psychology & Health, 23*(8), 909–934.

Cottingham, J., & Ravindran, T. (2008). Gender aspects of sexual & reproductive health. In S. Quah & K. Heggenhougen (Ed.), *International Encyclopedia of Public Health* (pp. 19–25). New York, NY: Academic Press.

Francis, J., Eccles, M., Johnston, M., Walker, A., Grimshaw, J., Foy, R. et al. (2004). *Constructing questionnaires based on the Theory of Planned Behavior: A manual for health service researchers.* University of Newcastle upon Tyne, UK: Centre for Health Services Research.

Horowitz, S. (2003). Applying the Transtheoretical Model to pregnancy and STD prevention: A review of the literature. *American Journal of Health Promotion, 17*(5), 304–328.

King Jones, T. (2010). 'It drives us to do it': Pregnant adolescents identify drivers for sexual risk-taking. *Issues in Comprehensive Pediatric Nursing, 33*, 82–100.

Maes, C., & Louis, M. (2003). Knowledge of AIDS, perceived risk of AIDS, and at-risk sexual behaviors among older adults. *Journal of the American Academy of Nurse Practitioners, 15*(11), 509–516.

Masters, N., Beadnell, B., Morrison, D., Hoppe, M., & Gillmore, M. (2008). The opposite of sex? Adolescents' thoughts about abstinence and sex, and their sexual behavior. *Perspectives on Sexual & Reproductive Health, 40*(2), 87–93.

Mausbacha, B., Semplea, S., Strathdeeb, S., & Patterson, T. (2009). Predictors of safer sex intentions and protected sex among heterosexual HIV-negative methamphetamine users: An expanded model of the Theory of Planned Behavior. *AIDS Care, 21*(1), 17–24.

Naar-King, S., Wright, K., Parsons, J., Frey, M., Templin, T., & Ondersma, S. (2006). Transtheoretical Model and condom use in HIV-positive youths. *Health Psychology, 25*(5), 648–652.

Neff, J., Crawford, S., & MacMaster, S. (2002). Ethnicity and multiple sex partners. *Journal of HIV/AIDS & Social Services, 1*(3), 41–65.

Ogden, J. (1996). *Health psychology: A textbook.* Buckingham, UK: Open University Press.

Prochaska, J., Redding, C., Harlow, L., Rossi, J., & Velicer, W. (1994). The Transtheoretical Model of change and HIV prevention: A review. *Health Education Quarterly, 21,* 471–486.

Ragsdale, K., Anders, J., & Philippakos, E. (2007). Migrant Latinas and brothel sex workers in Belize: Sexual agency and sexual risk. *Journal of Cultural Diversity, 14*(1), 26–34.

Rosenstock, I. (1974). Historical origins of the health belief model. *Health Education Monographs, 2*(4), 328–335.

Strecher, V., Champion, V., & Rosenstock, I. (1997). The Health Belief Model and health behavior. In D. S. Gochman (Ed.), *Handbook of health behavior research I: Personal and social determinants* (pp. 71–91). New York, NY: Plenum Press

Tambling, R., & Johnson, L. (2008). The relationship between stages of change and outcome in couple therapy. *The American Journal of Family Therapy, 36,* 229–241.

Taylor-Seehafer, M., Johnson, R., Rew, L., Fouladi, R., Land, L., & Abel, E. (2007). Attachment and sexual health behaviors in homeless youth. *Journal for Specialists in Pediatric Nursing, 12*(1), 37–48.

chapter four

FEMALE SEXUAL/ REPRODUCTIVE ANATOMY & PHYSIOLOGY

CHAPTER OBJECTIVES

On completion of this chapter, students will be able to:

- understand the difference between primary and secondary sexual characteristics;
- identify the structures of the internal female sexual/reproductive anatomy;
- explain the female reproductive process;
- name the structures of the external female genitalia;
- distinguish the cancers that can occur in the female reproductive system.

ABBREVIATIONS AND ACRONYMS USED IN THIS CHAPTER

ACOG	American Congress of Obstetricians and Gynecologists
CDC	Centers for Disease Control and Prevention
cm	centimeters
DNA	deoxyribonucleic acid
FSH	follicle-stimulating hormone
HIV	human immunodeficiency virus
HPV	human papillomavirus
IUD	intra-uterine device
LH	luteinizing hormone
PMS	premenstrual syndrome
WHO	World Health Organization

PRIMARY AND SECONDARY SEXUAL CHARACTERISTICS

Both females and males have primary and secondary sexual characteristics. The *primary sexual characteristics* present in the human body are directly involved in reproductive function. For example, ovaries in females and testes in males are needed for procreation. *Secondary sexual characteristics* are physical aspects not part of the reproductive process and are typically associated with one sex but not the other (Jones & Lopez, 2006). Both primary and secondary sexual characteristics are developed or begin performing their function during puberty for both females and males (Jones & Lopez, 2006).

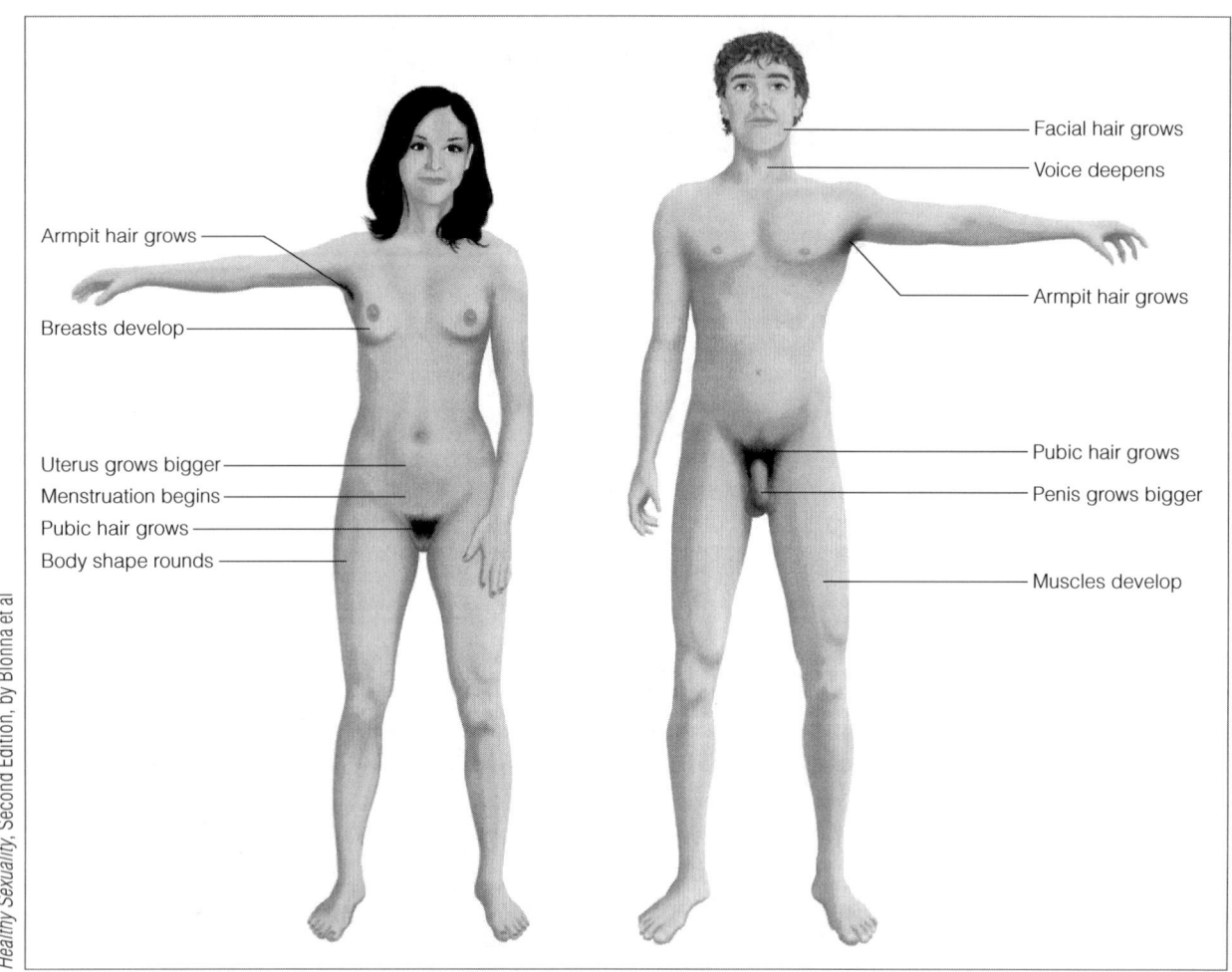

As illustrated above women are more likely to have increased fat deposits around the hips, whereas men are more likely to have broader shoulders (other male secondary sexual characteristics are discussed in chapter 5). Even though many countries (but not all) around the world have placed a sexual meaning on female breasts, they are not considered part of the reproductive process because they are not needed for procreation to occur. In females, the vagina, cervix, uterus, and fallopian tubes all have a role to play in reproduction, and thus are considered primary sexual characteristics. Their specific functions are discussed below.

Internal Female Reproductive/Sexual Anatomy

The internal reproductive anatomy consists of the vagina, cervix, uterus, fallopian tubes, and ovaries. The vagina and cervix are considered parts of the lower reproductive tract and the uterus, fallopian tubes, and ovaries are considered parts of the upper reproductive tract.

The Vagina

The vagina is a 4-inch elastic muscular canal that functions as a passageway for the menstrual flow, as a receptacle for the penis during coitus (vaginal-penile intercourse), and as part of the birth canal (Jones & Lopez, 2006). The vagina is located behind the bladder and in front of the rectum. The vaginal walls are composed of soft elastic folds of mucous membrane that are normally collapsed, but can stretch or contract (with support from pelvic muscles) during penetration and during a vaginal birth (Jones & Lopez, 2006).

The vagina has a balanced amount of "good" and "bad" bacteria to maintain an acidic environment that helps decrease microorganisms ascending into the upper reproductive tract (Ricci & Kyle, 2009). Any fluid with a pH level of 7 or lower is considered to be acidic. When a woman is not aroused, the vaginal pH level is approximately 4.5. When a woman is aroused, the vaginal pH level increases to 6.0 (Levin, 2003). Even though the vagina becomes less acidic when a woman is sexually aroused, as you will read in subsequent chapters, this organ's strong defense system kills the majority of sperm.

When a woman is sexually aroused, the vaginal walls begin to lubricate and become dark purple as this area engorges with blood (Meston, 2002). Estrogen receptors throughout the vaginal lining are responsible for maintaining vaginal lubrication, as well as the thickness and ridges of the vagina (Hirsch, 1998). Vaginal discharge occurs throughout the menstrual cycle (regardless of sexual activity). This is normal and should be seen as the vagina getting rid of cellular debris. During menstruation and after (unprotected) coitus, the vaginal walls push any fluid out of the *introitus* (vaginal opening).

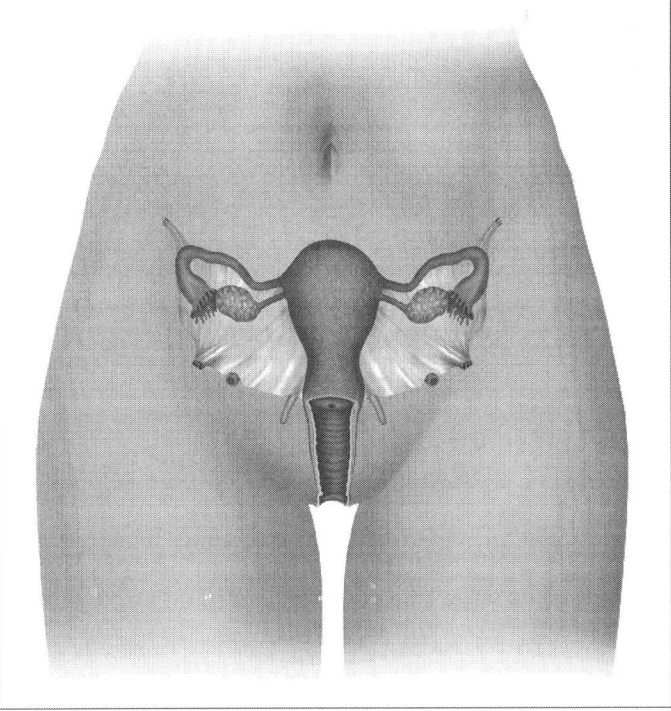

Many women are advised by well-meaning relatives and friends to douche to get rid of unwanted odor or fluid from the vagina. Martino and Vermund (2002) have found vaginal cleansing, such as douching, to harm the pH balance that could predispose women to vaginal infections like bacterial vaginosis (discussed in chapter 7). The vagina needs to be seen as a "self-cleaning oven"—we leave it alone and let it do its job! Any abnormal discharge that isn't consistent with a woman's normal secretions should be seen by a doctor instead of trying to self-medicate with over-the-counter feminine hygiene products.

Glands near the vaginal opening secrete fluid to keep the vaginal lining moist. The vaginal lining can tear if the vagina is not properly lubricated during coitus. This increases the risk of infection so care should be taken before penetration to ensure the vaginal lining will not be injured. Water-based lubricants that may be used to facilitate penetration will not harm the vaginal lining and can be used frequently. Only the first 1–2 centimeters (cm) in the vagina are believed to encompass numerous nerve receptors, which would make this area sensitive to the touch (Ginger & Yang, 2011). If penetration is painful, regardless of adequate lubrication, then such activity should cease until the cause is found

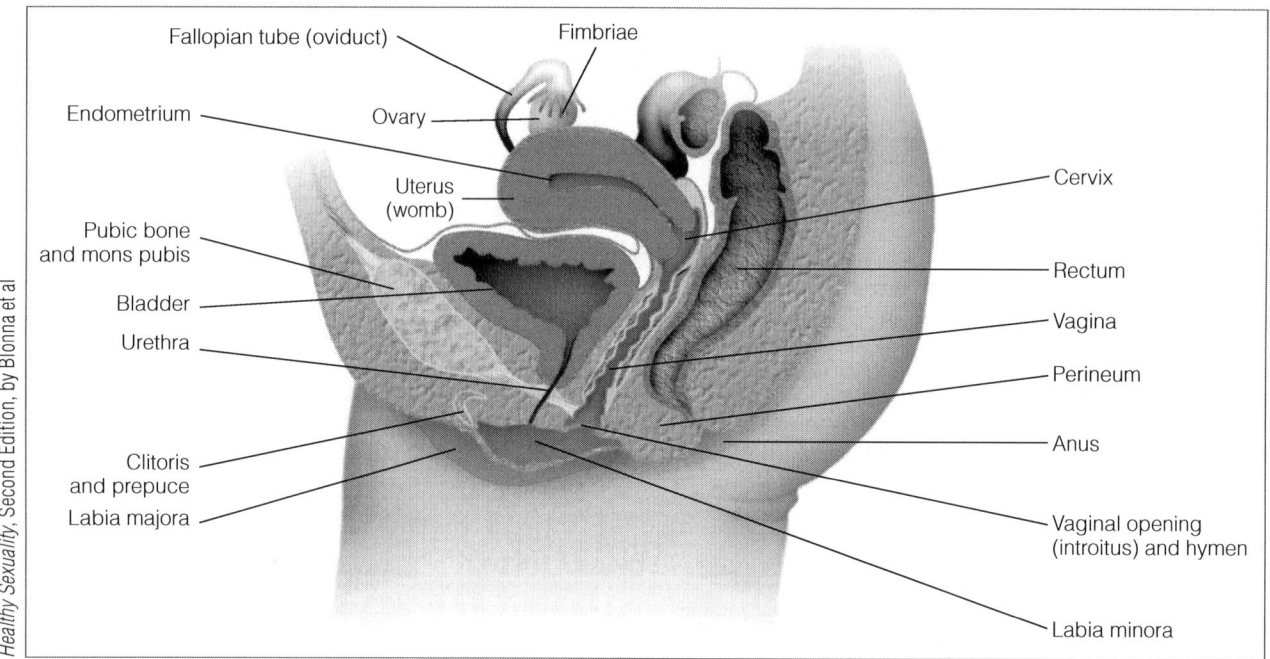

and rectified. Keep in mind that there are numerous other sensual activities possible (i.e., mutual masturbation and oral sex) that are pleasurable for both partners and do not require penetration.

How Deep Can a Penis Go in a Vagina?

The vagina is around 4 inches long and becomes a bit elongated when a woman is sexually aroused. During sexual arousal, the cervix decreases in length making it seem as if the vagina is even longer. The penis, which is around 5–6 inches when erect, cannot pass through the cervix so it will never be inside a uterus even though some women experience sensations as if the penis were in their abdomen. The size of an erect penis differs more than the length of a woman's vagina. For example, adult film star Lexington Steele's erect penis measures 13½ inches! A longer penis doesn't mean a better sexual experience, though. As mentioned above, only the first 1–2 cm of the vagina have nerve receptors, thus concentrating on this area can be pleasurable to the woman. Moreover, for

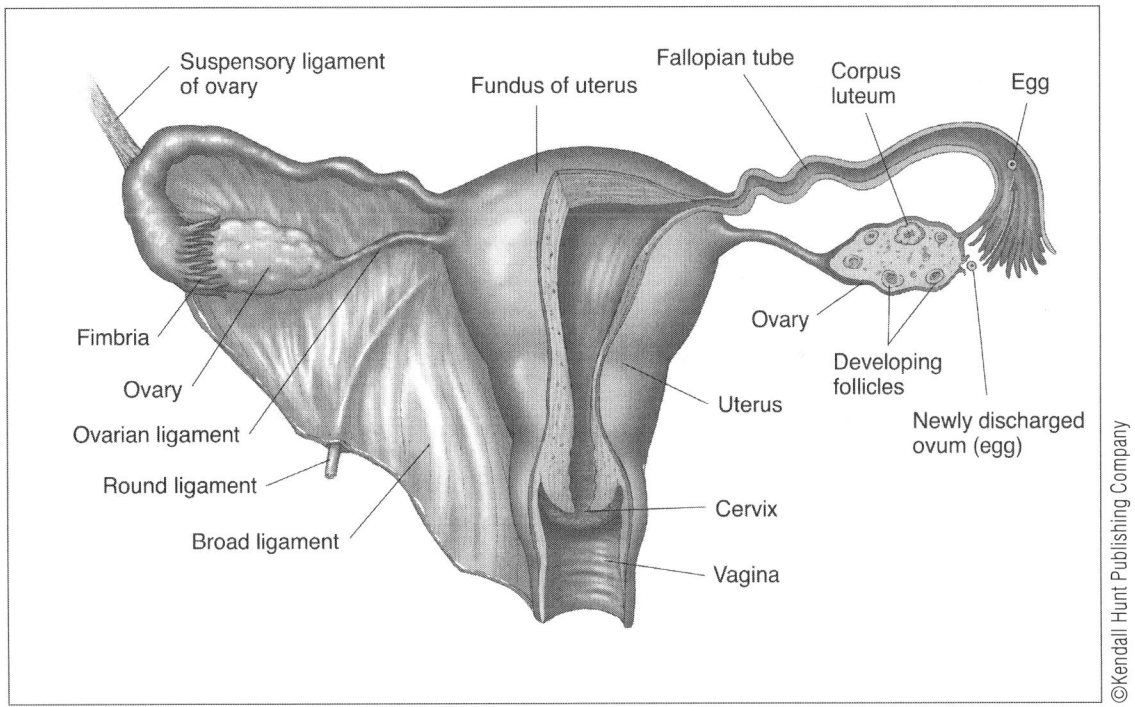

some women a longer penis means they will experience pain since the penis can constantly hit the cervix during thrusting, which in turn can shift the internal reproductive organs. The ovaries are homologous to the testes. As men painfully know, any unwanted shifting of the testes can hurt, and similarly, so can the ovaries if they are "moved" around.

The Cervix

The *cervix* is considered to be the lower part of the uterus (*cervix* means neck in Latin). The cervix connects the body of the uterus to the vagina. The *endocervix* is the part of the cervix closest to the uterus. The part next to the vagina is called the *ectocervix*. The ectocervix has a small opening called the *os*. During menstruation, the shedding of the endometrial lining emerges from the os to the vagina. To decrease infection of the upper reproductive tract, the cervix contains glands that secrete acidic mucus to plug the cervix (and the os) to prevent sperm or other microorganisms from entering the uterus (Jones & Lopez, 2006). When ovulation occurs (a mature ovarian follicle containing an oocyte is released from an ovary), the acidic mucus is released and discharged through the vagina. The cervix then produces mucus that is hospitable to sperm, allowing any live sperm (that have survived the vagina!) to travel through it to enter the uterus to make their way to the fallopian tubes to find the ovum (or egg) to fertilize it (Ricci & Kyle, 2009).

As soon as a pregnancy is established, the cervix creates a special antibacterial mucosal plug to block passage of microorganisms to the upper reproductive tract (Jones & Lopez, 2006). This reduces the risk of infection ascending into the uterus and harming the fetus. The cervix plays a vital role during the first stage of labor, as well. Contractions are focused on thinning out and dilating the cervix to 10 cm (around 4 inches) to allow the fetus to go through the vaginal canal and to be pushed out by the mother (the birth process is discussed in chapter 11). If a vaginal birth has not occurred, then the os has an oval opening. After a vaginal birth, the os is converted into a transverse slit (Ricci & Kyle, 2009).

The Uterus

The *uterus* is an inverted pear-shaped organ held in place by ligaments that stretch (as can the uterus) when a woman is pregnant (Jones & Lopez, 2006). The uterus is located in front of the rectum and behind the bladder. The body of the uterus is called the *corpus*. When a female is not pregnant, the uterus is around the size of her fist.

The uterus has three layers of tissue (Ricci & Kyle, 2009). The external surface of the uterus is called the *perimetrium*. Inside the perimetrium is a thick layer of smooth muscle called the *myometrium*. The strong uterine contractions a pregnant woman feels during labor come from the myometrium. Also, this layer contracts when a woman experiences an orgasm. The layer of the uterus that lines the uterine cavity is called the *endometrium*. This layer is shed during menstruation and it is the layer in which the blastocyst (discussed in chapter 11) implants itself to become a pregnancy (Jones & Lopez, 2006). Unlike the other layers of the uterus, the endometrium is under the control of progesterone and it endures a distinct transformation in structure and function throughout the menstrual cycle. The endometrial lining is at its thinnest just after menstruation and it is at its thickest during the part of the menstrual cycle in which the blastocyst would be expected to enter the uterus (Ricci & Kyle, 2009).

The surgical removal of the uterus is called a *hysterectomy* (his-tur-EK-tuh-mee). The uterus is usually removed through an incision in the lower abdomen, close to the pubic area. This procedure is usually performed in women in their early to mid 40s (Fogel & Woods, 2008). A partial hysterectomy removes only the uterus. This procedure is performed because of *endometriosis* (a medical condition in which the endometrial lining grows in other areas of the body), uterine cancer, chronic pelvic pain, and excessive menstrual bleeding (Bayram & Beji, 2010). A total hysterectomy removes the uterus and the cervix. A radical hysterectomy removes the uterus, cervix, fallopian tubes, ovaries, *and* the upper portion of the vagina. A radical hysterectomy is usually performed because of the spread of cancer to more than one of the reproductive organs.

A woman's menstrual cycle averages 28 days, but can range from 21 to 35 days and can vary every month. A woman experiences uterine bleeding for an average of 4 days, but that can vary from 2–6 days (Nelson & Baldwin, 2007). In the United States, the monthly flow of blood and cellular debris (called menses) usually starts around the age of 12½. Women experience menopause (discussed later in this chapter) around age 51 (Alexander LaRosa, Bader, & Garfield, 2007). During this timeframe, women will bleed around 13 times a year for almost 40 years. Given such statistics, more women should seriously consider buying feminine hygiene products in bulk!

Menstrual Difficulties

Dysmenorrhea is a condition in which a female experiences painful uterine cramping during menstruation. This can be caused by increased levels of the

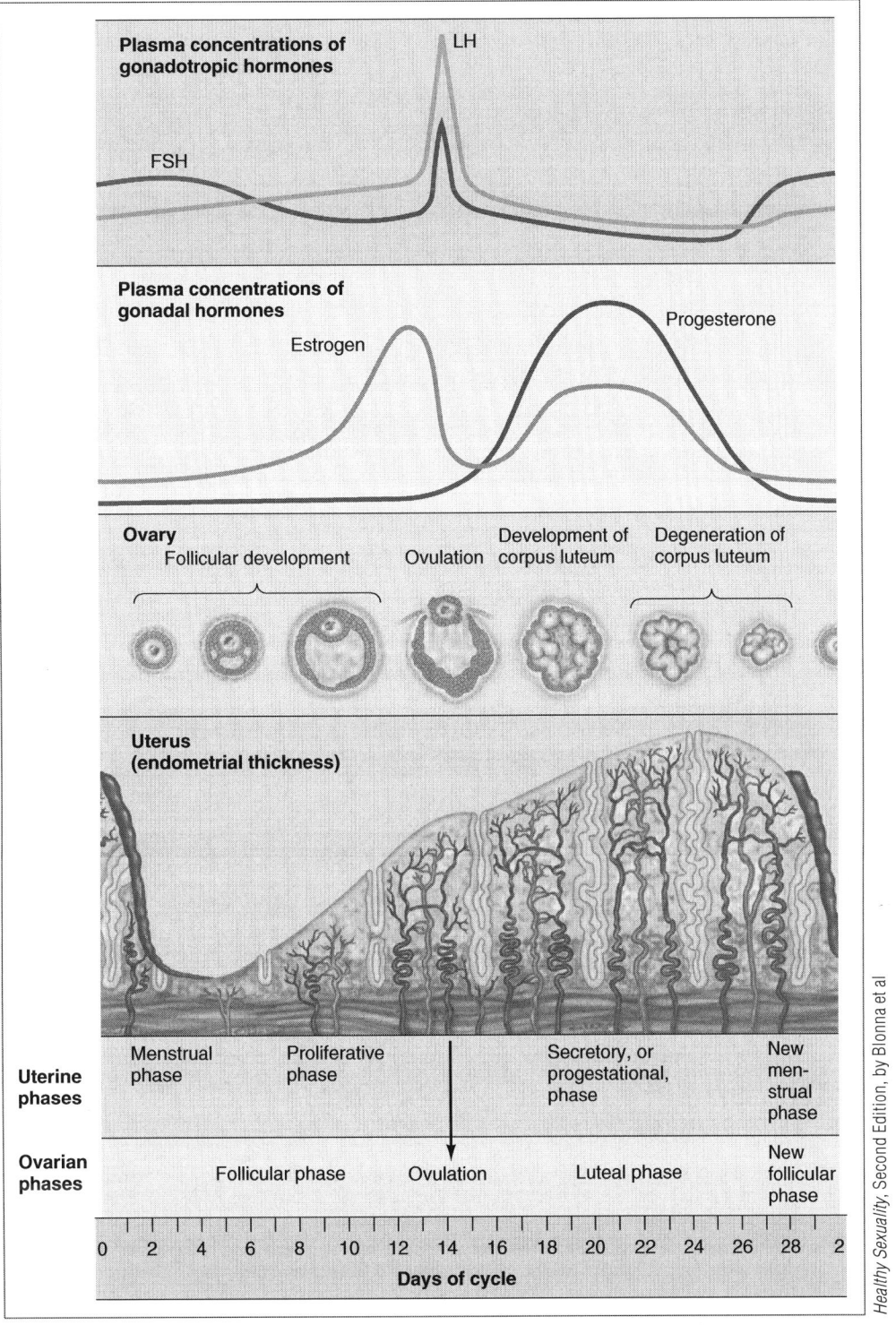

hormone, prostaglandins, an intra-uterine device (IUD), pelvic infection, endometriosis, and uterine tumors (Jones & Lopez, 2006). Women are asked to modify their dietary intake of caffeine and sodium, stop smoking, participate in daily physical activity, and use a heating pad when the cramping begins, as well as take over-the-counter pain medications to alleviate the pain.

Menorrhagia is a condition in which a female experiences very heavy menstrual bleeding. This can be caused by a hormonal imbalance, abnormal blood clotting, endometriosis, and uterine tumors. Menorrhagia may cause frequent absences from school, work, or other activities because of the constant heavy flow. Some women are prescribed a hormonal contraceptive to help control the amount of and days spent bleeding.

Oligomenorrhea is a condition in which a female misses or has infrequent menstrual periods, even though she has been menstruating for a while and is not pregnant (Jones & Lopez, 2006). This condition can be genetic or caused by stress, certain medications, or another uterine disorder. The cause needs to be ascertained because a treatment approach is recommended.

Amenorrhea is a condition in which a female has not started menstruating either by the time she is 16 years old or three years after starting puberty, has not developed signs of puberty by age 14, or has had normal menstrual periods but has stopped menstruating for some reason other than pregnancy (Jones & Lopez, 2006). This could be due to a hormonal imbalance, excessive exercise, an extremely low body fat (an adult woman's body needs around 22 percent body fat for menstrual cycles to continue) or an eating disorder.

The Fallopian Tubes

The *fallopian tubes*, named after the 16th century anatomist Fallopius, are about four inches in length and have a diameter about the size of a drinking straw (Jones & Lopez, 2006). The fallopian tubes are lined with *cilia* (hair-like extensions on cells) that beat toward the uterus. When ovulation occurs, the ovum is captured by the ends of the fallopian tube called the *fimbriae*. Fertilization (union of one egg and one sperm) must take place near the end of the fallopian tube to increase the chances of a successful implantation in the uterus in about a week's time. Unfortunately, the fallopian tubes can be harmed by bacterial infections such as chlamydia and gonorrhea (which are sexually transmitted) and bacterial vaginosis (which is not sexually transmitted). The irreversible damage to the fallopian tubes caused by any of these reproductive tract infections can lead to an ectopic pregnancy (a life-threatening condition that requires immediate medical attention). These reproductive tract infections are discussed in chapter 7.

The Ovaries

The *ovaries* are almond-shaped organs connected to the uterus and pelvic wall by supportive ligaments. They serve two functions in female reproduction: the development and maturation of *oocytes* (eggs), and the production of three hormones (Jones & Lopez, 2006). These hormones are estrogen, progesterone, and testosterone.

Females are born with a lifetime supply of eggs. According to the American Congress of Obstetricians and Gynecologists (ACOG), by the fifth month of pregnancy, the eggs have formed in the ovaries of a female fetus (ACOG, 2010). At birth, a female infant is born with about 5 million immature ovarian follicles that decrease to about 500,000 at puberty (Speroff & Fritz, 2005). That number continues to decline as females get older. By the age of 35, there will be fewer than 100,000 and by menopause the follicular supply will be nearly depleted (Jones & Lopez, 2006). Most women will ovulate one ovum (ova is plural) once a month over a 40-year reproductive life span. That means women will ovulate

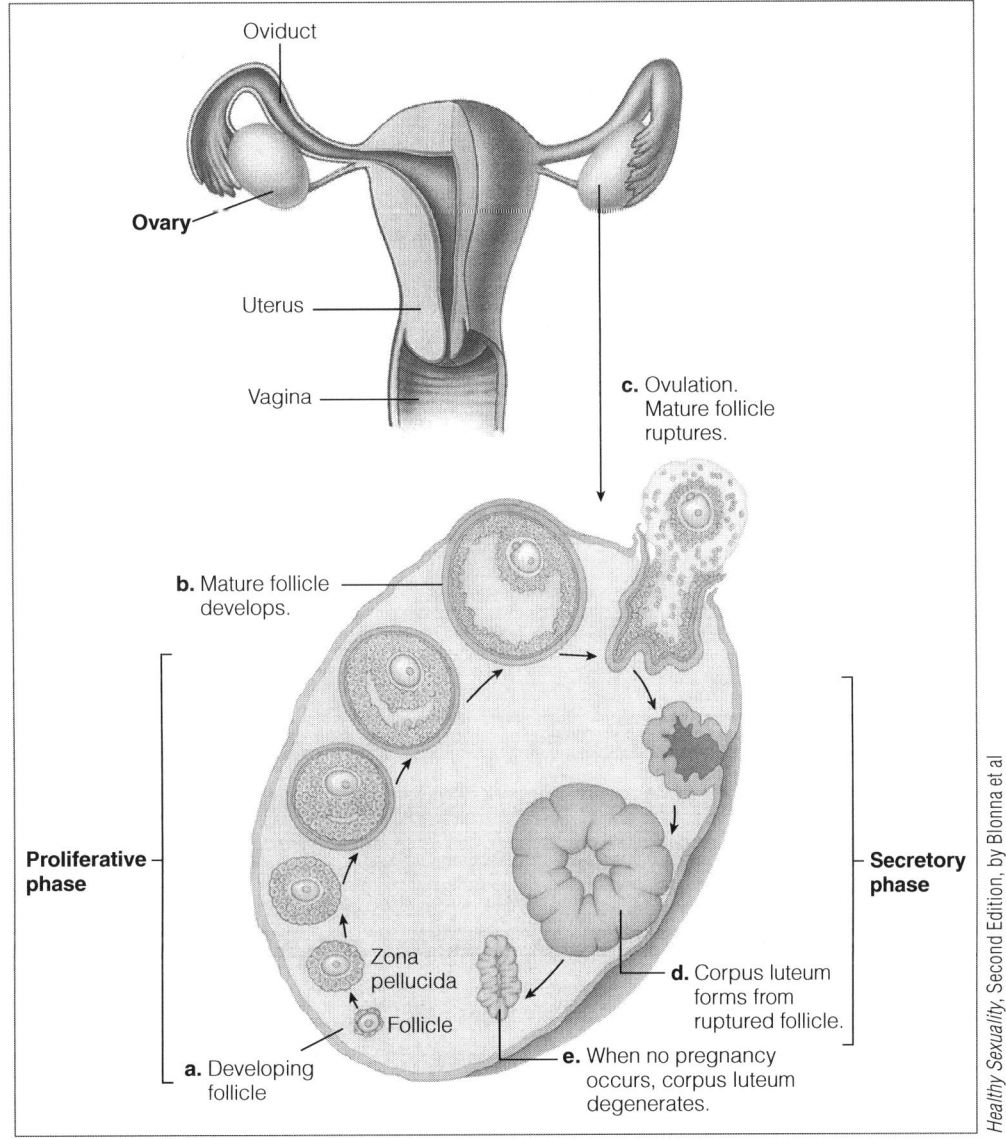

around 400–500 times during their fertile years. An ovum is viable for fertilization for around 24–48 hours (Ricci & Kyle, 2009). Most of these ova are not fertilized and women will bleed anywhere from 14–20 days *after* ovulation occurs (Ricci & Kyle, 2009).

Women's fertile years in the United States have changed dramatically relative to our hunter-gatherer ancestors (Jones & Lopez, 2006). For example, thousands of years ago, females experienced menarche (their first menstrual period) around the age of 16. Girls now start menstruating 3½ years earlier. We used to give birth to our first child around the age of 19. Now we give birth for the first time around the age of 25 (the oldest average age for a first birth on record for this country). An average completed family size used to include five children. Now, on average, women have around two children in their lifetime. Thousands of years ago, women breast-fed their baby for three years. Today, women breast-feed their baby for three months (CDC, 2007). Why are females menstruating earlier, starting a family later in life, having a smaller family size,

Chapter Four **47**

and breast-feeding for considerably less time? We can attribute the "birth" of modern industrialized societies to the changes in fertility. Like many societies similar to ours, the United States has changed significantly by the advances of agricultural, industrial, and medical industries (Jones & Lopez, 2006). That is not to say these advances have not been beneficial to society. Our life expectancy has increased and our maternal/infant mortality has decreased, and for this our societal advances can take much of the credit.

FEMALE REPRODUCTIVE PROCESS

Cholesterol is needed for the development and secretion of the hormones by the ovaries (Jones & Lopez, 2006). Cholesterol is made by the liver. Women do not need extra cholesterol from the food they eat because their bodies make all that

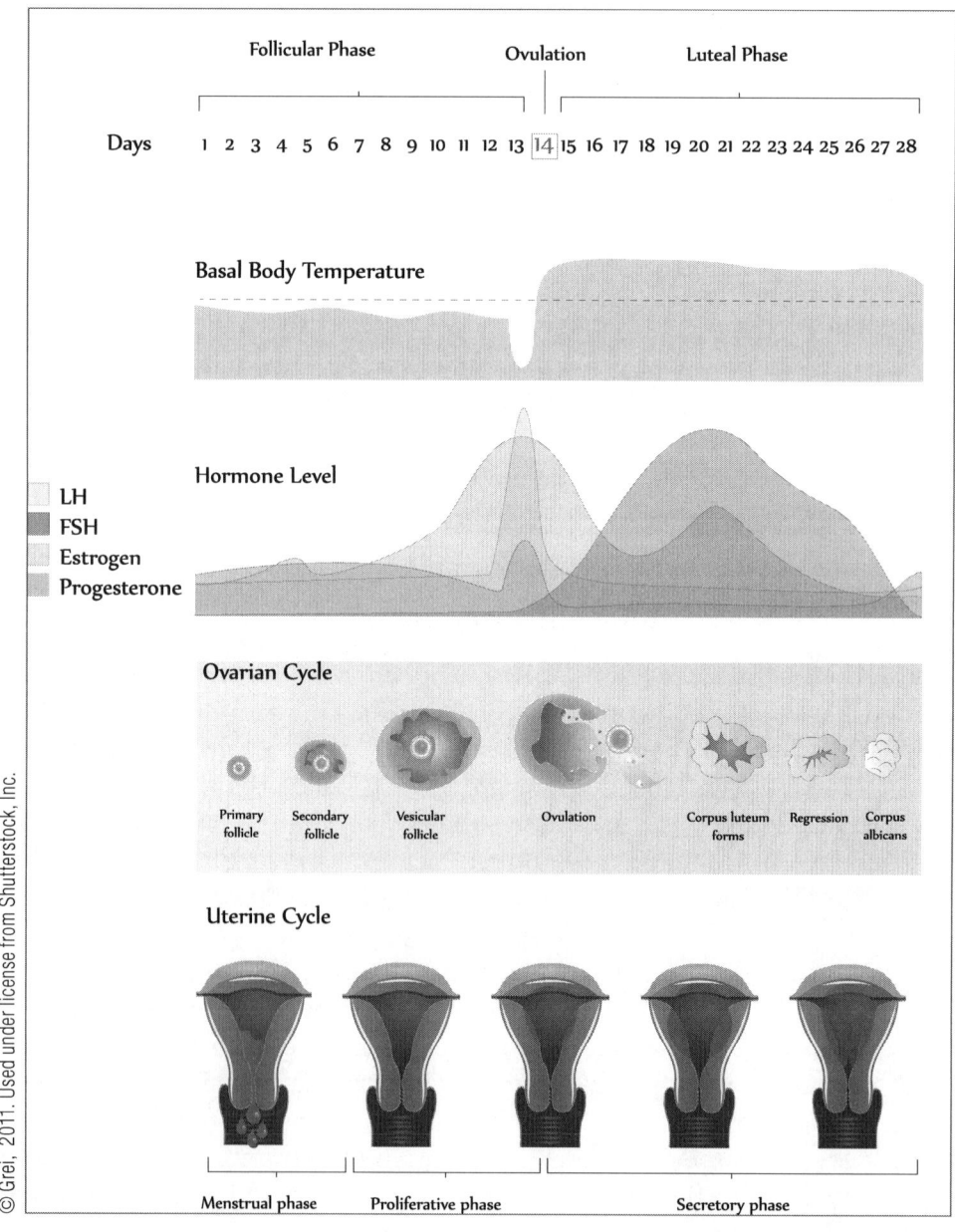

they need. As previously mentioned, these hormones are estrogen, progesterone, and testosterone. Testosterone is also made by the female's adrenal glands. The secretion of these hormones and the maturation of the ovarian follicles are controlled by the release of follicle-stimulating hormone (FSH) and luteinizing hormone (LH) in the pituitary gland (Harvard Medical School, 2005; Jones & Lopez, 2006). The following figure illustrates how these two hormones orchestrate the menstrual cycle:

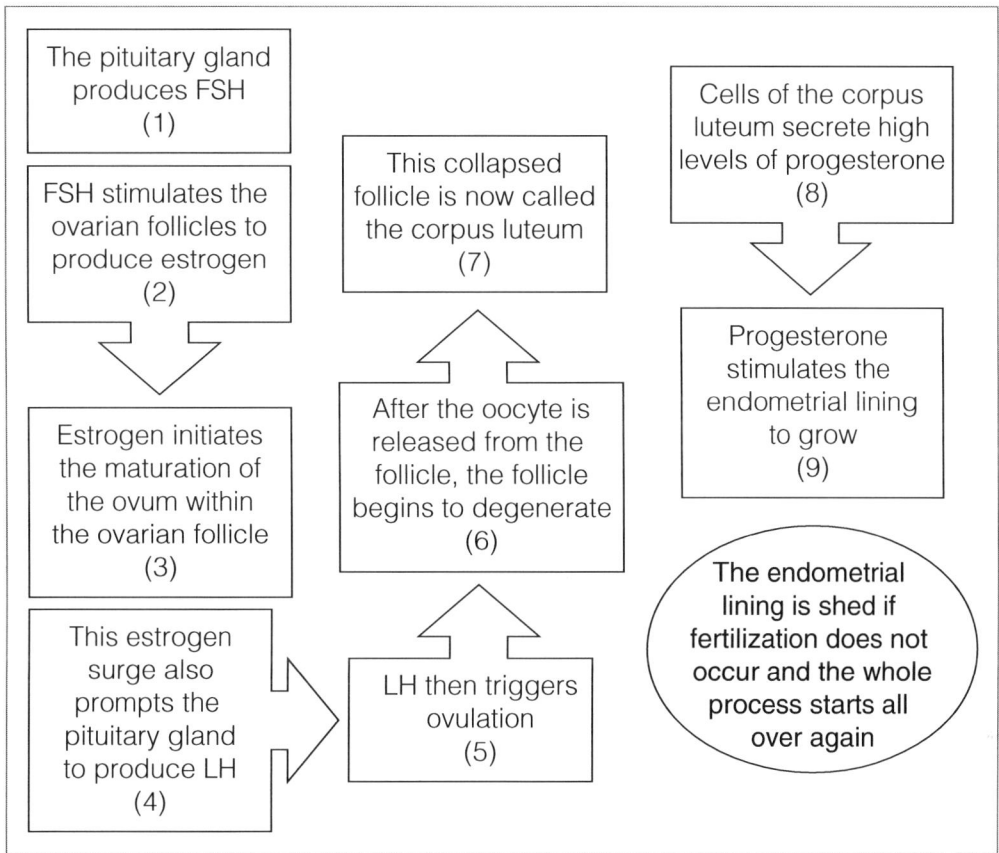

Figure 5.1   The Menstruel Cycle

During a female's reproductive years (in the United States, that range is from 12½ to 51 years of age), hormonal fluctuations occur across the menstrual cycle. The rise and fall of certain hormones can affect a woman's mood, appetite, and sex drive. For example, estrogen and testosterone affect energy levels, and progesterone induces a sense of relaxation and calmness (Douma, Husband, O'Donnelly, Baruin, & Wooden, 2005; Santoro et al., 2005). Every menstrual cycle begins on the first day a female starts bleeding. Levels of estrogen, progesterone, and testosterone are low early in the cycle. Thus, it is no surprise that many women experience a low libido and have low energy. Right before ovulation, estrogen and testosterone levels peak. Many women feel a surge in energy, as well as sex drive (Douma et al., 2005). After ovulation, hormonal production of progesterone begins to surge as testosterone and estrogen levels decline. Many women feel a sense of tranquility during this time (Santoro et al., 2005). Mood, though, is affected by a woman's surroundings, so if she is experiencing high levels of stress due to external factors, then her sex drive or sense of well-being could be compromised, regardless of what stage she is in during her menstrual cycle.

One or two weeks before the onset of menstruation, women may begin experiencing *premenstrual syndrome* (PMS). PMS occurs because the sharp drop in hormonal levels triggers a sense of withdrawal, which can produce an array of symptoms. Some women begin craving certain foods, experience bloating, headaches, mood swings, breast tenderness, and even a surge in their sex drive (Freeman et al., 2011). Interestingly, many of these symptoms can occur throughout the menstrual cycle. To alleviate the symptoms, women are asked to

1. participate in daily physical activity;
2. reduce their intake of high-calorie, low nutrient dense foods and liquids (i.e., junk food);
3. increase their intake of water;
4. decrease their consumption of salty foods;
5. improve their sleeping habits;
6. try to reduce stress (ACOG, 2001).

Females can also experience a range of emotional (i.e., mood swings), behavioral (i.e., food cravings), and physical (i.e., breast tenderness) symptoms during key life transitions, such as during puberty, premenstrual, postpartum, and perimenopausal periods (Howland, 2010).

Menopause

According to the North American Menopause Society, menopause is considered the permanent end of menstruation and fertility. All women eventually experience menopause. It is a normal, natural event when the ovaries cease producing the hormones estrogen, progesterone, and testosterone, and they no longer release an ovum from an ovary (Nelson & Stewart, 2007). During the reproductive years, these hormones are critical in the maintenance of the tissue structure and function of the genitals. The loss of these hormones alters the genital tissue in structure (i.e., thins out the vaginal walls and shortens the vagina), which adversely affects the response to sexual stimulation. Moreover, the lowered levels of estrogen and testosterone are associated with reduced genital blood flow and lubrication (Goldstein & Silberstein, 2011).

Even so, women can continue to experience sexual pleasure and satisfying sexual relationships after menopause (Katz-Bearnot, 2010). Women and their sexual partners need to realize these physical changes are normal and that there are numerous ways to alleviate any anxiety, frustration, or pain by exploring numerous ways that sexual pleasure can be achieved. For example, for reduced vaginal lubrication, buying a water-based lubricant helps keep the introitus and vagina wet for penetration. Using a vibrator can also help women experience an orgasm if other forms of stimulation are not as intense as they used to be. Moreover, considering other forms of pleasure (i.e., lying naked together, giving each other body massages, and washing each other's body in the shower) that may not lead to orgasm for either partner can be pleasing as well.

As previously mentioned, women in the Unites States go through menopause around the age of 51 (Alexander et al., 2007). One percent of women are menopausal before the age of 40 and around 2 percent of women have not experienced menopause by the age of 55. Half of all women will not experience any symptoms associated with menopause, such as hot flashes (the scientific name is vasomotor symptoms), night sweats, sleep disturbances, and irritability (Harvard Medical School, 2005). Vasomotor instability occurs because estrogen levels fluctuate erratically and fall during menopause, thus disrupting a woman's internal thermostat causing hot flashes. Research has found that women who are overweight or obese, smoke, and are stressed out are more likely to experience hot flashes. For months or years leading up to menopause, women can experience many of the symptoms listed above, as well as menstruating irregularly or bleeding more heavily than usual. This is known as *perimenopause*. Many women start producing less progesterone in their late 30s (Nelson & Stewart, 2007). This is believed to be a cause for menstrual problems during this life transition. If a woman's menstrual cycle becomes irregular, she should visit her doctor to confirm if she is experiencing perimenopause or menopause, or if her cycle is being affected by some other medical condition. A woman might have her blood tested to determine her hormonal levels, an internal exam (where her doctor inserts a few of her/his fingers into her vagina to feel her uterus and her ovaries), and/or an ultrasound to obtain a better view of a woman's uterus and ovaries. The latter two screenings are to rule out ovarian cysts (pockets of fluid in an ovary), uterine fibroids (noncancerous tumors that grow in the uterus), endometriosis (when the endometrial lining grows outside of the uterus), and uterine cancer.

EXTERNAL FEMALE GENITALIA

Girls and women in the United States find it easier to recall the clinical terms to the internal female reproductive anatomy than a female's external genitals. Even though many of us do not know the clinical terms to this external area of the female body, we were raised with colorful words for the female genitalia. Why do you think that's the case? Along with discussing what's really "down there," this section reviews female cosmetic genital surgeries, such as hymenoplasty, labiaplasty, perineoplasty, and vaginoplasty. Keep in mind that the American Congress of Obstetrics and Gynecology (ACOG, 2007) advises against many of these cosmetic procedures due to lack of safety and efficacy data, as well as potential complications, including infection, altered sensation, chronic genital pain, adhesions, and scarring.

Vulva

The *vulva* is the clinical term that covers all of the female external genitals. Some of us were raised calling this area the "vagina," but that part of the female anatomy is internal, not external. The vulva varies greatly in appearance. There is no set standard as to what is considered "normal." Moreover, sexual pleasure is not determined by the size or shape of the vulva. The vulva includes the following:

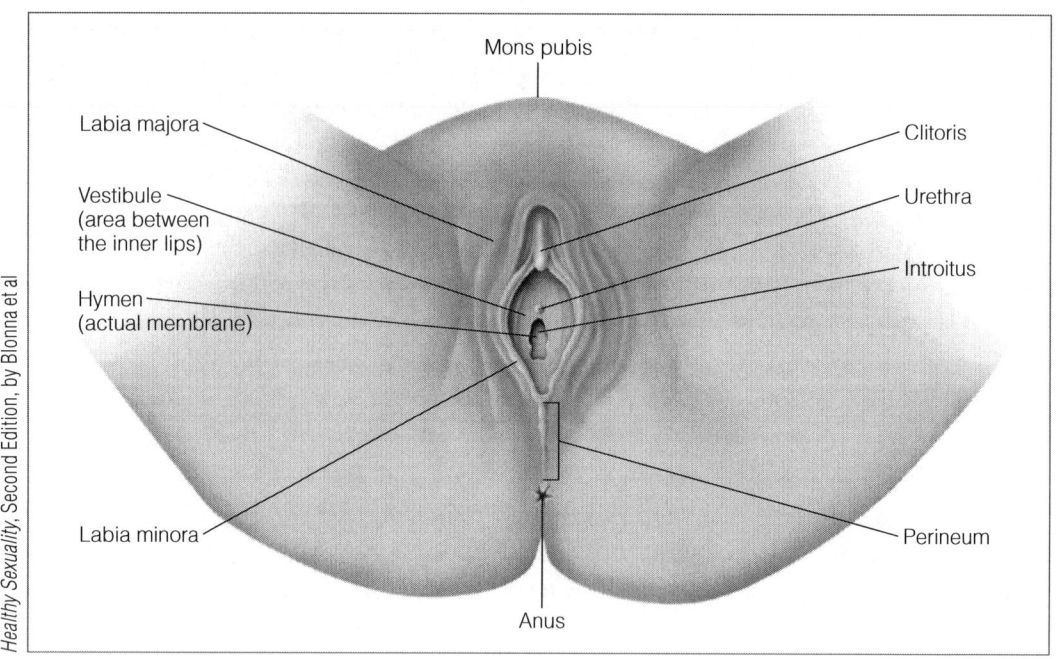

Mons Pubis

The *mons pubis*, which has also been called the mons veneris, is a cushion of fatty tissue, covered by skin and pubic hair forming an inverted pyramid. This area contains numerous touch receptors, which means the mons pubis can be sensitive to the touch (Ricci & Kyle, 2009).

Labia Majora

The *labia majora* are fleshy folds of tissue that extend down from the mons pubis and surround the vaginal and urethral openings. This area contains fat, sweat and oil glands, as well as pubic hair on the pigmented skin. This area is not as sensitive to the touch as the mons pubis (Jones & Lopez, 2006).

Labia Minora

The *labia minora* are paired folds of smooth tissue underlying the labia majora and outlining the vaginal opening (Ginger & Yang, 2011). They are fleshy-looking in color and are hairless, but contain oil glands. Smegma (natural secretions that moisten the area) can accumulate and cause discomfort and infection. To avoid smegma buildup, a female can gently clean the vulva with water and a washcloth or her fingers on a daily basis. The labia minora are abundant with nerve endings, making this area highly sensitive. When a woman becomes sexually aroused, they engorge with blood and turn a darker color (Ricci & Kyle, 2008). They vary in size and have become a focal point in women who are dissatisfied with the appearance of their genitals or experience discomfort due to their size (Cartwright & Cardozo, 2008). Women with this negative attitude can opt to have their labia minora surgically altered, a practice called *labiaplasty*. This relatively new cosmetic surgical procedure is known to decrease vulvar sensitivity and there are few validated long-term safety or outcome data presently available, thus caution is strongly encouraged (Goodman, 2009). Interestingly, in Rwanda, females are raised in the practice of elongating their labia minora. To do so is meant to increase female and male pleasure (Koster & Leimar Price, 2008).

Glans of the Clitoris

Most people believe that the external part of the clitoris is the only part of the clitoris. The whole clitoris is found both internally and externally, and encompasses thousands of nerve endings and contains erectile tissue (spongy tissue with blood vessels that engorge with blood to cause an erection). The whole clitoris (both internal and external) measures around 10 cm in length. The internal body of the clitoris extends over both sides of the mons pubis and the vaginal walls (Ginger & Yang, 2011). The external part is located approximately 1 cm above the urethral opening (Ginger & Yang, 2011). It increases in size when a woman becomes sexually aroused. This is the only organ in the human body whose sole purpose is to transmit sexual pleasure (Katz, 2007). Conversely, there is no part of the male body whose sole purpose is for sexual pleasure. Touching the glans of the clitoris can also be uncomfortable, if not painful to the touch. When this area is stimulated effectively, though, a woman can experience an array of pleasurable sensations.

Clitoral Hood

The clitoral hood is a fold of skin that covers and protects the glans of the clitoris (Jones & Lopez, 2006). During sexual arousal, as the glans of the clitoris engorges with blood it "hides" behind the clitoral hood.

Urethral Opening

The vulva has three openings that lead to outside the body. The urethral opening allows liquid waste to leave a female's body. The *Skene's glands* are located on either side of the urethral opening. These glands secrete fluid to keep the urethral opening moist and lubricated for the passage of urine (Schuiling & Likis, 2006). The Skene's glands are also believed to ejaculate a fluid in some women during orgasm (it is unknown why some women ejaculate and why some women don't). This fluid does not contain urine and is similar to the fluid developed by a male's prostate gland (discussed in chapter 5). The Skene's glands are homologous to the prostate gland. The Skene's glands have been referred to as the "female prostate," but it is erroneous to identify these glands as such even if both the Skene's and

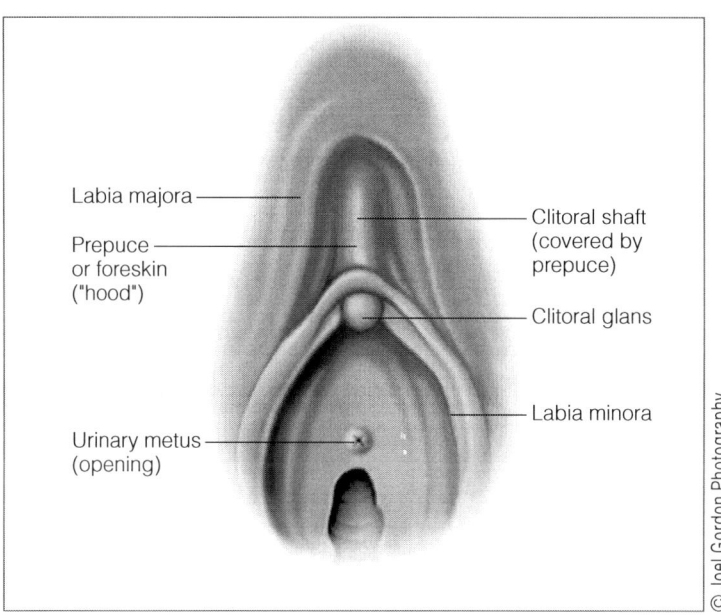

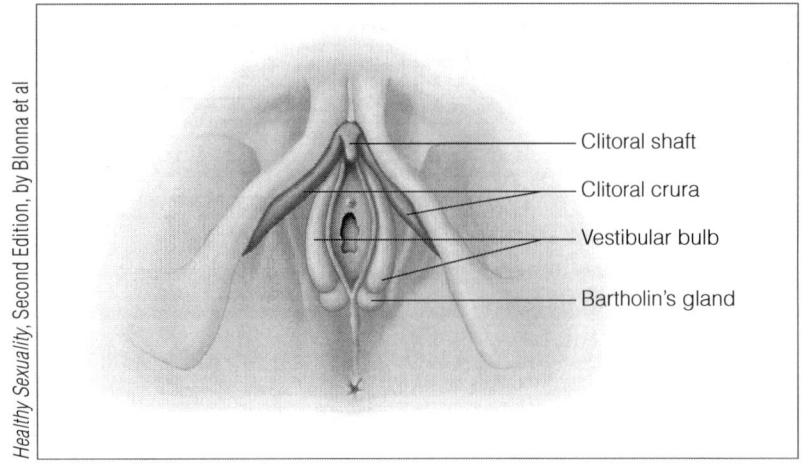

prostate glands were developed from the same embryonic tissue. They were provided different names because their function is not exactly the same and their physical structure does not carry much resemblance.

Introitus

The opening to the vagina is called the *introitus*. This area contains numerous touch receptors, which means the vaginal opening can be sensitive to the touch (Ginger & Yang, 2011). This is the opening through which menstrual blood will flow out of the body, a baby can be born, and an erect penis can enter. Through tiny ducts beside the lower portion of the introitus, the Bartholin's glands secrete fluid that provides vaginal lubrication when a woman is sexually aroused (Schuiling & Likis, 2006).

The reconstruction of a vagina is called *vaginoplasty* (Goodman, 2009). It has been used on women who were born with genetic abnormalities (e.g., androgen insensitivity syndrome, congenital adrenal hyperplasia, vaginal agenesis, and müllerian agenesis) that affected the development of a "functional" vagina. For some of these women, the vagina has limited vaginal dimensions (depth and width), thus hindering the participation in coitus (if wanted). Females who were born with ambiguous genitals have also undergone this procedure even though the Intersex Society of North America questions the need for such surgery. Women who have experienced trauma to the lower reproductive tract due to cervical, vaginal, or vulvar cancer have also taken advantage of this surgical cosmetic procedure to reshape their vagina. A vaginoplasty can also be performed during male to female sex reassignment surgery. This unique procedure is discussed in chapter 8.

Hymen

The *hymen* is a fold of mucous membrane that surrounds or partially covers the introitus at birth. Its purpose is unknown, even though many cultures throughout history have used the (perceived) absence of the hymen as indication that a woman has previously participated in coitus. However, any tearing of the hymen is not an indication that a female has had a penis in her vagina (Mattson & Smith, 2004). The hymen can also tear by participating in any number of physical activities, such as strenuous sports and even horseback riding. That does not mean horseback riding should be prohibited. The point is to realize that the hymen can tear for reasons unrelated to sexual activity. Moreover, the hymen can remain intact, though stretched, after penile penetration. The hymen is not completely removed until a vaginal birth has occurred.

Hymenoplasty is a surgical procedure in which the hymen is restored to mimic the appearance that the vagina had not been penetrated, thus attempting to

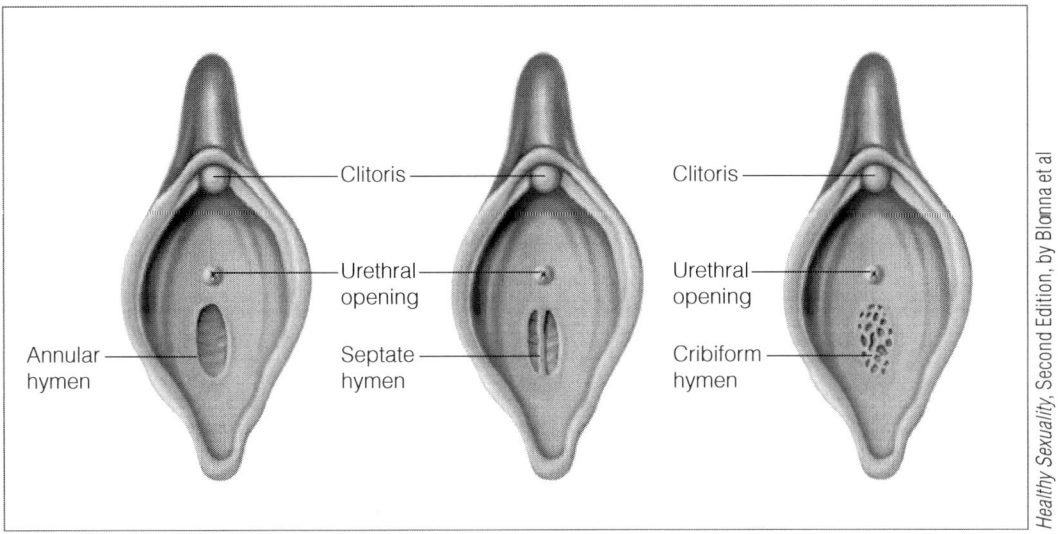

erase evidence of the sexual history of a woman (O'Conner, 2008). Such practice is sought after by women (or their families) contemplating marriage in cultures where a high value is placed on (female) virginity (defined as never having had participated in coitus). Thus, this controversial practice is seen to perpetuate misogynist myths about virginity (Cartwright & Cardozo, 2008). Moreover, there is no evidence to suggest hymenoplasty has a high success rate, but scarring, infection, and chronic pain are a reality for many women who have undergone this procedure.

Perineum

The area of the *perineum* is located between the introitus and the anus. It contains numerous nerve endings and is sensitive to the touch (Ricci & Kyle, 2009). Males also have a perineum and it is also called a perineum! A surgical incision to this area can be performed to widen the vaginal opening if a pregnant woman is having difficulty pushing the baby out. This procedure is called an *episiotomy*.

Sometimes after a vaginal birth or an episiotomy, the perineum is damaged and becomes loose over time. A surgical procedure known as *perineoplasty* is sometimes used to remedy this affliction by tightening the perineal muscles (Goodman, 2009). Actually, perineum repair is the most common use of perineoplasty. Perineoplasty is also used to treat *vaginismus* (involuntary contraction of the perineal muscles) and *dyspareunia* (painful coitus). To alleviate these medical conditions, this procedure can also be used to loosen the tight perineal muscles and introitus (Goodman, 2009).

Anus

The anus is the external opening of the rectum. There is no difference between a female and a male anus. This area allows solid waste (i.e., feces) to be expelled from the body. The area has a relatively high concentration of nerve endings that suggests sensitivity to the touch. The anus does not contain glands to moisten the area, so a water-based lubricant is required if penetration is expected. Moreover, the anal sphincter does not stretch like the introitus, thus moistening the area may reduce any tearing. To reduce pain that may occur when participating in anal sex for the first time, the anus should be penetrated gently by a finger or sex toys specifically designed for the anus. Anal/penile penetration should only be initiated when the receptive (and insertive) partner is willing to participate in this sexual activity. Also, a condom should always be worn to reduce the risk of sexually transmitted infections and coming into contact with feces.

FEMALE GENITAL MODIFICATION

For hundreds, if not thousands of years, girls and women have had their external genitals modified to decrease sexual desire and deter nonmarital sexual activity (Talle, 2001). All of these societies condemn (to some extent) female sexual pleasure. Boys and men in these countries (or any country for that matter) never had to endure having their genitals modified for the same reasons (male genital modification is discussed in chapter 5). Most of these countries are in Africa and parts of the Middle East (Smith Oboler, 2001). It has also occurred in Southeast Asia, and been reported in some tribes in South America and Australia. According to the World Health Organization (WHO), some of the countries with high rates of female genital modification are India, Chad, Côte d'Ivoire, Eritrea, Ethiopia, Gambia, Guinea, Kenya, Mali, Sierra Leone, northern Saudi Arabia, Sudan, Djibouti, southern Jordan, and Iraq Kurdistan, Indonesia, Central African Republic, Burkina Faso, and Mauritania.

The majority of the time these girls' genitals are not modified under hygienic conditions in sterile environments and, thus, risk of infection is high. The equipment used for these procedures are usually scissors, shard glass, and a razor blade. There is rarely, if ever, any local or general anesthesia used to help the female experience less pain.

Circumcision

The "least invasive" genital modification procedure is called a circumcision (Smith Oboler, 2001). It is somewhat similar to the modification performed on males in which their foreskin and frenulum are removed. In this procedure for girls, the clitoral hood is removed, permanently exposing the glans of the clitoris. Depending on the culture, this procedure may be performed during infancy or childhood.

Clitoridectomy

A clitoridectomy removes the clitoral hood and the glans of the clitoris (Smith Oboler, 2001). In some societies, this procedure is performed on girls between 7–11 years of age. Before the procedure, a girl is given special attention to highlight the significance of the event. Depending on the culture, other women may not be present during the clitoridectomy. Many times a man (usually a relative) holds the girl's legs and spreads them as she sits on him. A "healer" from the community, which, depending on the culture, may only be a man, takes a pair of scissors and cuts the girl's clitoral hood and glans of the clitoris. The girl will experience extreme pain. The healer will bandage the area tightly to reduce bleeding. The girl is allowed a few days to rest at home. Again, depending on the culture, she may be made to wear her glans of the clitoris (which is wrapped in a bandage) on her wrist during her resting period. Why would a girl be made to wear a part of her body that was recently removed? Many believe it is a way for the girl (and others around her) to realize that is she is now "pure" and she will not succumb to the immoral thoughts and behaviors that occur in females whose clitoral glans have not been removed.

Genital Infibulation

Genital infibulation is the most invasive procedure done, and death has occurred from the loss of blood and infection (Smith Oboler, 2001). The girl is held by other women as the procedure is performed, and she is usually around the age of 9–11. Keep in mind that *no* anesthesia is provided to the girl, thus extreme pain is experienced throughout the procedure and for days or weeks after. First, a clitoridectomy is performed, either with scissors or shard glass. Then her labia minora and labia majora are cut off, usually using shard glass. The area is sewn together and a small wooden stick is placed in her vaginal opening. The insertion of a wooden stick in the introitus helps keep the opening from closing completely. The area of the genitals where the urethral opening resides is now sewn up, but not the urethral opening itself. When a female with this procedure urinates, the urine is expelled through the opening left for the introitus. That means the urine has to flow down to the vaginal opening to leave the body. It is possible for urine and menstrual blood to pool within this opening instead of flowing freely through the vaginal opening.

The United Nations Human Rights Committee and the American Academy of Pediatrics consider female genital modification unethical. After a few infamous cases in which girls' genitals were modified in this country, the U.S. passed a law in 1995 that makes the practice illegal to anyone under the age of 18. What is not well known is that from 1890 to the late 1930s, the U.S. allowed various forms of female genital modification to "cure" masturbation (Hamilton, 2002). Even today, there are African and Muslim immigrant families in the U.S. that condone this practice for cultural and religious reasons (Elwood, 2005). Moreover, the U.S. continues to allow the controversial practice of removing the clitoral glans of baby girls born with a larger than normal clitoris (Crooks & Baur, 2011). The United Kingdom bans this practice for all females, regardless of age. Many countries with residents who practice female genital modification have laws against it as well, mostly pressured by the United States. These laws, though, are rarely enforced and, thus, female genital modification continues (Smith Oboler, 2001).

CANCER OF THE FEMALE REPRODUCTIVE SYSTEM

When women think about cancer, many think of breast cancer and/or cervical cancer (depending on age and media exposure). Other than skin cancer, breast cancer is the most common cancer in American women and most of them will be diagnosed over the age of 60 (American Cancer Society, 2011). Breast cancer is the second leading cause of cancer deaths in American women, behind only lung cancer. Additionally, women are plagued by cervical cancer, cancer of the vulva, vagina, uterus, and ovaries. Each of these cancers is discussed below. Three out of the five cancers discussed in this chapter are primarily caused by human papillomavirus, or HPV, a sexually transmitted infection (zur Hausen, 2009).

Cancer Statistics

The American Cancer Society's most recent estimates for cancers of the female reproductive organs in the United States are for 2011. Keep in mind that women are more likely to be diagnosed with heart disease (1 in 2 women), sexually transmitted infections (1 in 4 women), or breast cancer (1 in 8 women) than a cancer of the reproductive organs. In 2011, 88,080 women were diagnosed with a cancer of one of five reproductive organs: cervical, ovarian, uterine, vaginal, or vulvar. Table 4.1 includes statistics on cancers of the female reproductive organs (American Cancer Society, 2011).

Table 4.1 STATISTICS ON CANCERS OF THE FEMALE REPRODUCTIVE ORGANS, 2011*

Cancer	2011 Estimated New Cases	2011 Estimated Deaths	2011 Lifetime Risk of Being Diagnosed	Percent of All Cancers of the Female Reproductive Organs
Uterus (corpus)	46,470	8,120	1 in 39	52.7%
Ovaries	21,990	15,460	1 in 70	24.9%
Cervix	12,710	4,290	1 in 147	14.4%
Vulva	4,340	940	**	4.9%
Vagina	2,570	780	**	2.9%

* American Cancer Society (2011). Cancer facts and figures 2011. Atlanta, GA: American Cancer Society.
** Rate is low because of how rare these cancers are.

Cancer of the Uterus

According to the American Cancer Society (2011), almost half of all cancers of the female reproductive organs were reported as developing in the uterus. Thus, cancer of the uterus (which includes cancer of the body of the uterus and the endometrial lining) is the most common cancer of the female reproductive organs in the United States. Why is that the case? After the person becomes an adult, most cells in the body divide only to replace worn-out or dying cells or to repair injuries. However, the cells of the inner lining of the uterus, the endometrium, divide based on a woman's monthly menstrual cycle. Constant cell division can increase the risk of one cell not dividing properly or not dying off when it is expected to. Moreover, the endometrium is influenced by the hormone estrogen that is supplied by the ovaries. As previously mentioned, the ovaries also produce progesterone, but a shift in the balance of these two hormones toward more estrogen increases a woman's risk for developing endometrial cancer. Endometrial cancer is rare in women under age 40. Most cases are found in women 50 years and older (American Cancer Society, 2011).

Some common symptoms of uterine cancer are abnormal vaginal bleeding, pain during coitus and/or in the pelvic area, as well pain when urinating. Depending on the stage of the cancer, a *partial hysterectomy* may have to be performed to reduce the risk of the cancer spreading to the lymph nodes or other parts of the body. A partial hysterectomy is the surgical removal of the uterus. If the cancer has spread to other reproductive organs, a radical hysterectomy removes the ovaries, fallopian tubes, uterus, cervix, and upper portion of the vagina.

Cancer of the Cervix

The incidence of new cases of cervical cancer in the United States was 7 per 100,000 women in 2004, about half the incidence globally. Given the media exposure of preventing cervical cancer, most women believe they are at a higher risk of cervical cancer than uterine cancer. But that is not the case, at least not here in the United States. In the United States, the risk is greater in that 1 in 39 women will be diagnosed with uterine cancer in her lifetime, but 1 in 147 women will be diagnosed with cervical cancer (American Cancer Society, 2011). That means more American women will be diagnosed with uterine cancer than cervical cancer. Worldwide, though, cancer of the cervix is the second most common cancer in women, with about 500,000 new cases and 250,000 deaths each year (zur Hausen, 2009).

The rate of cervical cancer has been declining in the United States since the 1940s when Dr. Georgios Papanikolaou invented the Papanicolaou test (also called the Pap Smear) to detect abnormal cells on the cervix (Winer & Koutsky, 2008). From that invention, doctors were able to discover which women were at risk of cervical cancer and they developed methods to stop the spread and/or formation of cancerous cells. Between 1955 and 1992, the death rate from cervical cancer declined by almost 80 percent (Balasubramanian, Palefsky, & Koutsky, 2008)! At one time, over 35,000 women *a year* were diagnosed with cervical cancer in this country.

UNDERSTANDING PREVENTION AND CERVICAL CANCER

Were you surprised to learn American women are more likely to experience uterine cancer instead of cervical cancer? Why do you think there is so much more media hype to cervical cancer than uterine cancer? Do you know how uterine cancer can be prevented? How about cervical cancer? Advances in medical technology have made cervical cancer easier to prevent than uterine cancer. Three types of prevention are discussed below using cervical cancer as an example in each type.

Primary Prevention

Primary prevention of cervical cancer means a woman does not place herself at risk of the factors known to cause this cancer. Ninety percent of cervical cancers are believed to be caused by HPV (American Cancer Society, 2011). As previously mentioned, HPV is a sexually transmitted infection (STI) that can be passed on by participating in (unprotected) coitus, anal intercourse, fellatio (oral sex on the external male genitals), cunniligus (oral sex on the external female genitals), and skin-to-skin contact by an infected partner. Abstinence is the best way to prevent exposure. Because the majority of us will (eventually) participate in sexual activity with another person, abstinence is not always a realistic option. Thus, condoms must be used consistently with every type of sexual act to prevent fluid transmission and skin-to-skin contact to *reduce the risk* of acquiring HPV. Unless it is known whether or not each sexual partner is infected with HPV (or any other STI), precautions must always be taken. Keep in mind that having no observable symptoms is *never* an indication that an individual is not infected, especially with the HPV types that increase one's risk of cancer. Also, the more sexual partners a person has, the more likely one will be exposed to HPV. Unlike other viral STIs (like genital herpes and HIV), a vaccine has been developed that can protect both women and men from some strains of HPV infection. This is discussed in detail in chapter 7.

The other 10 percent of cervical cancers are believed to be caused by smoking. According to the American Cancer Society (2011), women who smoke are twice as likely as nonsmokers to develop cervical cancer. Smoking carries many cancer-causing substances that affect organs all over the body. Interestingly, tobacco byproducts have been found in the cervical mucus of women who smoke. Researchers believe that these harmful chemicals damage the DNA (a nucleic acid that contains genetic instructions) of cervical cells and may contribute to the development of cervical cancer. Never picking up a cigarette or cigar can help prevent cervical cancer caused by this addictive behavior.

According to the American Cancer Society (2011), there are other factors that may influence (but are not known to cause) abnormal changes in the cervical cells due to HPV or smoking. One factor is having a family history of cervical cancer. This may mean that a woman inherited defective genes that do not help the body fight off abnormal cervical changes. Having a compromised immune system is another factor. This can happen if a woman is HIV+ or has already been diagnosed with another cancer. Both of these medical conditions can slow a body's ability to fend off abnormal cervical changes. Having had three or more full-term pregnancies is also a factor, but it is unknown why this is the case. Giving birth before the age of 17 is another factor that may increase a woman's risk of cervical cancer. This may be partly due to participating in sexual activities at an early age which could lead to more sexual partners in one's lifetime and increased likelihood of being exposed to HPV. Also, a young woman's cervix is more susceptible to infection, which could lead to the growth of abnormal cervical cells. Using oral contraceptives for more than five years is also believed to be a factor. This could be partly due to the decreased use of condoms while being on "the pill," but hormonal methods may also change the ability of the cervical cells to fight off abnormal cervical changes. Living in poverty also increases a woman's chances of developing cervical cancer later in life. This is partly due to the lack of access to quality medical care that could otherwise have helped prevent abnormal cervical cell growth from developing into cervical cancer (American Cancer Society, 2011).

Secondary Prevention

Secondary prevention of cervical cancer means a woman is screened to diagnose and treat abnormal cervical cells in its early stages before it progresses to cervical dysplasia (precancerous cells) and cancer. Most women do not exhibit symptoms to alert them to harmful cervical changes. Some women, though, may bleed from their cervix or vagina, especially after participating in coitus (Dizon & Abu-Rustum, 2009). A visit to a doctor is warranted to ascertain the reason for the unexpected bleeding.

A Pap smear is performed when a doctor removes a sample of cells and mucus by gently scraping the ectocervix (part of the cervix closest to the vagina) with a special instrument. ACOG (2009) recommends all women to begin receiving a Pap smear (every three years) starting at the age of 21 (regardless of sexual activity with men). If abnormal cervical cells are detected, newer tests look for the genes identifying the presence of HPV in the cervical cells (Cox, 2006). This test is called the HPV DNA test. Because most women who develop cervical cancer will not do so until after age 30, the HPV DNA test is recommended for women only over age 30. Any woman, regardless of age, can ask her medical provider if this test is right for her.

The cervix is covered by two main types of cells. The *ectocervix* is covered by a layer of flat cells called squamous cells and the *endocervix* is covered by glandular cells (cells that secrete mucus). Both cells meet in an area called the transformation zone. According to the American Cancer Society (2011), most cervical cancers begin in the transformation zone. About 80–90 percent of cervical cancers are squamous cell carcinomas. These cancers are from the squamous cells that cover the surface of the ectocervix. About two-thirds of all cervical cancers are caused by HPV 16 and 18 (zur Hausen, 2009).

In the United Sates, most cervical cancers are diagnosed in women under age 50. Around 20 percent are found in women over the age of 65. Cervical cancer rarely develops in women under age 20. African American women develop cervical cancer about 50 percent more often than non-Hispanic white women. Hispanic women are twice as likely as non-Hispanic white women to be diagnosed with cervical cancer (American Cancer Society, 2011).

Tertiary Prevention

Tertiary prevention of cervical cancer aims to reduce the negative impact of this established disease by restoring function and reducing disease-related

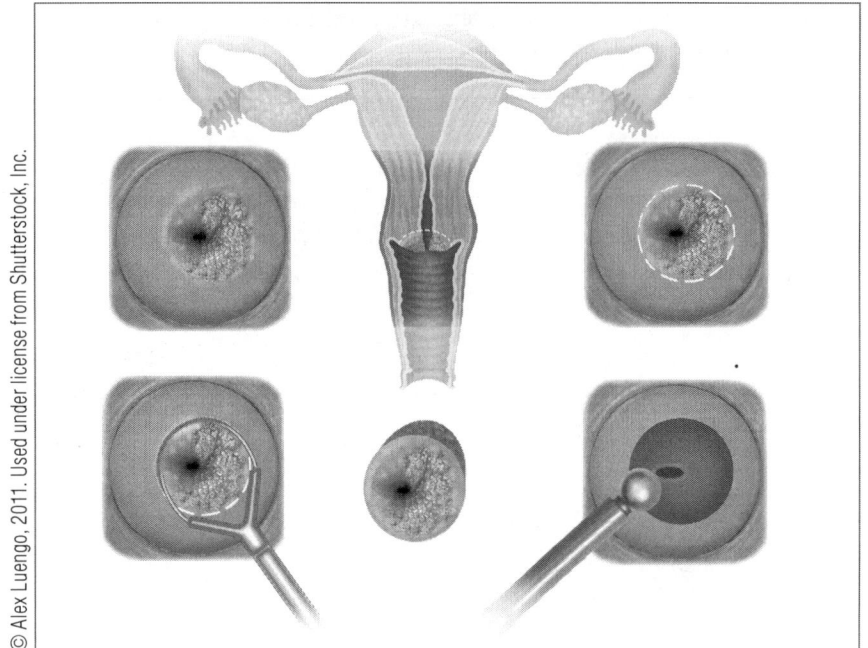

complications. If a woman is suspected of having precancerous or cancer cells on her cervix, she will have her cervix biopsied (Dizon & Abu-Rustum, 2009). What this means is that tissue from either the ectocervix or endocervix (or both) is removed for further testing. Some women may have a cone biopsy done in which a cone-shaped piece of tissue is removed from the cervix. Cells from the ectocervix, endocervix, and in the transformation zone are contained within the tissue and removed for further analysis and to remove suspicious cervical cells (Balasubramanian, Palefsky, & Koutsky, 2008).

Abnormal cells can be destroyed with cryosurgery or laser surgery. With cryosurgery, liquid nitrogen is used to kill the abnormal cells on the cervix by freezing them. With laser surgery, a focused beam of high-energy light is used to burn off the abnormal tissue from the cervix (Dizon & Abu-Rustum, 2009). Depending on the severity of the damage to the cervix and the chances of a full recovery, future pregnancies may not be able to be carried to term.

Cancer of the Ovaries

According to the American Cancer Society (2011), ovarian cancer is the ninth most common cancer among women, excluding nonmelanoma skin cancers. It ranks fifth in cancer deaths among women, accounting for more deaths than any other cancer of the female reproductive system. This cancer mainly develops in older women (American Cancer Society, 2011). Ovarian cancer is rare in women younger than 40. About half the women who are diagnosed with ovarian cancer are 60 years or older.

Symptoms that might occur are bloating, pressure or pain in the abdomen or pelvis, frequent urination, and feeling full very quickly during meals (Dizon & Abu-Rustum, 2009). Women who are considered obese (women with a body mass index of at least 30) have a higher risk of developing this cancer. Women with a family history of breast and ovarian cancer also have a higher risk of developing this cancer. If necessary, the ovary or ovaries can be surgically removed to decrease the chance of the cancer spreading to the lymph nodes or other parts of the body. This procedure is called an *oophorectomy*.

Certain protective factors have been found to decrease a woman's chance of developing ovarian cancer later in life. Women who have given birth, breastfed, were on a hormonal contraceptive for at least five years during their lifetime, or had a hysterectomy were found to be less likely to experience ovarian cancer.

Keep in mind that not all of these protective factors need to be met for a woman to decrease her chances of being diagnosed with ovarian cancer.

Cancer of the Vulva

Eighty percent of vulvar cancers are caused by HPV (zur Hausen, 2009). Even though the vulva consists of many structures of the external female genitals, this cancer usually implies that the labia majora, labia minora, or glans of the clitoris have been invaded by cancerous cells. The labia majora is the most common site and accounts for about 50 percent of cases, with the labia minora coming in second with 15–20 percent of cases (Winer & Koutsky, 2008). Many women exhibit no symptoms for cancer of the vulva. Some women, though, may feel or see a growth on their vulva. This warrants a visit to the doctor to ascertain the reason for the growth.

Cancer of the Vagina

The vagina is lined by a layer of flat cells called squamous cells. Seventy percent of vaginal cancers begin in the squamous cells. These cancers are more common in the upper area of the vagina near the cervix. Fifteen percent of vaginal cancers begin in the glandular cells of the vagina (called adenocarcinoma) and are found near the vaginal opening. This cancer typically develops in women older than 50. Even though most of us think of skin cancer when we hear the term "melanoma," 9 percent of vaginal cancers that develop in the lower portion of the vagina are believed to be melanoma. Up to 4 percent of vaginal cancers are sarcomas. A sarcoma is a cancer that begins in the cells of bones, muscles, or connective tissue. These cancers form deep in the wall of the vagina, not on its surface (American Cancer Society, 2011).

According to the American Cancer Society (2011), up to 90 percent of vaginal cancers are caused by HPV. Almost half the cases occur in women who are 70 years old or older. Only 15 percent of cases are found in women younger than 40. Similar to cervical cancer, the other 10 percent is thought to be caused by smoking. Most vaginal cancers do not cause symptoms until after they have reached an advanced stage. Symptoms that might occur include feeling a lump in the vagina, bleeding unrelated to menstruation, or pain during coitus and/or in the pelvic area (Dizon & Abu-Rustum, 2009). A Pap smear test can detect abnormal cells in the cervix that could have ascended from the vagina. More testing is performed to locate what areas are cancerous and need to be treated.

Factors other than HPV or smoking that may influence (but are not known to cause) abnormal changes in the vaginal cells are having personally experienced cervical cancer, having a compromised immune system, and a family history of vaginal cancer. Studies have shown that there is an abnormality of chromosome 3 in many vaginal cancers, which could indicate an inherited genetic defect that can increase a woman's risk of cancer of the vagina (American Cancer Society, 2011).

Cancer of the reproductive organs or the treatment to cure or reduce the spread of these cancers can affect the sexual response that women experience. The ability to experience an orgasm, the intensity of an orgasm, and the level of sexual desire or arousal can all be affected by direct injury or removal of specific reproductive organs or certain areas of the external genitals. These cancers and/or their treatment can also indirectly negatively affect sexual response by disrupting the blood flow to the genitals, the nerves surrounding any of these reproductive organs, or the hormones supplied to the genitals (Ginger & Yang, 2011).

It should be noted that many of the symptoms listed in each cancer section above can alternatively be related to health conditions other than cancer. If any symptoms occur that are cause for concern, then a visit to a doctor is prudent to ascertain the underlying cause of the symptoms. The earlier (in progression) any of these cancers are detected, though, the higher the rate of success for a cure should be expected.

Reflections

The purpose of this chapter was to familiarize students with the female sexual and reproductive anatomy and the cancers that can occur within the female reproductive system. This is particularly important as many women are unacquainted with their genitals and/or their internal reproductive structures. Gaining knowledge and understanding of our bodies is an important aspect of maintaining women's and men's sexual well-being and sexual intelligence.

Critical Thinking Questions

1. How can women decrease their risk of cancer in their reproductive organs?
2. Genital piercing and cosmetic labiaplasty are becoming more common in the Western world. How are these procedures similar to and different from the genital cutting done to women and girls in parts of Africa, the Middle East, and Asia?
3. What messages about menstruation do you observe in advertising and television programs?
4. Why do you think some adults lack basic knowledge of the female sexual/reproductive anatomy? Could it be that they consider it taboo, embarrassing, or too "dirty" to learn?
5. When do you think sexual/reproductive anatomy should be taught to kids and by whom?
6. Do you think boys should be informed as well as girls on the female sexual/reproductive anatomy?

How Much Do You Remember from the Chapter?

(1–7) • Match the structure with its correct definition/function:

1. Endometrium   __e__
2. Myometrium   __c__
3. Perimetrium   __a__
4. Cervix   __g__
5. Fallopian tubes   __f__
6. Ovaries   __d__
7. Vagina   __b__

a. external layer of the uterus
b. this area is very acidic
c. allows the uterus to contract during labor
d. hormone production occurs here
e. shed during menstruation/site of implantation
f. fertilization must take place here
g. creates mucus throughout the menstrual cycle as a barrier to the upper reproductive organs

(8–13) • Match the rate with the health risk for women:

8. Ovarian cancer   __e__
9. Heart disease   __a__
10. Breast cancer   __c__
11. Cervical cancer   __f__
12. STIs   __b__
13. Uterine cancer   __d__

a. 1 in 2
b. 1 in 4
c. 1 in 8
d. 1 in 37
e. 1 in 70
f. 1 in 147

14. What female body part below is *not* considered a primary sexual characteristic?
    a. vagina
    b. cervix
    c. ovaries
    d. breasts ✓

15. An ovum (egg) is viable for fertilization for around _____.
    a. 24–48 hours ✓
    b. 7 days
    c. 5 days
    d. 2 hours

Chapter Four 65

Challenge Yourself!

Label each structure that is part of the external female genitalia:

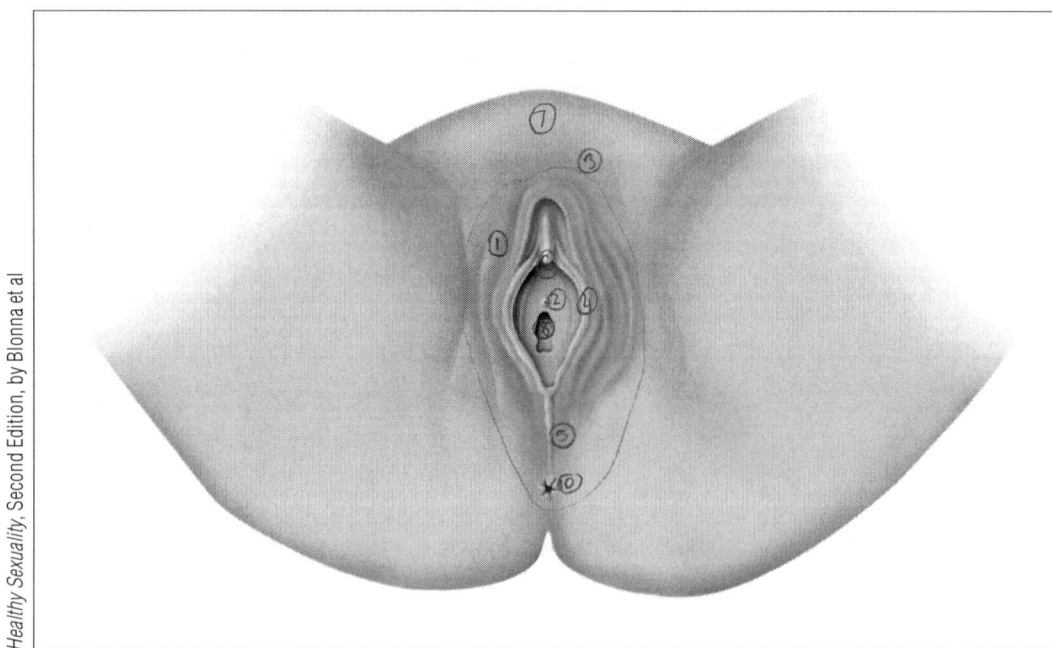

1. Labia majora
2. Urethral opening
3. Vulva
4. Labia minora
5. Perineum
6. Glans of the clitoris
7. Mons pubis
8. Vaginal opening (introitus)
9. Clitoris
10. Anus

Websites

www.cancer.gov
The American Cancer Society

www.menopause.org
The North American Menopause Society

www.ourbodiesourselves.org/
Our Bodies Ourselves

References

Alexander, L., LaRosa, J., Bader, H., & Garfield, S. (2007). *New dimensions in women's health* (3rd Ed.). Sudbury, MA: Jones & Bartlett Publishers.

American Cancer Society. (2011). *Cancer facts and figures 2011*. Atlanta, GA: Author.

American Congress of Obstetricians and Gynecologists (ACOG). (2001). Practice bulletin: Premenstrual syndrome. *International Journal of Gynecology & Obstetrics, 73*, 183–191.

American Congress of Obstetricians and Gynecologists (ACOG). (2007). ACOG committee opinion, no. 378: Vaginal "rejuvenation" and cosmetic vaginal procedures. *Obstetrics & Gynecology, 110*(3), 737–738.

American Congress of Obstetricians and Gynecologists (ACOG). (2009). ACOG practice bulletin no. 109: Cervical cytology screening. *Obstetrics & Gynecology, 114*, 1409–1420.

American Congress of Obstetricians and Gynecologists (ACOG). (2010). *How your baby grows during pregnancy.* Danvers, MA: Author

Balasubramanian, A., Palefsky, J., & Koutsky, L. (2008). Cervical neoplasia and other STD-related genital tract neoplasias. In K. Holmes, P. Sparling, W. Stamm, P. Piot, J. Wasserheit, L. Corey, & M. Cohen (Eds.), *Sexually transmitted diseases* (4th ed., pp. 1051–1074). New York, NY: McGraw-Hill, Inc.

Bayram, G., & Beji, N. (2010). Psychosexual adaptation and quality of life after hysterectomy. *Sexuality & Disability, 28*, 3–13.

Cartwright, R., & Cardozo, L. (2008). Cosmetic vulvovaginal surgery. *Obstetrics, Gynecology & Reproductive Medicine, 18*(10), 285–286.

Centers for Disease Control and Prevention (CDC). (2007). Breastfeeding trends and updated national health objectives for exclusive breastfeeding–United States, birth years 2000–2004. *Morbidity & Mortality Weekly Report, 56*, 760–763.

Cox, J. (2006). Human papillomavirus testing in primary cervical screening and abnormal Papanicolaou management. *Obstetrical & Gynecological Survey, 61*, (Supplemental 1), S15–S25.

Crooks, R., & Baur, K. (2011). *Our sexuality.* Belmont, CA: Wadsworth/Cengage.

Dizon, D., & Abu-Rustum, N. (2009). *Gynecologic tumor board. Clinical cases in diagnosis and management of cancer of the female reproductive system.* Sudbury, MA: Jones & Bartlett Publishers.

Douma, S., Husband, C., O'Donnelly, R., Baruin, R., & Wooden, A. (2005). Estrogen-related mood disorders reproductive life cycle factors. *Advances in Nursing Science, 28*(4), 364–375.

Elwood, A. (2005). Female genital cutting, "circumcision" and mutilation: Physical, psychological and cultural perspectives. *Contemporary Sexuality, 39*, i–v.

Fogel, C., & Woods, N. (2008). *Women's health care in advanced practice nursing.* New York, NY: Springer.

Freeman, E., Halberstadt, S., Rickels, K., Legler, J., Lin, H., & Samme, M. (2011). Core symptoms that discriminate premenstrual syndrome. *Journal of Women's Health, 20*(1), 29–35.

Ginger, V., & Yang, C. (2011). Function anatomy of the female sex organs. In P. Mulhall, L. Incrocci, I. Goldstein, & R. Rosen (Eds.), *Cancer & sexual health* (pp. 13–24). New York, NY: Springer-Science.

Goldstein, I., & Silberstein, J. (2011). Physiology of female genital sexual arousal. In P. Mulhall, L. Incrocci, I. Goldstein, & R. Rosen (Eds.), *Cancer & sexual health* (pp. 51–68). New York, NY: Springer-Science.

Goodman, M. (2009). Female cosmetic genital surgery. *Obstetrics & Gynecology, 113*(1), 154–159.

Hamilton, T. (2002). *Skin flutes and velvet gloves: A collection of facts and fancies, legends and oddities about the body's private parts*. New York, NY: St. Martin's Press.

Harvard Medical School (2005). Perimenopause: Rocky road to menopause: Symptoms we call "menopausal" often precede menopause by years. *Harvard Women's Health Watch, 12*(12), 1–4.

Hirsch, M. (1998, October 23–25). Functional neurovascular anatomy. *Paper presented at Boston University School of Medicine and the Department of Urology Conference on New Perspectives in the Management of Female Sexual Dysfunction*, Burlington, MA.

Howland, R. (2010). Use of endocrine hormones for treating depression. *Journal of Psychosocial Nursing, 48*(12), 13–16.

Jones, R., & Lopez, K. (2006). *Human reproductive biology* (3rd Ed.). Burlington, MA: Elsevier.

Katz, A. (2007). Sexuality and women. *Nursing for Women's Health, 11*(1), 37–43.

Katz-Bearnot, S. (2010). Menopause, depression, and loss of sexual desire: A psychodynamic contribution. *Journal of the American Academy of Psychoanalysis & Dynamic Psychiatry, 38*(1), 99–116.

Koster, M., & Leimar Price, L. (2008). Rwandan female genital modification: Elongation of the labia minora and the use of local botanical species. *Culture, Health & Sexuality, 10*(2), 191–204.

Levin, R. (2003). A journey through two lumens! *International Journal of Impotence Research, 15*, 2–9.

Martino, J., & Vermund, S. (2002). Vaginal douching: Evidence for risks or benefits to women's health. *Epidemiologic Reviews, 24*(2), 109–124.

Mattson, S., & Smith, J. (2004). *Core curriculum for maternal newborn nursing* (3rd Ed.). St. Louis, MO: Elsevier Saunders.

Meston, C. (2002). The psychophysiological assessment of female sexual function. *Journal of Sex Education & Therapy, 25*(1), 6–16.

Nelson, A., & Baldwin, S. (2007). Menstrual disorders and related concerns. In R. Hatcher, J. Trussell, A. Nelson, W. Cates, F. Stewart, & D. Kowal (Eds.), *Contraceptive technology*, (19th Ed., pp. 451–498). New York, NY: Ardent Media.

Nelson, A., & Stewart F. (2007). Menopause and perimenopausal health. In R. Hatcher, J. Trussell, A. Nelson, W. Cates, F. Stewart, & D. Kowal (Eds.), *Contraceptive technology*, (19th Ed., pp. 699–746). New York, NY: Ardent Media.

O'Connor, M. (2008). Reconstructing the hymen: Mutilation or restoration? *Journal of Law & Medicine, 16*(1), 161–175.

Ricci, S., & Kyle, T. (2009). *Maternity and pediatric nursing*. Philadelphia, PA: Lippincott Williams & Wilkins.

Santoro, N., Torrens, J., Crawford, S., Allsworth, J., Finkelstein, J., Gold, E. et al. (2005). Correlates of circulating androgens in midlife women: The study of women's health across the nation. *Journal of Clinical Endocrinology & Metabolism, 90*, 4836–4845.

Schuiling, K., & Likis, F. (2006). *Women's gynecologic health*. Sudbury, MA: Jones & Barlett Publishers.

Smith Oboler, R. (2001). Law and persuasion in the elimination of female genital modification. *Society for Applied Anthropology, 60*(4), 311–318.

Speroff, L., & Fritz, M. (2005). *Clinical gynecologic endocrinology & infertility* (7th Ed.). Philadelphia, PA: Lippincott Williams & Wilkins.

Talle, A. (2001). Female genital mutilation. In N. Smelser & P. Baltes (Eds.), *International Encyclopedia of the Social & Behavioral Sciences* (pp. 5447–5451). Oxford, UK: Elsevier Science Ltd.

Winer, R., & Koutsky, L. (2008). Genital human papillomavirus infection (2008). In K. Holmes, P. Sparling, W. Stamm, P. Piot, J. Wasserheit, L. Corey, & M. Cohen (Eds.), *Sexually transmitted diseases* (4th Ed., pp. 489–508). New York, NY: McGraw-Hill.

zur Hausen, H. (2009). Papillomaviruses in the causation of human cancers—A brief historical account. *Virology, 384*, 260–265.

chapter five

MALE SEXUAL/ REPRODUCTIVE ANATOMY & PHYSIOLOGY

CHAPTER OBJECTIVES

On completion of this chapter, students will be able to:

- understand the difference between primary and secondary sexual characteristics;
- name the structures of the external male genitalia;
- identify the structures of the internal male sexual/reproductive anatomy;
- explain the male reproductive process;
- distinguish the cancers that can occur in the male reproductive system.

ABBREVIATIONS AND ACRONYMS USED IN THIS CHAPTER

cm	centimeters
HIV	human immunodeficiency virus
HPV	human papillomavirus
PSA	prostate-specific antigen

PRIMARY AND SECONDARY SEXUAL CHARACTERISTICS

As was discussed in the previous chapter, primary sexual characteristics are directly involved in reproductive function. Even though the penis serves as the conduit for urination, it is seen as a primary sexual characteristic because it also serves the purpose of expelling semen (sperm and seminal fluid) into the vagina that may lead to procreation. Secondary sexual characteristics are physical aspects typically associated with one sex but not the other. Examples in men would be facial hair growth, deepening of the voice, increased body hair growth, and increased muscle development. These physical attributes occur during puberty, resulting from the production of testosterone, the hormone developed in abundance in the testes (Jones & Lopez, 2006).

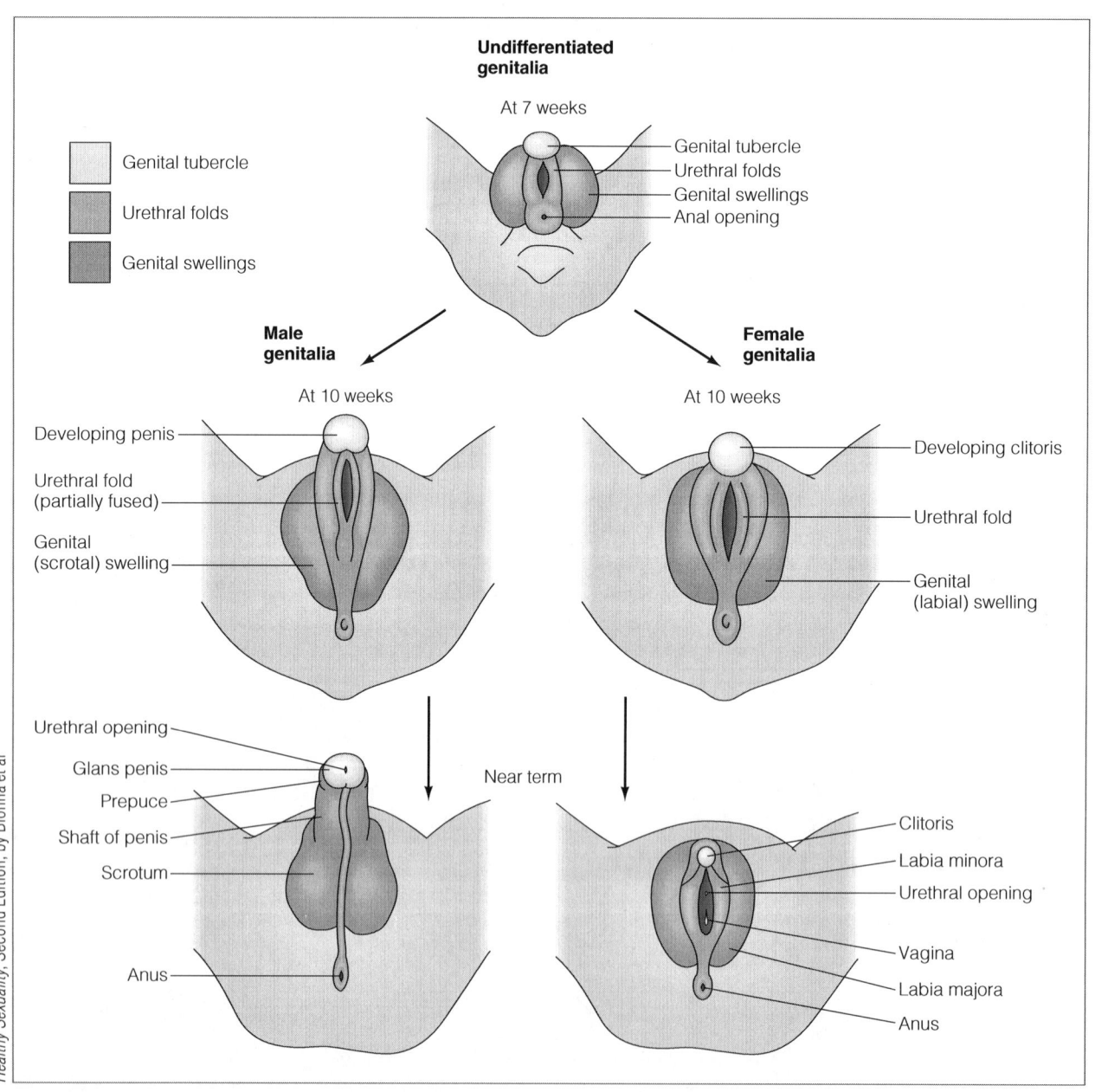

SEXUAL/REPRODUCTIVE ANATOMY

Even though the female and male sexual/reproductive anatomies are perceived to be different, these areas developed from the same embryonic tissue during pregnancy. Initial fetal genital formation occurs around 8–9 weeks after conception (Jones & Lopez, 2006). The process continues throughout the pregnancy until all internal and external structures are fully developed by the 38th week of pregnancy (Heffner & Schust, 2006).

Here is a list of anatomically homologous structures shared between the two sexes:

Table 5.1

Male	Female
Testes	Ovaries
Scrotum	Labia majora
Shaft of the penis	Labia minora
Glans of the penis	Glans of the clitoris
Foreskin	Clitoral hood
Cowper's gland	Bartholin's gland
Prostate gland	Skene's gland

EXTERNAL MALE GENITALIA

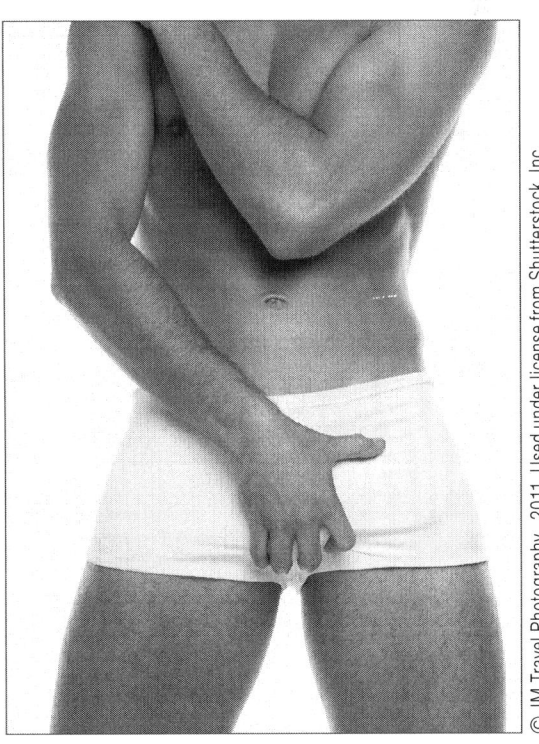

Unlike girls and women in the United States who are more likely to have difficulty in recalling the clinical terms of their external genitalia, boys and men find it easier to remember the clinical terms of their external male genitals than their internal reproductive anatomy. Even so, creative phrases abound to describe a male's external genitalia! For the majority of us, we call our hand, "hand," our leg, "leg," so why don't we all call the penis, "penis"?

The Penis

At birth, the penis consists of the shaft of the penis, the glans of the penis, the corona, the frenulum, and the foreskin. A male is born with the glans of the penis and the foreskin connected. Unless the male is circumcised (discussed below), these structures do not separate

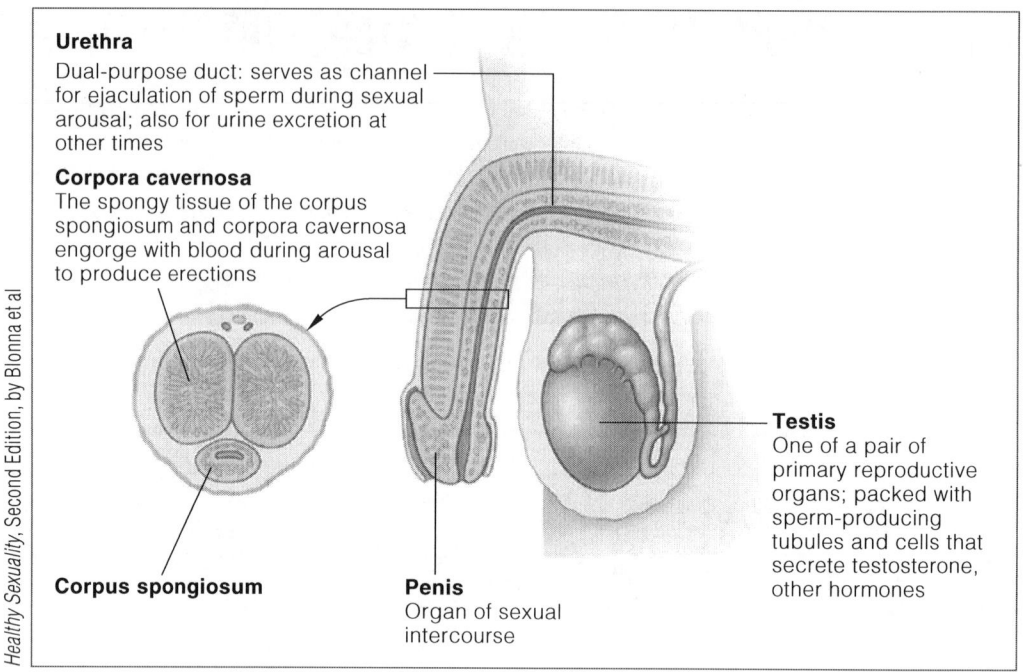

naturally until a few years later. At that time, the male needs to learn to retract the foreskin to clean inside of it to avoid the buildup of smegma (natural secretions that moisten the glans of the penis) which may lead to infection (Burgu, Aydogdu, Tangal, & Soygur, 2010).

The penis is a rod-shaped male reproductive organ that passes semen and urine from the body (Jones & Lopez, 2006). It contains two types of spongy erectile tissue. The *corpora cavernosa* consists of two cylinders of erectile tissue that form most of the penis. The *corpus spongiosum* is a single column of erectile tissue that forms a small portion of the penis and surrounds the urethra (Ricci & Kyle, 2009). The urethra extends from the neck of the bladder to the tip of the glans of the penis and is around 20 cm in length (Bella & Shamloul, 2011). The erectile tissue surrounding the urethra is wrapped in connective tissue and covered with skin, but no pubic hair. The cylinders are each surrounded by an elastic membrane called the *tunica albuginea*. The penis does not contain any bones or muscles.

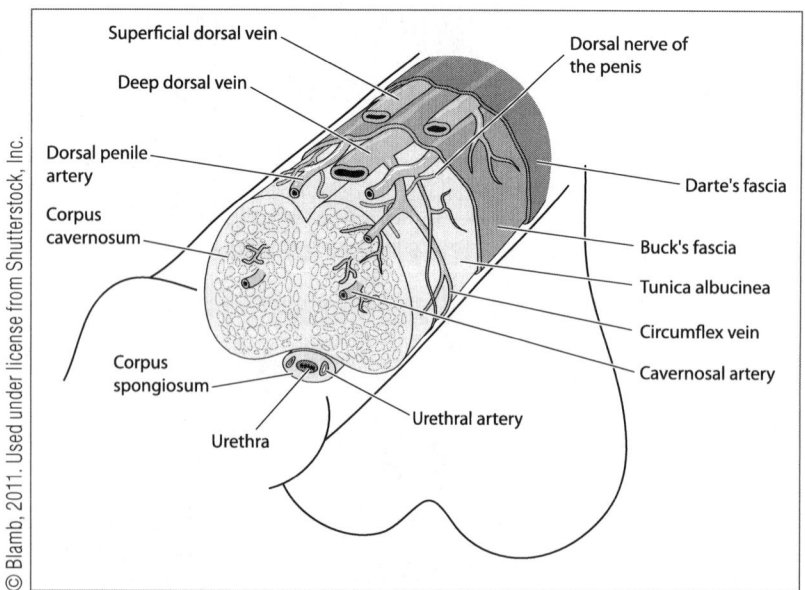

When a man is sexually aroused, nerve impulses from the autonomic nervous system dilate the arteries of the penis, allowing arterial blood to flow into the corpora cavernosa and causing the penis to become enlarged and firm (Ricci & Kyle, 2009). The blood flow to the cylinders increases by about seven times the normal amount. The tunica albuginea compresses the veins that normally drain blood away from the penis, thereby trapping the blood and maintaining the erection. The glans of the penis has the greatest concentration of nerve endings, believed to consist of thousands of nerve endings. At birth, the glans of the penis is covered with loose skin called the foreskin. The *frenulum* helps contract the foreskin over the glans. The *corona* is at the base of the glans of the penis, which forms a rounded projecting border.

The Scrotum

The *scrotum* is external and its purpose is to regulate the temperature of and provide protection to the testicles (Ceo,

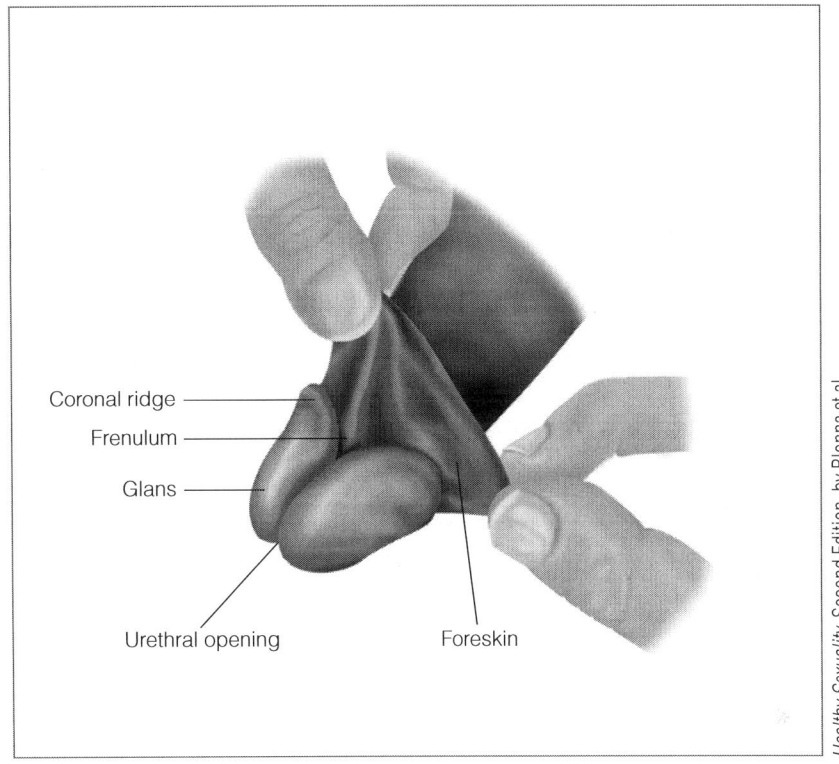

2006). For instance, when the ambient temperature is cold, the scrotum moves the testicles closer to the body to maintain optimal temperature for the testicles to produce sperm. Optimal temperature for sperm production is 94 degrees Fahrenheit, just below normal body temperature. The scrotum does not hold the testes in place. The testes are suspended from the body wall by the spermatic cord (Jones & Lopez, 2006).

The Perineum

The area of the *perineum* is located between the scrotum and the anus. It contains numerous nerve endings that indicate it is sensitive to the touch (Ricci & Kyle, 2009). The perineum has nerves and blood vessels responsible for an erection. Prolonged pressure on this area may cause perineal numbness and damage to the blood vessels and nerves, which can lead to temporary erectile dysfunction (Dettori, Koepsell, Cummings, & Corman, 2004). Damage to the area can occur from sitting for excessive amounts of time in the same position, such as on the saddle while cycling. The risk of erectile dysfunction can be reduced by adhering to these preventive strategies: (1) wearing padded bicycle shorts; (2) raising the handlebars to sit upright while riding a bicycle, which shifts the pressure from the perineum to the buttocks; (3) using a well-padded gel seat rather than a narrow one; and (4) by positioning the seat so a man does not have to extend his legs fully at the bottom of his pedal stroke (Nixon-Cobb & Bonillas, 2011). Other risk factors for erectile dysfunction are discussed in chapter 6.

The Anus

The anus is the external opening of the rectum. As discussed in chapter 4, there is no difference between a female and a male anus. This area allows solid waste to be expelled from the body. The area has a relatively high concentration of nerve endings that suggest sensitivity to the touch. The anus does not contain glands to moisten the area so a water-based lubricant is required if penetration is expected. Men do not have to identify a specific sexual orientation to enjoy having their anus penetrated by their sexual partner. The male anus is more likely to be ignored by female sexual partners than a female's anus by male sexual partners. If an anus is the same, regardless of biological sex and sexual orientation, why is a men's anus not penetrated as often when they have female sexual partners?

INTERNAL MALE REPRODUCTIVE SYSTEM

As previously stated, the external sexual/reproductive anatomies for both females and males initially develop in the same form. The same is true for the internal sexual/reproductive anatomy for both sexes (Heffner & Schust, 2006). An embryo develops two pairs of parallel ducts, the *Wolffian* and *Müllerian ducts*. The expression of specific genes is needed in males (with the sex chromosomes, XY) and females (with the sex chromosomes, XX) for embryonic external genital formation to begin, as well as the transformation of the Wolffian and Müllerian ducts (Sinclair et al., 1990). In males, the Müllerian ducts are suppressed and the Wolffian ducts develop into the vas deferens, seminal vesicles, and ejaculatory duct. In females, the regression of the Wolffian ducts occurs and the Müllerian ducts form the fallopian tubes, uterus (including the cervix), and inner third of the vagina (Heffner & Schust, 2006). Table 5.2 distinguishes the ducts and what they transform into during embryonic sexual/reproductive development. Unlike the structures presented in Table 5.1, these structures are *not* homologous (that is, they are not created from the same embryonic tissue).

Table 5.2

Wolffian ducts	Müllerian ducts
Ejaculatory ducts	Fallopian tubes
Seminal vesicles	Inner third of the vagina
Vas deferens	Uterus (including the cervix)

The Testes

According to the American Congress of Obstetricians and Gynecologists, the testicles begin to descend from the abdomen into the scrotum around the fifth month of pregnancy (ACOG, 2010). This is the only organ located outside the body. Each testis begins sperm production (known as *spermatogenesis*) and secretion of testosterone and estrogen at puberty. The production of testosterone and estrogen (which is mostly converted to testosterone) takes place in the tissue located between the seminiferous tubules, known as the Leydig cells (Krieger & Graney, 2008). In addition to being responsible for the development of primary and secondary male sexual characteristics, testosterone influences a male's sex drive, health, and the prevention of osteoporosis (Tuck & Francis, 2009). A man produces about 10 times more testosterone than a female body, but a woman is more sensitive to the hormone (Dabbs & Dabbs, 2000).

Production and secretion of testosterone into the bloodstream reach a peak around puberty, resulting in the development of male secondary sexual characteristics discussed above. From around the age of 30 until death, though, the amount of testosterone produced declines (Harman, Metter, Tobin, Pearson, & Blackman, 2001). This may occur because of a decline in the number of Leydig cells in the testes (Krieger & Graney, 2008) or it may be a secondary effect resulting from dysfunction in the controlling mechanism of the hypothalamus and pituitary gland in the brain (Harman et al., 2001). The hypothalamus controls the pituitary, which secretes *gonadotrophins* (a follicle-stimulating hormone and a luteinizing hormone) that, in turn, stimulate sperm and testosterone production by the testes.

Sperm is also produced in the seminiferous tubules within the testes (Krieger & Graney, 2008). On average, 1,000 sperm a second are produced from puberty until death. The entire process of sperm production takes 65–75 days (Jones & Lopez, 2006).

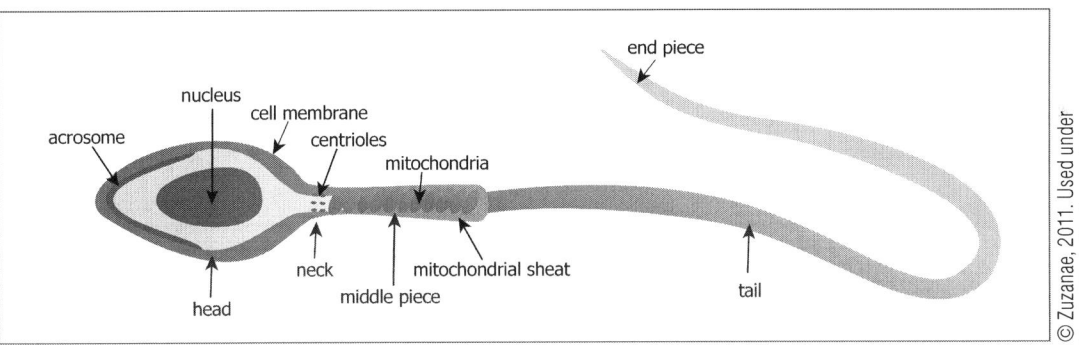

The average amount of sperm in a single ejaculation is around 200 million, ranging from 40 million to 500 million. Yet, only 1 percent of the seminal fluid ejaculated is sperm! The rest consists of substances (discussed below) needed for the maintenance, maturation, and transport of sperm (Clement & Giuliano, 2011). If ejaculation occurs in a vagina, the sperm are viable for around five days in the female reproductive tract (Ricci & Kyle, 2009).

The Epididymis

The *epididymis* is located on the posterior side of the testes. Sperm are stored in the epididymis until ejaculation. In the epididymis, sperm undergo the final stages of maturation and obtain the capability to fertilize an egg (Clement & Giuliano, 2011). If this comma-shaped organ were stretched out it would be

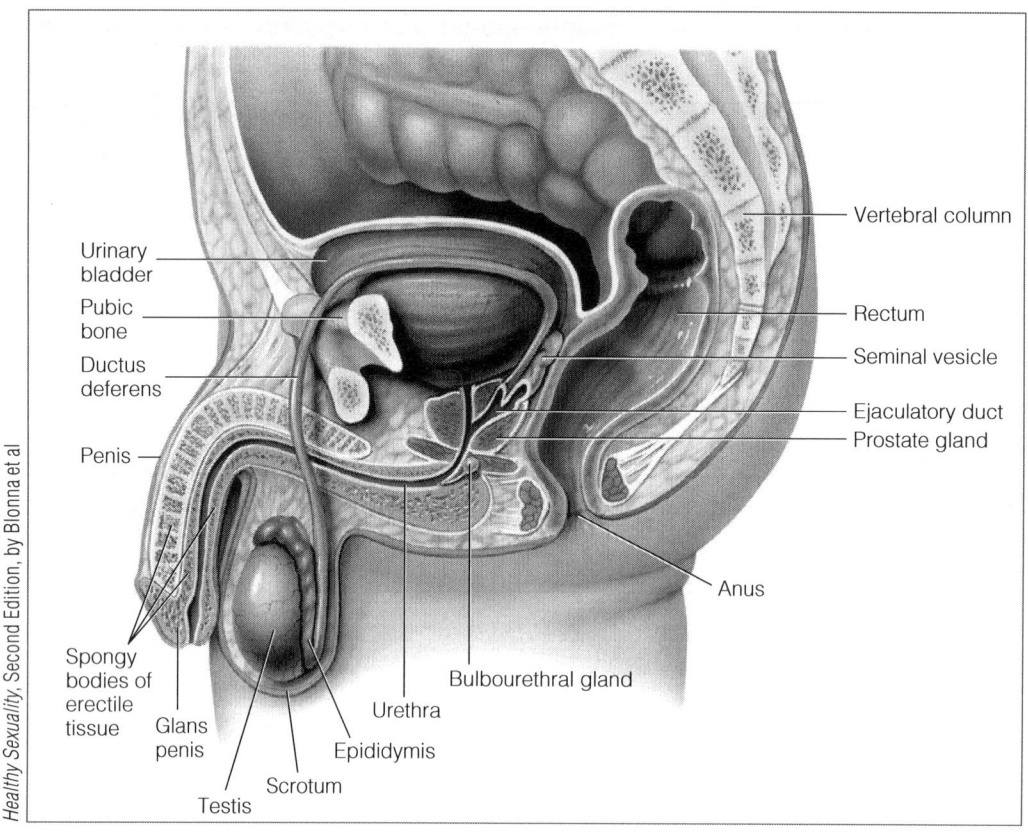

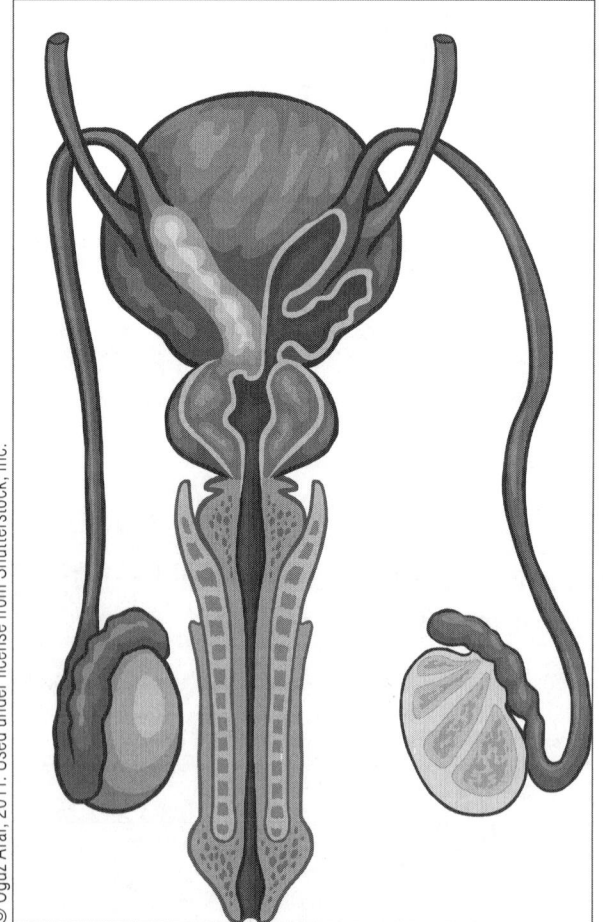

almost 20 feet long (Ricci & Kyle, 2009). If ejaculation does not occur before more sperm are ready to enter the epididymis from the testes, they are reabsorbed into the body.

The Vas Deferens

The *vas deferens* or *vasa deferentia* (plural) are coiled ducts (around 35 cm in length) that transport sperm from the epididymis to the seminal vesicles (Krieger & Graney, 2008). When a man wishes to be sterilized, each vas deferens is severed. This procedure is called a *vasectomy* (discussed in chapter 12). There is no noticeable depletion in an ejaculation after a vasectomy because the seminal fluid in the semen is not affected. Seminal fluid is produced in the seminal vesicles, the prostate gland, and a small amount in the Cowper's gland (Ceo, 2006).

The Seminal Vesicles

The *seminal vesicles* are glands (around 5 cm in length) that lie posterior to the bladder. They produce around 70 percent of the seminal fluid found in semen (Jones & Lopez, 2006). This substance contains water, is rich in two nutrients—sugar fructose (main source of energy for sperm) and citric acid—and consists of chemicals and enzymes that help neutralize the acidity in the male urethra and vagina, prolonging the lifespan of sperm (Clement & Giuliano, 2011).

The Ejaculatory Duct

The seminal fluid from the seminal vesicles is transported to the *ejaculatory duct*. These ducts (around 2 cm long) deliver the seminal fluid to the prostate gland by contracting during the emission phase of an orgasm (Clement & Giuliano, 2011).

The Prostate Gland

The *prostate gland* (slightly larger than a chestnut) is in front of the rectum, located under the bladder, and it completely encircles around 3 cm of the urethra (Jones & Lopez, 2006). This part of the urethra is considered to be the widest (Bella & Shamloul, 2011). Around 30 percent of the seminal fluid is secreted by the prostate gland through 20 ducts that open into the urethra. Similar to the secretions from the seminal vesicles, this fluid helps neutralize the acidity of the urethra and the vagina. Moreover, the prostatic fluid contains high concentrations of sugars and zinc to help sperm become strong swimmers and live longer in the female reproductive tract (Clement & Giuliano, 2011). During an orgasm, the prostate gland contracts to propel the semen out of the penis and to close the part of the urethra by the bladder to prevent urine from being expelled during ejaculation (Krieger & Graney, 2008).

The Cowper's Gland

The *Cowper's gland* is also called the *bulbourethral gland*. These pea-sized glands secrete a small amount of clear fluid when a male becomes sexually aroused (Krieger & Graney, 2008). Males may notice the fluid on the urethral opening at erection, right before ejaculation or not at all. This alkaline fluid is believed to coat the urethra before ejaculation to decrease the acidity of the vagina and the male urethra, which is mostly used for urination (and urine is acidic) (Clement & Giuliano, 2011). This fluid can also carry live sperm to the urethral opening that were not expelled during a recent ejaculation (Jones & Lopez, 2006). Thus, caution should be taken if condoms are not used consistently or the withdrawal method is used for contraception.

Andropause

Andropause, or "age-related hypogonadism," can be categorized as the slow, but steady reduction of testosterone production in the testicles beginning in middle age. Half of all men will experience physiological and physical changes due to low testosterone in the latter third of their lives (Morales, Heaton, & Carson, 2000). The decline in testosterone can delay the onset of sexual desire and/or arousal, can prolong the time to achieve an erection, and can decrease semen production (Jones & Lopez, 2006). Compared to a 20-year-old whose erections (and ejaculations) can occur quickly and without much stimulation, a

60-year-old man may require more direct stimulation and erotic fantasy to get an erection. However, the older man is likely to maintain the erection for a longer time, even though it may require over a day to achieve another erection. Secondary male sexual characteristics that might also change due to andropause are: facial hair growth may decrease, muscle mass and strength may decline, and the penis and scrotum may shrink. Men may also find it difficult to manage weight gain and may experience diminished energy, depressed mood, and decreased cognitive function (Matsumoto, 2002).

Whereas menopause usually occurs over a period of a few months or years in women (discussed in chapter 4), andropause seems to occur over a period of decades (Jones & Lopez, 2006). Unlike menopause, men experiencing andropause do not undergo a complete and permanent physiological shut-down of the reproductive system as a normal event. Thus a man can impregnate a woman even at an advanced age.

FACTORS AFFECTING EJACULATION

An average ejaculation, which consists of sperm and seminal fluid from the seminal vesicles, prostate gland, and a bit from the Cowper's gland can fill a teaspoon. The amount of semen ejaculated can be affected by anything that interferes with testosterone production. For example, according to Corona and colleagues (2011), the amount of semen ejaculated can be affected by erectile dysfunction (discussed chapter 6), diabetes, certain medications, smoking, older age, obesity, hypoactive sexual desire (decreased sexual interest, discussed in chapter 6), and hypogonadism (condition in which the testes produce little, if any, hormones).

Many of you have probably heard the saying, "you are what you eat." Well, it seems to apply to semen, too! At least to the taste of it. Most body parts, including vaginas and rectums could care less about the taste, but someone' mouth,

Table 5.3 Factors Affecting Taste of Ejaculate

Taste	Source of Taste
Bitter	Alcohol, cigarettes, coffee, and marijuana (can also be due to prostate or urinary infections)
Sharp	Asparagus, broccoli, chocolate, dairy products, greasy foods, red meats, and spinach
Mild	Vegetarian diet, celery, fruit (such as pineapple and apple), parsley, peppermint, and spearmint
Moderate	Having none of the bitter factors and only one or two from the sharp list
Sweet	Naturally fermented beverages or someone who is diabetic or borderline diabetic

well, that's a different story! Table 5.3 includes a list of factors that affect the taste of the ejaculate (Hamilton, 2002; Steele, 2011; Tarkovsky, 2006). So if fellatio is expected, then a man should consider what foods could affect how his semen will taste to his sexual partner.

MALE GENITAL MODIFICATIONS

For thousands of years males have had their external genitals modified for various reasons. Males' genitals may be modified to look like their fathers' genitals, because of cultural tradition or religion, and for hygienic reasons. Males' genitals can also be modified for the purpose of punishment, to decrease procreation in targeted populations, to prevent a cancer from spreading to vital organs, and for male to female sex reassignment surgery.

Circumcision

A *circumcision*, a procedure in which the foreskin and frenulum are removed from the penis, is rarely performed to deter sexual pleasure or nonmarital sexual activity. In fact, there is strong evidence to suggest that circumcised men's level of sexual pleasure does not differ to that of uncircumcised men (Masters & Johnson, 1966). After a circumcision, the glans of the penis and corona remain permanently exposed. A circumcision occurs to follow religious doctrine (in Judaism and Islam, for example), for hygienic reasons, because of cultural tradition, and as a ritual to welcome the boy into manhood (Totaro et al., 2011).

Globally, around 30 percent of males are circumcised. These males usually have this procedure done before late adolescence. This procedure is rarely performed in countries in Europe (Burgu et al., 2010). Over 60 percent of males in the United States are circumcised (Burgu et al., 2010). These procedures usually occur soon after birth, with little fanfare in the hospital or doctor's office.

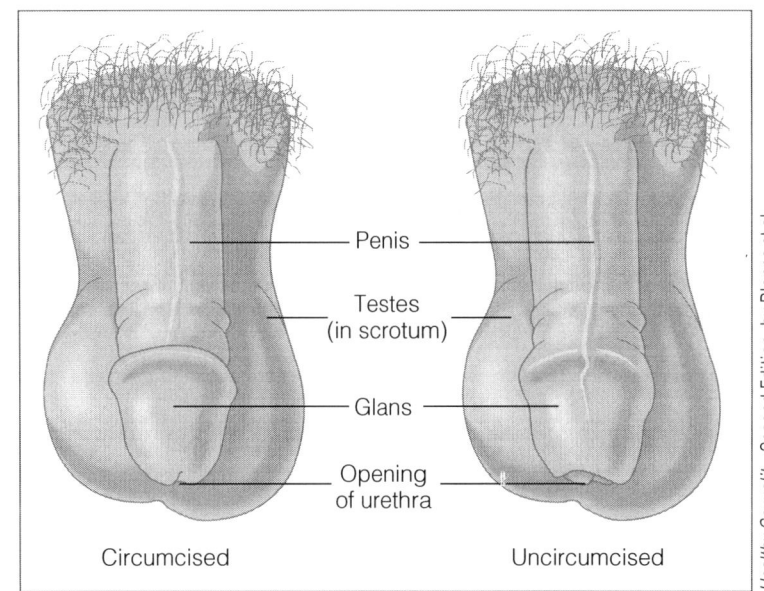

Depending on the setting, the baby is either held by a parent or tied down to prevent unnecessary movement that could interfere with the procedure. The baby is not given general anesthesia, but will be provided with local pain medication on the penis (Ridings & Amaya, 2007). A baby does not start producing vitamin K until around the eighth day after birth. This vitamin is needed to help blood clotting. Because most circumcisions are performed before the eighth day, most babies have to receive a shot of vitamin K before the procedure. The American Academy of Pediatrics takes a neutral stance to male circumcision (Burgu et al.,

2010). There is no scientific basis to justify a circumcision for hygienic reasons, even though there is mounting evidence that circumcised men have a decreased risk to HIV infection (Golden & Wasserheit, 2009).

Castration

Throughout the centuries, males have been castrated. *Castration* is defined as the removal of the testes. Removing the testicles can severely reduce the sex drive and eliminate the ability to procreate (Higano, 2003). Thus, throughout history this procedure has been used to punish convicted sex offenders and create a new class of men called *eunuchs* who were used to staff harems (Wassersug & Johnson, 2007). Castration has also been performed on individuals considered "unfit" to procreate. In the early 1900s, the eugenics (meaning well-born) movement castrated thousands of men because of the belief they were alcoholics, illiterate, impoverished, or suffering from a mental disorder, and thus were considered a threat to society by producing "unhealthy" offspring (Taylor, 2000).

There are currently two methods to castrate a male. The first is one where he has his testes surgically removed. This is a permanent form of castration. Surgical castration is used today to slow the progression of a cancerous tumor located in the prostate gland (Kumar, Barqawi, & Crawford, 2005). Testosterone has been found to influence the size of a tumor of the prostate gland so removing the testes would cease the production of this hormone and its effect on the tumor. Males who have testicular cancer may also undergo surgical castration (Dahl, Mykletun, & Fossa, 2005). If the cancer has not spread to both testes only the cancerous testis will be removed. Many males who experience surgical castration can have testicular implants inserted for aesthetic reasons. Also, males who identify as females undergo surgical castration as part of the process in male to female sex reassignment surgery.

The second form of castration is medical (also known as chemical). The man is given an anti-androgen to suppress ability of his testes to produce testosterone, thus ceasing sperm production and reducing libido (Kumar, Barqawi, & Crawford, 2005). Depo-Provera, a contraceptive injection given to women every 12 weeks, has also been used as a form of medical castration in males. This is not a permanent form of castration, and hormone and sperm production will resume after the anti-androgen drugs are no longer administered. Medical castration is used today on convicted sex offenders who volunteer for this procedure (if available in that state), and in return they usually obtain a lower prison sentence (Weinberger, Sreenivasan, Garrick, & Osran, 2005). They remain medically castrated for a set period of time after they have been released from prison as part of their plea deal.

CANCER OF THE MALE REPRODUCTIVE SYSTEM

The American Cancer Society estimates 250,540 cases of cancer of the male reproductive organs in the United States occurred in 2011. Along with prostate cancer, cancer of the penis and testicles are also possible. Only penile cancer is known to be primarily caused by HPV. Prostate and testicular cancers have other risk factors mentioned below.

Cancer of the Prostate

When men think about cancer, many think of prostate cancer. There's no surprise there because one in six men will be diagnosed with prostate cancer, but two-thirds of them will be over the age of 65. Other than skin cancer, prostate cancer is the most common cancer in American men (American Cancer Society, 2011). More than 2 million men in the United States who have been diagnosed with prostate cancer at some point are still alive today.

For prostate cancer, about 240,890 men were diagnosed and about 33,720 men died from it (American Cancer Society, 2011). Prostate cancer is the second leading cause of cancer deaths in American men, behind only lung cancer. While the risk of prostate cancer is 1 in 6, the risk of death due to metastasis is 1 in 30 (American Cancer Society, 2011). Prostate cancer can be detected by taking a simple annual screening test that measures levels of a protein called prostate-specific antigen (PSA) in the blood. The prostate gland can easily be felt by inserting a finger (or two) in the rectum. Clinicians use this approach to detect any tumor growing on the prostate gland.

The risk of prostate cancer increases with age, family history, and race (Cutler, 2008). For example, the disease is more prevalent in African American men and less so in Asian men. By the age of 60, one out of every 16 Caucasian men and one out of every 10 African American men will be diagnosed with prostate cancer. A strong family history (i.e., at least one first-degree relative such as a father or brother) of prostate cancer increases the risk to the disease (American Cancer Society, 2011).

Treatment may include radical prostatectomy, a procedure in which the prostate gland and surrounding tissue are removed; external beam radiation; brachytherapy, a form of radiation therapy where small, radioactive pellets are placed in the prostate gland; or androgen deprivation therapy (discussed above as medical castration), which is the administration of anti-androgen medications to decrease the production of testosterone (American Cancer Society, 2011).

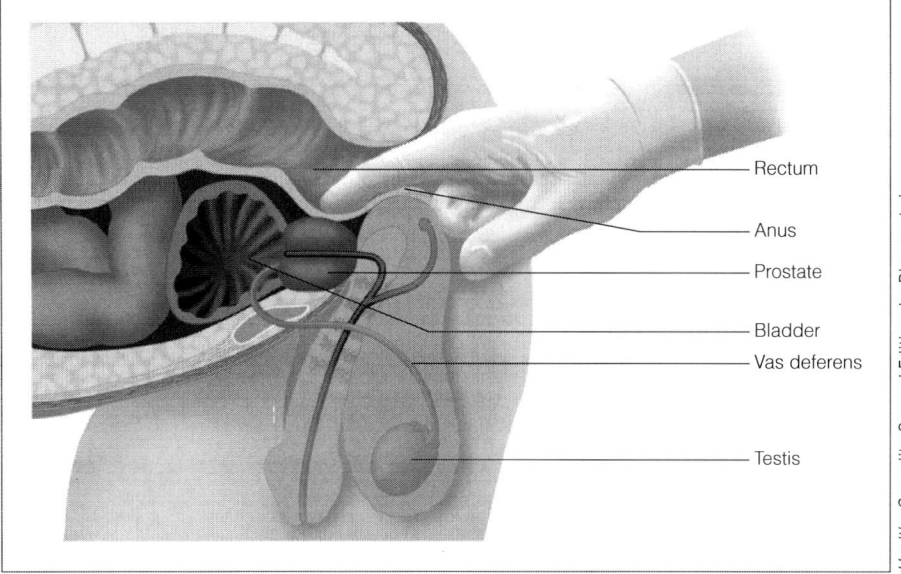

Cancer of the Testicles

In 2011, about 8,290 new cases of testicular cancer were diagnosed and about 350 men died from it (American Cancer Society, 2011). Even though only around 3 percent of cancers of the male reproductive organs occur in the testes, the rate of testicular cancer has been increasing in many countries, including the United States. The increase is mostly in the cancer originating in the seminiferous tubules, the area in the testes where sperm production occurs (called seminoma). Experts have not been able to find reasons for this increase.

Most cancers occur in individuals over the age of 55. Yet, testicular cancer is the most common form of cancer in men between the ages of 15–35 (American Cancer Society, 2011). The main risk factors for testicular cancer are family history and being born with undescended testes (the testicles remain in the abdomen at birth). A slower growing form of testicular cancer (seminoma) is usually found in men in their 30s and 40s (American Cancer Society, 2011). Even so, testicular cancer is not common compared to other types of cancer. A man's lifetime chance of developing testicular cancer is about 1 in 300. In 2011, the U.S. Preventive Services Task Force reaffirmed its 2004 recommendation against screening for testicular cancer in adolescent and adult males without any symptoms. Because treatment is so successful, the risk of dying from this cancer is very low—about 1 in 5,000. Radiation and chemotherapy have been successful in keeping this cancer from spreading. If necessary, a testicle will be surgically removed, a procedure called an *orchiectomy*.

Symptoms include discomfort or pain in the testicle, or a feeling of heaviness in the scrotum, pain in the back or lower abdomen, enlargement of a testicle, or a change in the way it feels, and a lump or swelling in either testicle.

Cancer of the Penis

In 2011, about 1,360 new cases of penile cancer were diagnosed and an estimated 320 men died from it (American Cancer Society, 2011). Penile cancer is rare in North America and Europe. It accounts for less than 1 percent of cancers in men in the United States. This cancer occurs in about 1 man in 100,000 in the United States. However, penile cancer is much more common in some parts of Asia, Africa, and South America, where it accounts for up to 10 percent of cancers in men. Penile cancer rarely occurs in young men. This cancer is more often diagnosed in men over the age of 60 (dePaula et al., 2007). According to Blanco-Yarosh (2007), risk factors of penile cancer are HPV infection, smoking, and *phimosis* (inability to retract the foreskin from the glans of the penis in uncircumcised males).

Cancers in Both Women and Men Linked to HPV

HPV oral infection is mainly sexually acquired, and the recent increase in the incidence of oral cancers (or *oropharyngeal carcinoma*) has been considered the result of changing sexual behaviors (Chaturvedi, Engels, Anderson, & Gillison, 2008). Not only are more couples in the United States participating in fellatio or cunniligus, but they are also not taking precautions to limit their exposure to the genital skin or vaginal/seminal secretions (Kreimer, Clifford, Boyle, & Franceschi, 2005). Precautions need to be taken when participating in sexual activities that increase fluid transmission. A condom should be worn on a penis (there are condoms specifically made for oral sex) if fellatio is expected. A condom can also be cut in half, opened up and used on the vulva if cunniligus will be performed.

For over a decade, the incidence of anal cancer has been increasing in women and men who participate in anal intercourse. There is a growing body of evidence to support the role of HPV in this disease (Balasubramanian, Palefsky, & Koutsky, 2008). Receptive partners (i.e., their anus is being penetrated) in anal sex are more at risk of acquiring HPV, but that does not mean insertive partners cannot be infected. Safer sex practices must be performed consistently to reduce the risk of HPV infection. Condoms worn for coitus can also be used for anal penetration. Moreover, the anus does not lubricate naturally, thus a water-based lubricant is needed to prevent abrasions and tearing of the skin surrounding the anus, which can increase HPV infection.

Reflections

The purpose of this chapter is to familiarize students with the male sexual/reproductive anatomy. Many men are unacquainted with their internal reproductive structures. Gaining knowledge and understanding of our bodies is an important aspect of sexual well-being and sexual intelligence. Numerous factors, such as culture, religion, and politics play influential roles in a society in determining what should or should not be disseminated on male sexual health. Every man has a right to know how to protect his sexual health, though. Our society, thus, has the responsibility to promote male sexual health with medically accurate information.

Critical Thinking Questions

1. How can men decrease their risk to cancer in their reproductive organs?

2. Around 60 percent of males in this country are circumcised at birth, although European countries rarely modify the genitals of their babies. Why do you think we do and they don't?

3. The majority of women and men who participate in anal or oral sex do not protect their genitals to reduce the risk of HPV infection. Why do you think that is the case? How can society increase the use of condoms during these practices to reduce the exposure of HPV and other STIs?

4. Why do you think there may be individuals in your class who do not know some of the terms for the internal male sexual/reproductive anatomy?

5. When do you think this information should be taught and by whom?

How Much Do You Remember from the Chapter?

1. The greatest concentration of nerve endings on the penis is found on the:
   - a. corona
   - b. glans of the penis
   - c. frenulum
   - d. shaft of the penis

2. What area(s) in the penis is/are removed during a circumcision?
   - a. foreskin and frenulum
   - b. foreskin only
   - c. glans of the penis only
   - d. glans of the penis and foreskin

3. Around 70 percent of the seminal fluid comes from the Cowper's gland.
   - a. True
   - b. False

4. Seminal fluid consists of secretions from:
   - a. seminal vesicles, Cowper's gland, vas deferens
   - b. epididymis, vas deferens, ejaculatory duct, Cowper's gland
   - c. seminal vesicles, prostate gland, ejaculatory duct
   - d. seminal vesicles, prostate gland, Cowper's gland

5. Between 15–35 is the age range in which a male is most likely to be diagnosed with testicular cancer.
   - a. True
   - b. False

6. At puberty until death, sperm are produced, on average, _____ sperm a second.
   - a. 1 million
   - b. 100,000
   - c. 100
   - d. 1,000

7. What is cut during a vasectomy?
   - a. epididymis
   - b. prostate gland
   - c. vas deferens
   - d. Cowper's gland

8. What cancer of the reproductive system is the most prevalent in men?
   - a. prostate cancer
   - b. penile cancer
   - c. testicular cancer
   - d. epididymal cancer

9. Anal and oral cancers in both women and men are increasing because of:
   - a. smoking
   - b. HPV infection
   - c. excessive alcohol use
   - d. Chlamydia infection

10. Where is sperm stored before ejaculation?
    - a. vas deferens
    - b. prostate gland
    - c. Cowper's gland
    - d. epididymis

11. What structure coats the urethra with an alkaline fluid before ejaculation?
    a. vas deferens
    b. prostate gland
    c. Cowper's gland
    d. epididymis

12. The Wolffian ducts develop into the:
    a. vas deferens, seminal vesicles, ejaculatory duct
    b. fallopian tubes, uterus, inner third of the vagina
    c. shaft of the penis, glans of the penis, scrotum
    d. glans of the clitoris, labia majora, labia minora

13. The Mullerian ducts develop into the:
    a. glans of the clitoris, labia majora, labia minora
    b. vas deferens, seminal vesicles, ejaculatory duct
    c. shaft of the penis, glans of the penis, scrotum
    d. fallopian tubes, uterus, inner third of the vagina

14. What hormonal contraceptive injection available for women has also been used to drastically reduce the amount of testosterone in men (as a means to treat sex offenders or prostate cancer) because this is an anti-androgen drug?
    a. Mirena
    b. Lunelle
    c. Depo-Provera
    d. Seasonale

15. Cycling has been found to be a risk factor for erectile dysfunction.
    a. True
    b. False

Challenge Yourself!

Label each structure that is part of the internal male genitalia:

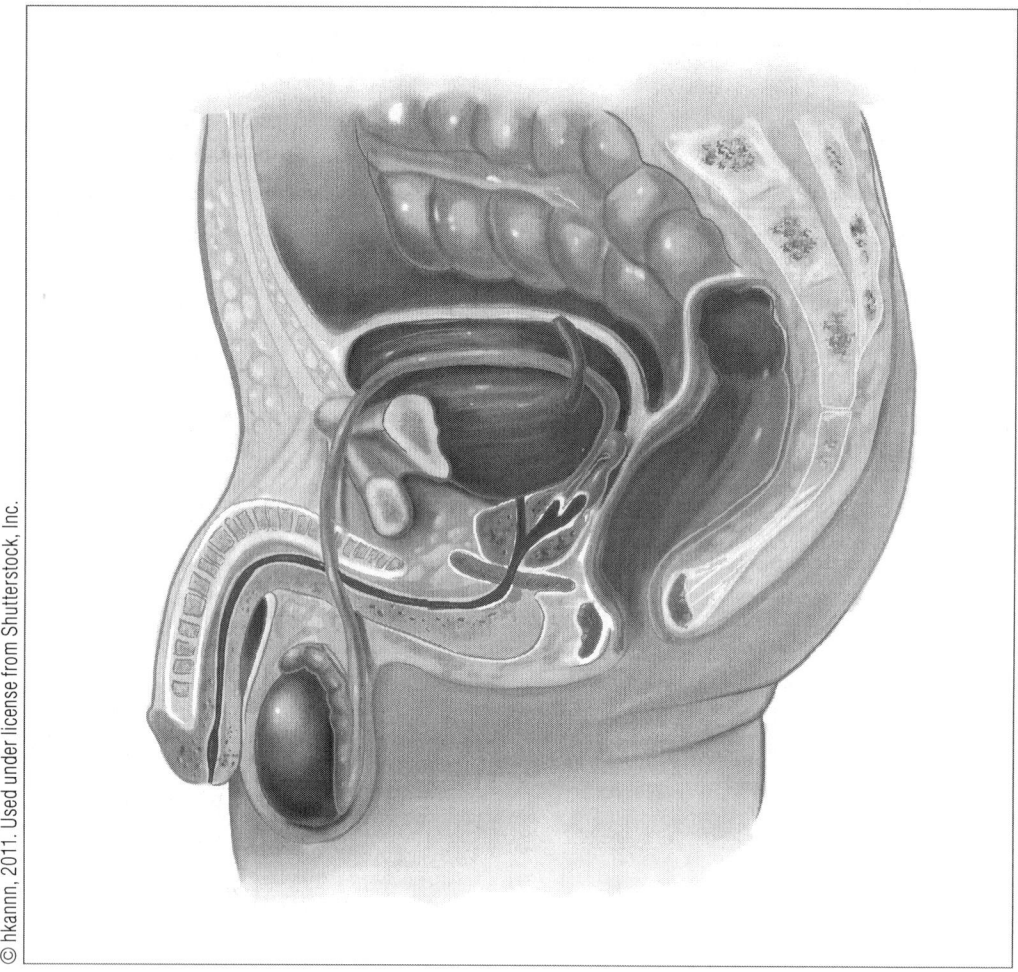

1. Vas deferens
2. Urethra
3. Testes
4. Bulbourethral/Cowper's gland
5. Scrotum
6. Ejaculatory
7. Seminal vesicles
8. Bladder
9. Epididymis
10. Prostate gland

Websites

www.goofyfootpress.com/
The Guide to Getting It On

www.womenshealth.gov/mens/sexual/
The National Women's Health Information Center

www.cdc.gov/cancer/
Centers for Disease Control and Prevention

References

American Cancer Society. (2011). *Cancer facts and figures 2011*. Atlanta, GA: Author.

American Congress of Obstetricians and Gynecologists (ACOG). (2010). *How your baby grows during pregnancy*. Danvers, MA: Author.

Balasubramanian, A., Palefsky, J., & Koutsky, L. (2008). Cervical neoplasia and other STD-related genital tract neoplasias. In K. Holmes, P. Sparling, W. Stamm, P. Piot, J. Wasserheit, L. Corey, & M. Cohen (Eds.), *Sexually transmitted diseases* (4th Ed., pp. 1051–1074). New York, NY: McGraw-Hill, Inc.

Bella, A., & Shamloul, R. (2011). Function anatomy of the male sex organs. In P. Mulhall, L. Incrocci, I. Goldstein, & R. Rosen (Eds.), *Cancer & sexual health* (pp. 3–12). New York, NY: Springer-Science.

Blanco-Yarosh, M. (2007). Penile cancer: An overview. *Urologic Nursing, 27*(4), 286–290.

Burgu, B., Aydogdu, O., Tangal, S., & Soygur, T. (2010). Circumcision: Pros and cons. *Indian Journal of Urology, 26*, 12–15.

Ceo, P. (2006). Assessment of the male reproductive system. *Urologic Nursing, 26*(4), 290–296.

Chaturvedi, A., Engels, A., Anderson, F., & Gillison, M. (2008). Incidence trends for human papillomavirus-related and -unrelated oral squamous cell carcinomas in the United States. *Journal of Clinical Oncology, 26*, 612–619.

Clement, P., & Giuliano, F. (2011). Physiology of ejaculation. In P. Mulhall, L. Incrocci, I. Goldstein, & R. Rosen (Eds.), *Cancer & sexual health* (pp. 77–92). New York: Springer-Science.

Corona, G., Boddi, V., Gacci, M., Sforza, A., Forti, G., Mannucci, E. et al. (2011). Perceived ejaculate volume reduction in patients with erectile dysfunction: Psychobiologic correlates. *Journal of Andrology, 32*(3), 333–339.

Cutler, D. (2008). Are we finally winning the war on cancer? *Journal of Economic Perspectives, 22*(4), 3–26.

Dabbs, M., & Dabbs, J. (2000). *Heroes, rogues, and lovers: Testosterone and behavior*. New York, NY: McGraw-Hill.

Dahl, A., Mykletun, A., & Fossa, S. (2005). Quality of life in survivors of testicular cancer. *Urologic Oncology: Seminars and Original Investigations, 23*, 193–200.

dePaula, A., Netto, J., Freitaas, R., dePaula, L., Mota, E., & Alencar, R. (2007). Penile carcinoma: The role of koilocytosis in groin metastasis and the association with disease-specific survival. *Journal of Urology, 177*(4), 1339–1343.

Dettori, J., Koepsell, T., Cummings, P., & Corman, J. (2004). Erectile dysfunction after a long-distance cycling event: Associations with bicycle characteristics. *The Journal of Urology, 172*(2), 637–641.

Golden, M., & Wasserheit, J. (2009). Prevention of viral sexually transmitted infections—Foreskin at the forefront. *New England Journal of Medicine, 360*, 1349–1351.

Hamilton, T. (2002). *Skin flutes and velvet gloves: A collection of facts and fancies, legends and oddities about the body's private parts*. New York, NY: St. Martin's Press.

Harman, S., Metter, E., Tobin, J., Pearson, J., & Blackman, M. (2001). Longitudinal effects of aging on serum total and free testosterone levels in healthy men: Baltimore longitudinal study of aging. *Journal of Endocrinology & Metabolism, 86,* 724–731.

Heffner, L., & Schust, D. (2006). *Reproductive systems at a glance* (2nd Ed.). Ames, IA: Blackwell Publishing Professional.

Higano, C. (2003). Side effects of androgen deprivation therapy: Monitoring and minimizing toxicity. *Urology, 61*(Suppl. 2A), 32–38.

Jones, R., & Lopez, K. (2006). *Human reproductive biology* (3rd Ed.). Burlington, MA: Elsevier.

Kreimer, A., Clifford, G., Boyle, P., & Franceschi, S. (2005). Human papillomavirus types in head and neck squamous cell carcinomas worldwide: A systematic review. *Cancer Epidemiology Biomarkers & Prevention, 14,* 467–475.

Krieger, J., & Graney, D. (2008). Clinical anatomy and physical examination of the male genital tract. In K. Holmes, P. Sparling, W. Stamm, P. Piot, J. Wasserheit, L. Corey, & M. Cohen (Eds.), *Sexually transmitted diseases* (4th ed., pp. 917–928). New York, NY: McGraw-Hill, Inc.

Kumar, R., Barqawi, A., & Crawford, E. (2005). Preventing and treating the complications of hormone therapy. *Current Urology Reports, 6*(3), 217–223.

Masters, W., & Johnson, V. (1966). *Human sexual response.* Boston, MA: Little Brown & Co.

Matsumoto, A. (2002). Andropause: Clinical implications of the decline in serum testosterone levels with aging in men. *Journals of Gerontology Series A: Biological Sciences and Medical Sciences, 57,* M76–M99.

Morales, A., Heaton, J., & Carson, C. (2000). Andropause: A misnomer for a true clinical entity. *Journal of Urology, 163,* 705–712.

Nixon-Cobb, E., & Bonillas, C. (2011). *Listen up! Student voices on critical issues and values in real life* (2nd Ed.). Dubuque, IA: Kendall Hunt Publishing.

Ricci, S., & Kyle, T. (2009). *Maternity and pediatric nursing.* Philadelphia, PA: Lippincott Williams & Wilkins.

Ridings, H., & Amaya, M. (2007). Male neonatal circumcision: An evidence-based review. *Journal of the American Academy of Physician Assistants, 20*(2), 32–36.

Sinclair, A., Berta, P., Palmer, M., Hawkins, J., Griffiths, B., Smith, M. et al. (1990). A gene from the human sex-determining region encodes a protein with homology to a conserved DNA-binding motif. *Nature, 346,* 240–244.

Steele, E. (2011, April 5). *Sperm tastes delicious—How to make your semen taste better.* Retrieved from www.ezinearticles.com/?Sperm-Tastes-Delicious---How-to-Make-Your-Semen-Taste-Better&id=6068195

Tarkovsky, S. (2006, February 2). *Your semen –A diet for better sperm taste.* Retrieved from www.ezinearticles.com/?Your-Semen---A--Diet--For-Better-Sperm-Taste&id=138648

Taylor, G. (2000). *Castration: An abbreviated history of western manhood.* New York, NY: Routledge.

Tuck, S., & Francis, R. (2009). Testosterone, bone and osteoporosis. *Frontiers of Hormone Research, 37,* 123–132.

Totaro, A., Volpe, A., Racioppi, M., Pinto, F., Sacco, E., & Bassi, P. F. (2011). Circumcision: History, religion and law. *Urologia, 78*(1), 1–9.

Wassersug, R., & Johnson, T. (2007). Modern day eunuchs: Motivations for and consequences of contemporary castration. *Perspectives in Biology & Medicine, 50,* 544-556.

Weinberger, L., Sreenivasan, S., Garrick, T., & Osran, H. (2005). The impact of surgical castration on sexual recidivism risk among sexually violent predatory offenders. *Journal of the American Academy of Psychiatry & Law, 33,* 16–36.

chapter six

FEMALE & MALE SEXUAL AROUSAL & RESPONSE

CHAPTER OBJECTIVES

On completion of this chapter, students will be able to:

- identify life changes that can affect one's sexual health;
- understand the different phases of the sexual response cycle;
- name the variety of behaviors experienced for sexual pleasure;
- explain the biological differences in the female and male sexual response cycles;
- distinguish the sexual dysfunctions experienced by females and males.

ABBREVIATIONS AND ACRONYMS USED IN THIS CHAPTER

APA	American Psychiatric Association
AUA	American Urological Association
ED	erectile dysfunction
FDA	Food and Drug Administration
HSDD	hypoactive sexual desire disorder
pH	potential hydrogen
PE	premature ejaculation
SSRI	selective serotonin reuptake inhibitors
STIs	sexually transmitted infections

THE SEXUAL RESPONSE CYCLE

Even though this chapter aims to simplify information about what we experience when we are sexually aroused, the state of arousal and what encompasses that response are complex (Bancroft, 2010; Giraldi, 2011; Hiller, 2004; Jones & Lopez, 2006). A number of factors—the interaction of our hormones, various body systems, what we learned (or did not learn) about sexuality from our family and our social environment, and the meanings we place on different aspects of sexuality—influence how we respond to a variety of sexual stimuli that we may encounter. Moreover, our sexual health will vary as we experience life changes, such as puberty, pregnancy, postpartum, an illness, stress, andropause, menopause, etc.

Masters and Johnson (1966, 1970) have completed extensive research on the sexual response cycle. They postulated that individuals experience four phases when sexually aroused: excitement, plateau, orgasm, and resolution. They asserted that people experience each phase in a linear fashion (i.e., excitement comes before plateau, plateau comes before orgasm, and orgasm comes before resolution). However, their theoretical underpinning of the sexual response cycle continues to be debated (Clement & Giuliano, 2011), and other researchers have either expanded or revised the sexual response cycle (Basson, 2001; Kaplan, 1979; Loulan, 1984). Individuals vary in the intensity of each phase, as well as the duration that an individual remains in a particular phase.

Excitement

Excitement can be explained as the phase in which individuals experience genital arousal (Masters & Johnson, 1966). For males, the penis becomes erect (known as vasocongestion) and if he is not circumcised the foreskin may seem to shorten to expose the glans of the penis. When erect, the male may notice small amounts of fluid on the urethral opening (from the Cowper's gland). He may also feel his scrotum tighten up, bringing the testicles (which have enlarged) closer to the body. For females, the vulva may begin to feel warm and if touched may feel fuller than when she is not aroused. During this phase, the labia majora, labia minora, and glans of the clitoris begin to engorge with blood. According to Meston (2002), within approximately 20 seconds of sexual stimulation, vaginal lubrication appears and the genitals increase in blood flow (known as vasocongestion). Vaginal lubrication originates from an inner layer of the vagina, as well as from secretions from the Bartholin's glands (Meston, 2000). During sexual activity, both sexes experience myotonia, or increased muscle tension that causes

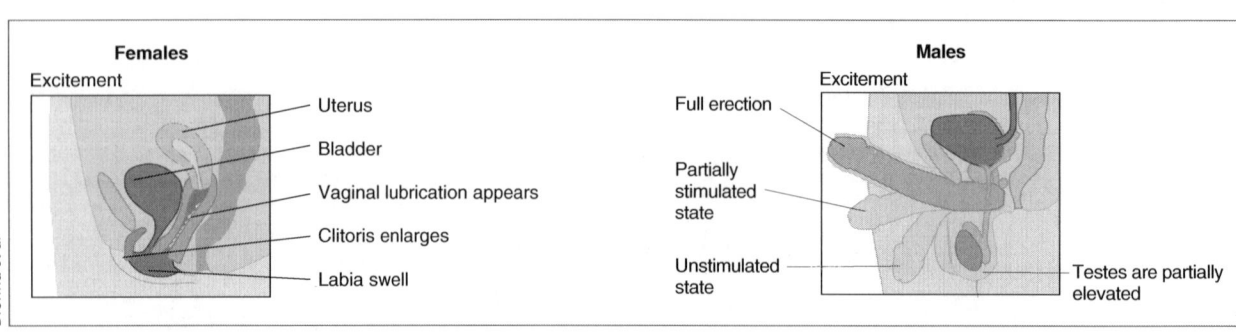

facial grimaces, spasms in the hands and feet, and then if stimulation is adequate, the spasms of orgasm (Masters & Johnson, 1966).

The following physiological changes occur in both females and males during the excitement phase and are experienced throughout the first three phases, with varying degrees of intensity: the pupils dilate, the heart rate increases, blood pressure rises, body temperature increases, nipples become erect, and both sexes experience something called the "sex flush" in which the color of the chest, areola (the pigmented skin surrounding the nipples), neck, and face darken or redden because of the increased body temperature and rise in blood pressure (Pfaus, 2011).

It is believed that the excitement phase helps an individual prepare the body and mind for sexual activity (Pfaus, 2011). Interestingly, individuals may not always be aware they are sexually aroused. While for males it can be hard not to notice an erection, studies have found some women experience difficulty in reporting feeling sexually aroused even though they physiologically are (Giraldi, 2011). Part of this discrepancy may be because some women do not detect subtle changes in vaginal blood flow, but instead become aware of their arousal when higher levels of physiological changes occur (Meston, 2002).

There is no set timeframe as to how long an individual remains in the excitement phase. Numerous factors need to be taken into account. For example, was the individual anticipating sexual activity when it occurred or was it spontaneous (and welcomed)? Was the stimulation pleasing enough to the individual to lead to arousal? What was the "goal" for this sexual encounter—for one individual to reach orgasm, for both, or for neither? Moreover, the level of excitement experienced by any individual can vary with each new sexual situation encountered (regardless if the person is alone, with a new sexual partner, or with a long-term sexual partner). If stimulation ends at this phase then the person will slowly enter the resolution phase.

Plateau

Plateau can be explained as the phase in which individuals cannot go beyond their sexual arousal. They have reached their peak of excitement before reaching orgasm (Masters & Johnson, 1966). At this phase, individuals can continue receiving the stimulation that has led to this level of arousal and for many they will enter the next phase and experience an orgasm. Couples can also reduce the amount of stimulation provided to "tease" each other to want more and to prolong the session before either of them experiences an orgasm. If stimulation ends during this phase then the person will not enter the next phase and reach orgasm, but will slowly enter the resolution phase.

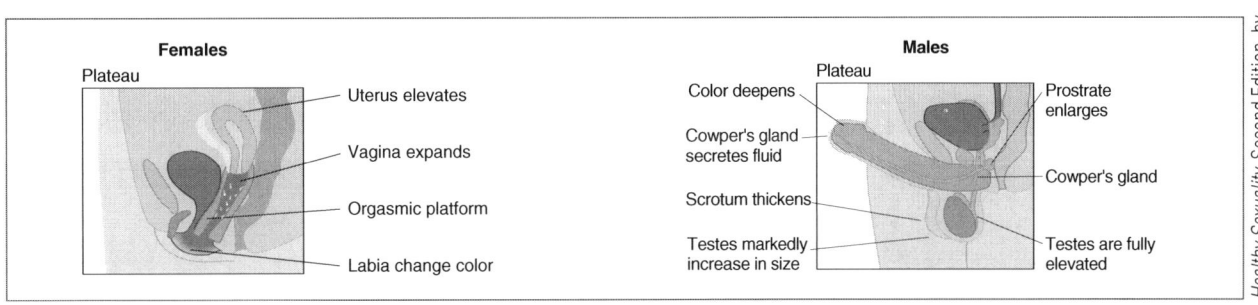

Orgasm

"Of all the various sexual responses, orgasm remains the most mysterious and least well-understood" (Bancroft, 2009, p. 84). Orgasm can be explained as the phase in which individuals reach a sexual peak with intense pleasurable sensations (Masters & Johnson, 1966). But what *is* an orgasm? For those who have experienced one, how would you describe it? Would you say it was one of the most intense, pleasurable feelings you have ever experienced? Where did you experience these intense pleasurable feelings—in the genitals, the internal sexual anatomy, or all over your body? Would you say that the world around you ceased to exist during those few seconds? What words would you use to describe an orgasm? Moreover, does an orgasm feel different if experienced through masturbation, oral sex, coitus, anal sex, or as you sleep? Even though women and men may describe an orgasm using different descriptive terms, it is believed that what men and women experience during an orgasm is similar (Levin, 2011). Some people (especially women) rarely experience this phase, though. If this phase is not reached, the individual will slowly enter the resolution phase.

Female Orgasm

For some women, experiencing an orgasm is as elusive as winning the lottery. This is not due to biological differences in women, but societal or personal expectations created to form a mental barrier to experiencing an orgasm (Stephenson, Ahrold, & Meston, 2011). For example, is a woman participating in sexual activity with a sexual partner to continue that relationship even if she doesn't want to be sexually intimate? Does she believe that women are supposed to feel pleasure vicariously through their sexual partner and so do not need to personally experience an orgasm? Does she find it hard to concentrate and enjoy the moment because she is concerned about a possible pregnancy or becoming infected with an STI?

For other women, experiencing an orgasm comes as easy as breathing! Women vary considerably in their orgasmic ability. For some women, an orgasm can only be attained by specific means—cunniligus, masturbation, using a vibrator, or being on top during coitus (Fugl-Meyer, Oberg, Lundberg, & Lewin, 2006). Any activity that focuses on stimulating the glans of the clitoris—usually indirectly because direct stimulation of the clitoral glans may be painful—can help a woman reach orgasm. Moreover, women have reported more intense orgasms after a longer stimulation phase prior to orgasm than after shorter time of stimulation (Laan, 2009). Even though most women need the glans of the clitoris stimulated in some fashion to reach orgasm, female orgasm by nipple stimulation alone has been reported (Paget, 2001). Also, women have reported experiencing "different-feeling" orgasms (but equally as intense), depending whether the glans of the clitoris is stimulated versus the cervix being stimulated versus vaginal stimulation. It is believed this is due to the distinctive nerves receiving sensory activity from each of these regions (Komisaruk, Beyer-Flores, & Whipple, 2006).

A female orgasm can be defined as brief, intense pleasure sensations partially concentrated on the genitals creating an altered state of consciousness. Strong, involuntary rhythmic contractions of the muscles beneath the perineum and the vulva occur, as well as contractions on the glans of the clitoris, the introitus, the uterus, and anus (Kinsey, Pomeroy, Martin, & Gebhard, 1953; Komisaruk & Whipple, 1991; Masters & Johnson, 1966; Meston, Levin, Sipski, Hull, & Heiman, 2004). This description does not do the experience justice, but is a point of reference.

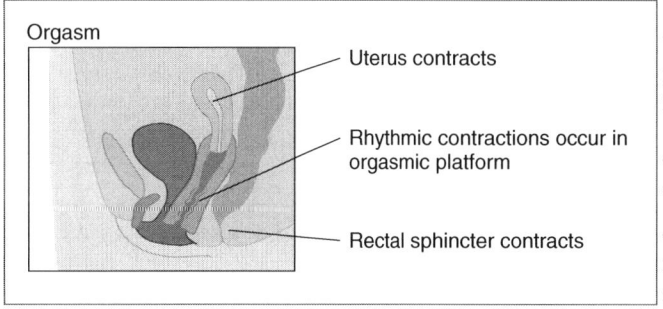

The Multiorgasmic Woman

A distinctive difference between the female and male sexual response cycle is that women have the capacity for multiple orgasms (Masters & Johnson, 1966). What that means is, after experiencing one orgasm, women can attain another one in a matter of seconds or minutes. Most men do not have that ability, even though research has found it can be possible for some men (Dunn & Trost, 1989). With adequate stimulation, women can move easily between the different levels of arousal, including orgasm.

For a woman to have a multiorgasmic experience, she should have an orgasm by any means that has worked for her in the past. After the first orgasm has been achieved, the woman has to maintain a certain degree of arousal—either by herself or with help from a sexual partner. The glans of the clitoris will be extremely sensitive after the first orgasm, so stimulation needs to be concentrated around the labia, introitus, vagina, or anus. The second orgasm can be achieved in the same manner as the first one or by using some other approach (Paget, 2001). A woman doesn't have to experience one orgasm after another. But the ability is generally there for women if they want to partake.

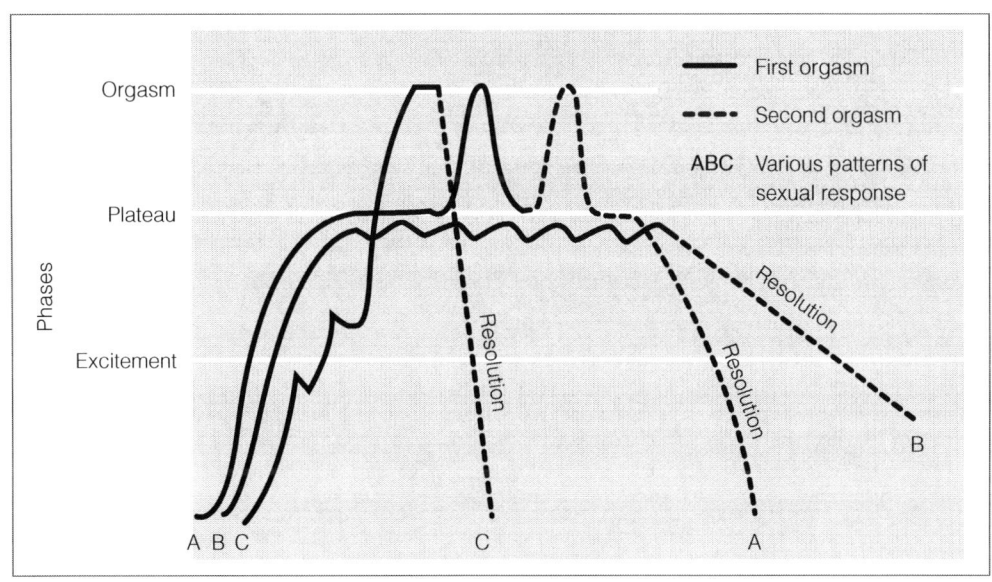

Chapter Six 97

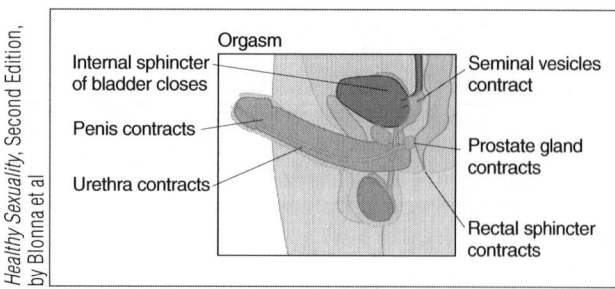

Male Orgasm

In males, orgasm and ejaculation are two separate physiological mechanisms, thus one can happen without the other. The orgasmic phase has two distinct phases: emission and expulsion (Clement & Giuliano, 2011). The emission phase can be identified by many men as the "point of no return"—orgasm will occur whether stimulation continues or not. If a male reaches the emission phase, that means he received enough stimulation that resulted in intense internal contractions. During the emission phase, the contractions are concentrated around the epididymis, vas deferens, the seminal vesicles, the ejaculatory duct, and the prostate gland (Clement & Giuliano, 2011). The portion of the urethra that surrounds the prostate gland expands in preparation for ejaculation. The internal urethral sphincter, located by the opening of the bladder, and the external urethral sphincter, located below the prostate gland, contract to prevent urine from entering the urethra and semen from entering the bladder (Bohlen, Hugonnet, Mills, Weise, & Schmid, 2000).

Ejaculation actually occurs during the expulsion phase. The male can experience an altered consciousness state as the penis and the muscles located at the base of the penis and the anal sphincter experience intense, rhythmic contractions. The majority of semen is expelled out of the urethra during the first 3–4 contractions (Jones & Lopez, 2006).

The (Male) Refractory Period

During the refractory period, a man cannot experience another orgasm, regardless of the stimulation provided. It has not been determined why after reaching orgasm men undergo a period in which they cannot maintain their level of sexual arousal at the same intensity as it was seconds or minutes prior to ejaculation. Even though the duration of the refractory period can be influenced

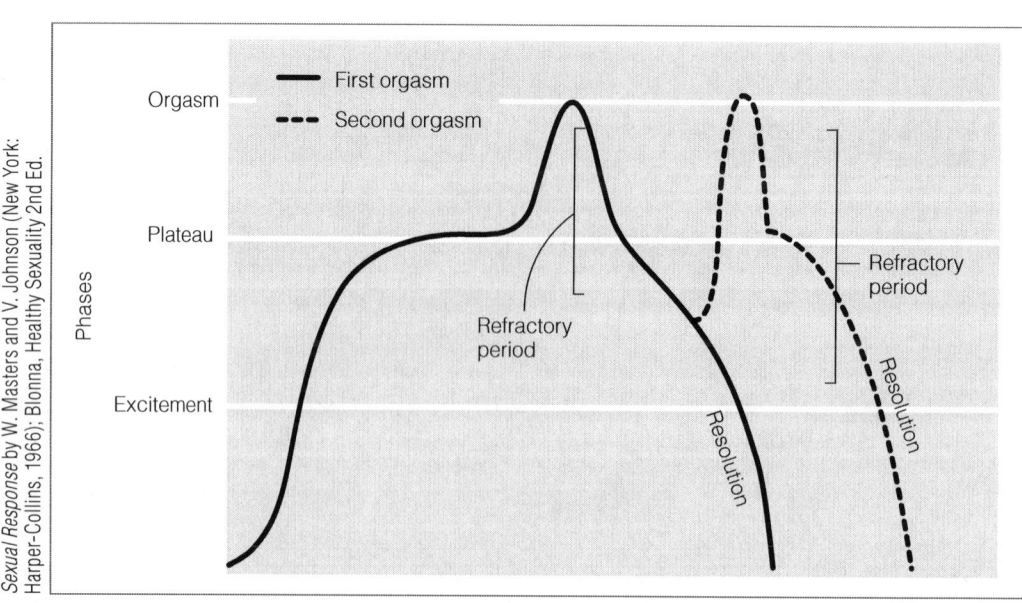

by many factors, such as stress, fatigue, overall health, and the amount of sexual stimulation, younger men seem to have a shorter refractory period than older men (Jones & Lopez, 2006).

Resolution

Resolution can be explained as the phase in which individuals return to their unaroused state (Masters & Johnson, 1966). This phase is reached quickly if orgasm is experienced because sexual release was achieved. The body (and the mind) may take longer to return to an unaroused state if orgasm is not reached (and depending on the intensity of the stimulation and state of arousal).

For females, resolution encompasses a decrease in blood flow to the vulva. Internally, the blood flow declines in the vagina and vaginal lubrication abates. The internal body of the clitoris returns to its non-erect state, as well. A woman's heart rate, body temperature, and pupils also return to normal.

For males, resolution encompasses a decrease in blood flow to the penis. For some men, the penis becomes flaccid almost immediately after ejaculation. For others, though, the penis remains erect after ejaculation (even if there is no intention to resume sexual activity). The scrotum begins to elongate, extending the testes (which have shrunk back to regular size) away from the abdomen. A man's heart rate, body temperature, and pupils also return to normal.

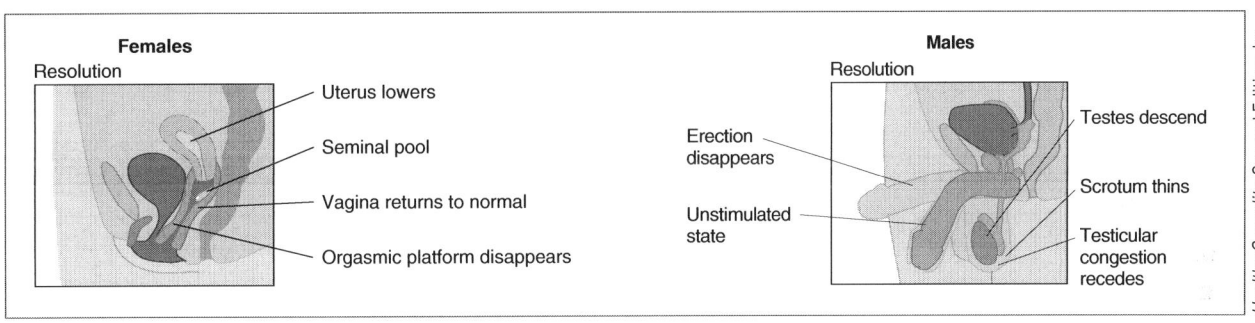

Healthy Sexuality, Second Edition, by Blonna et al

SEXUAL BEHAVIORS

A variety of sexual behaviors can be experienced for sexual pleasure. All of these can be used to enhance sexual arousal, to experience an orgasm, or to release sexual tension (to name a few). There is no correct order in which one behavior needs to follow another. Nor is the subsequent list below an exhaustive one on what activities lead to sexual pleasure. Even though many couples consider the "end" of a sexual session by experiencing orgasm (by one or both of the partners), there are individuals who "begin" with experiencing an orgasm and continue with other sexual behaviors that offer additional sexual pleasure. With any behavior in which fluid transmission or genital skin-to-skin contact can occur, strict precautions need to be taken to reduce the risk of sexually transmitted infections (STIs). This is discussed in detail in chapter 7.

Self-stimulation of the genitals is called *masturbation* (*Merriam-Webster's Collegiate Dictionary*, 2008). A male can use his hands (or a pillow or other object) to

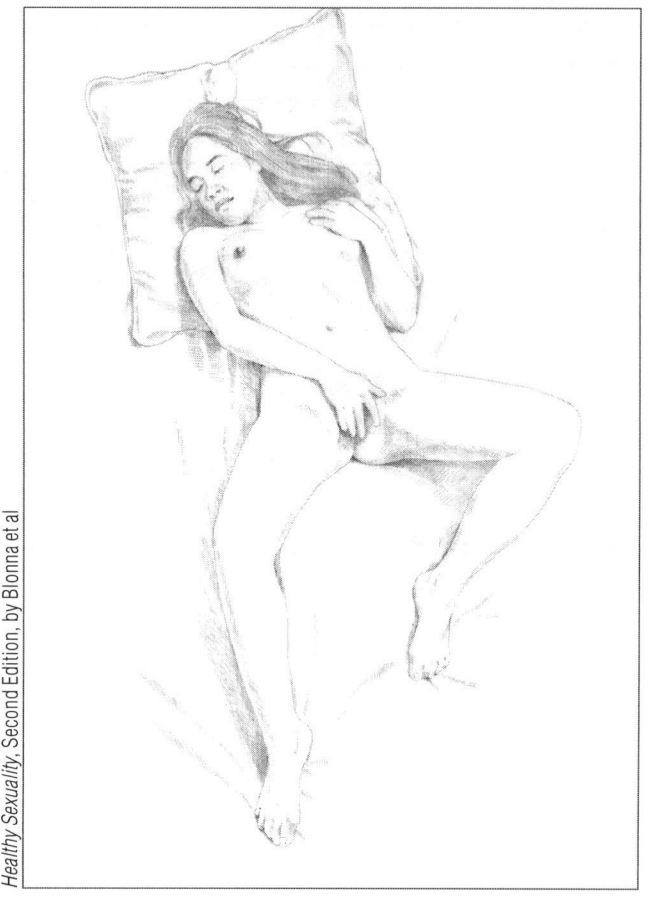
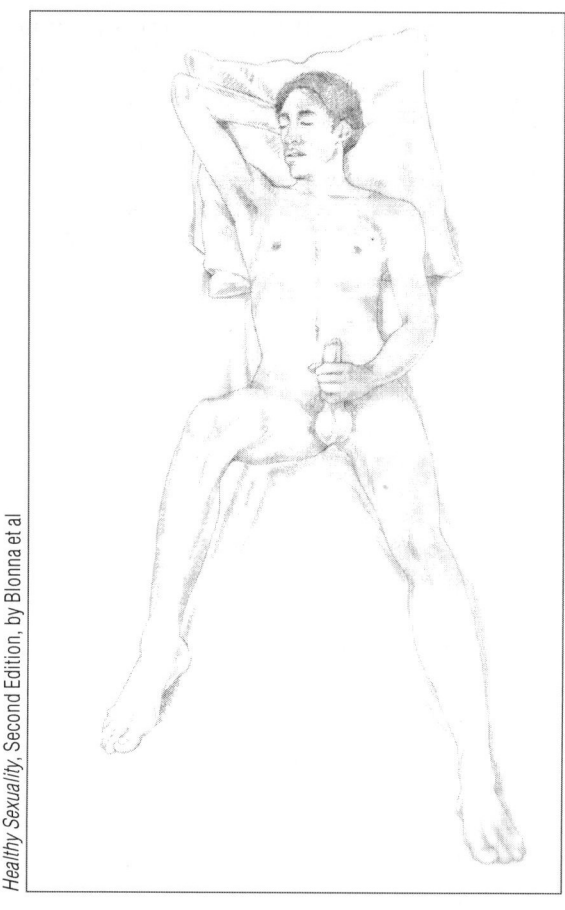

rub the shaft of the penis, the glans of the penis, and if not circumcised, the foreskin. A female can use her hands (or a pillow or other object) to rub the glans of the clitoris, the labia minora, or introitus. Both women and men can also use a variety of sex toys, such as dildos or vibrators to intensify the sensations (Davis, Black, Liu, & Bonillas, 1996). Individuals may or may not fantasize while they are masturbating. They can also watch and/or listen to sexually explicit material while they masturbate. Mutual masturbation is also possible in which a couple stimulates the genitals of each other for sexual pleasure.

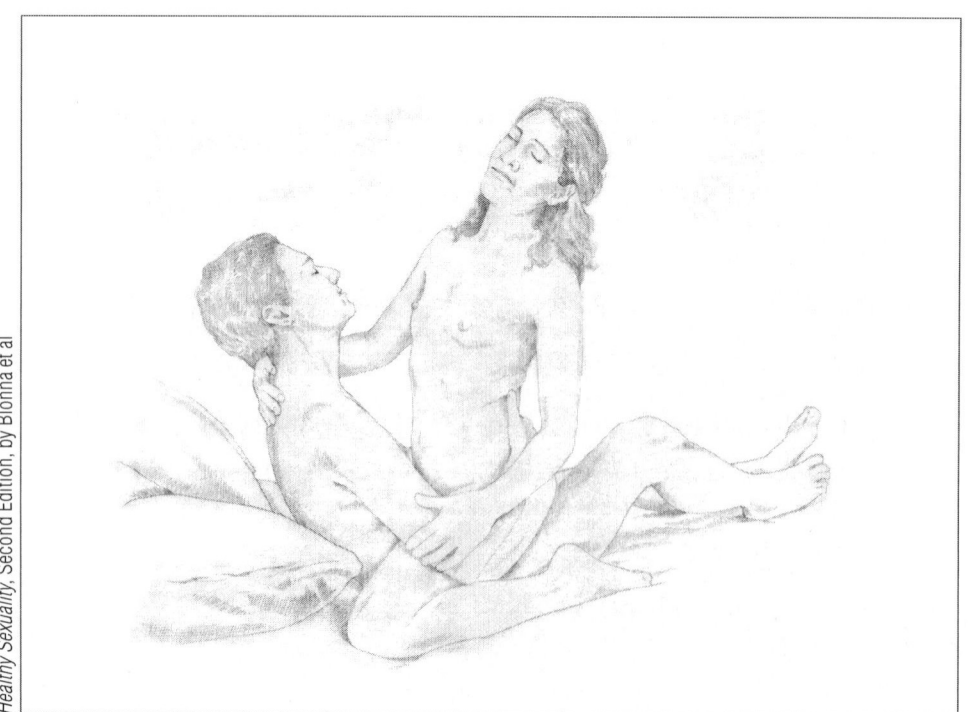

The clinical term for the insertion of a penis in a vagina is *coitus* (*Merriam-Webster's Collegiate Dictionary*, 2008). In Latin, coitus means "coming together" (Jones & Lopez, 2006). The term coitus (koi-təs) is used throughout this textbook to specifically refer to vaginal-penile intercourse. With this sexual behavior, the introitus, vagina, and cervix may be stimulated by the penetration and thrusting of the penis. The glans and shaft of the penis are stimulated by entering the introitus (i.e., vaginal opening), by being enveloped by the vaginal walls, and/or by the glans of the penis coming into contact with the cervix. Whereas men may find coitus an easy way to reach orgasm, this activity has been found to be one of the hardest ways for a woman to experience an orgasm (Levin, 2011). This is usually due to the lack of adequate stimulation (i.e., focus, duration, and intensity) that needs to be provided to the glans of the clitoris. Coital positions that stimulate the glans of the clitoris (such as "woman on top") can improve a woman's chances of reaching orgasm. Using a vibrator or masturbating while participating in coitus can also assist women in reaching orgasm (Davis et al., 1996).

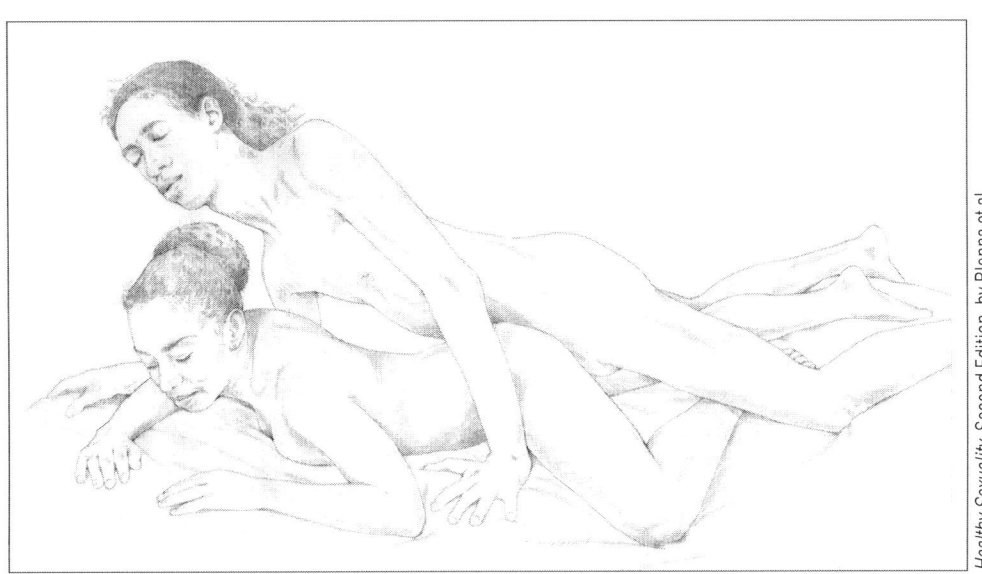

Anal sex is a sexual behavior in which a penis is (usually) inserted in an anus. Fingers, dildos, and other objects made specifically to penetrate the anus can also be used for this activity. With this sexual behavior, the anus and rectum are stimulated by the penetration and thrusting of the penis. The glans and shaft of the penis are stimulated by entering the anus and by being enveloped by the walls of the rectum. As was discussed in a previous chapter, the anus and rectum do not lubricate, thus a water-based

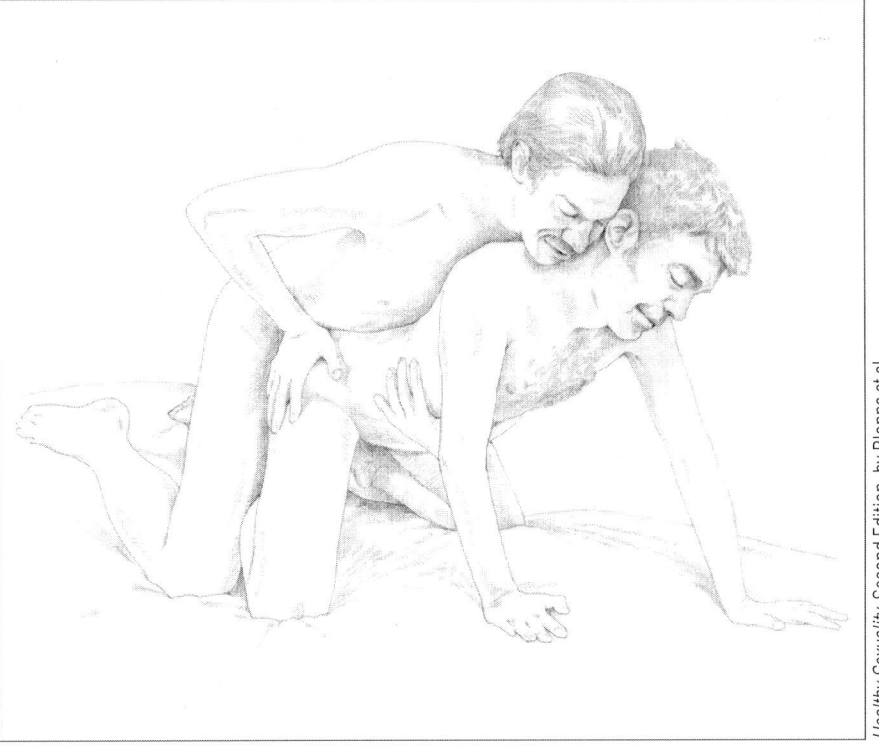

lubricant or saliva is needed for penetration to occur without pain and tearing of the skin around the anus (Jones & Lopez, 2006). Because the anus does not differ in sensitivity for either sex, anal sex can be pleasurable for men and women, regardless of sexual orientation.

Oral sex is a sexual behavior in which the genitals of one individual are stimulated by another person's lips, tongue, or mouth (*Merriam-Webster's Collegiate Dictionary*, 2008). The clinical term for oral stimulation of a female's genitals is *cunniligus* (kun'əling'gəs). In Latin, *cunnus* means vulva and *lingere* means to lick (Jones & Lopez, 2006). Cunniligus could encompass oral stimulation of the labia minora, the introitus, the clitoral hood, and the glans of the clitoris. Cunniligus has been found to be one of the easiest ways for a woman to experience an orgasm. This is due to the focus, duration, and intensity of the stimulation provided to the glans of the clitoris.

The clinical term for the oral stimulation of a male's genitals is *fellatio* (Merriam-Webster's Collegiate Dictionary, 2008). In Latin, *fellare* means to suck (Jones & Lopez, 2006). Fellatio (fĕ-la'she-o) could encompass oral stimulation of the shaft of the penis, the testes, the glans of the penis, the corona, and if not circumcised, the foreskin. Some men find experiencing an orgasm difficult, not because the sensations do not necessarily feel pleasurable, but because the stimulation is not focused properly (i.e., sucking on the shaft of the penis instead of the glans of the penis), the techniques being used do not provide the right stimulation, or teeth may inadvertently scrape against the shaft or glans of the penis. First and foremost, verbal communication is imperative for both partners to express their desire to participate (or not!) in this sexual behavior but also to

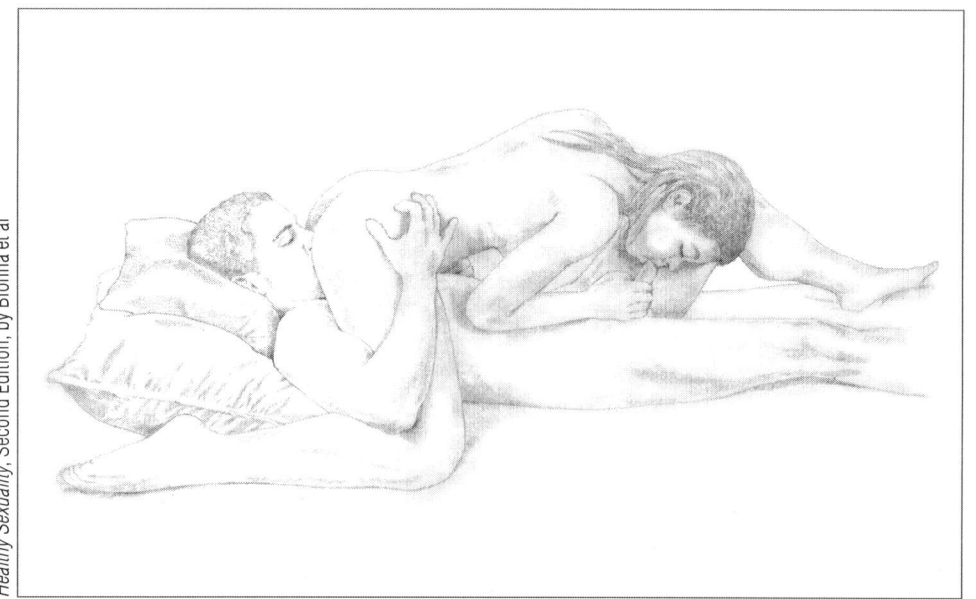

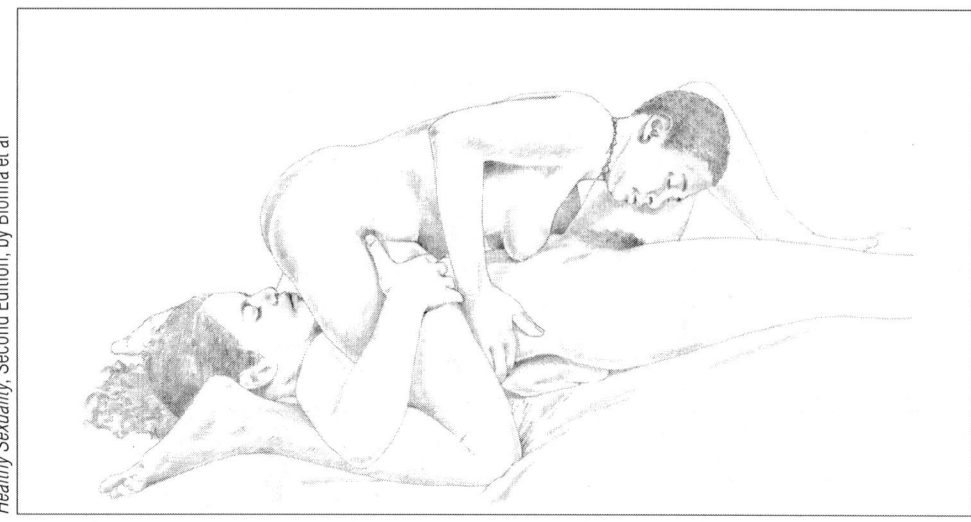

provide guidance in how to improve the pleasurable sensations experienced by both. For example, the "69" sexual position is where two people turn their bodies such that each person's genitals is aligned with the other's mouth and oral stimulation can be performed simultaneously.

Analingus (ā'niling'gəs) is the clinical term for the oral stimulation of an anus (Merriam-Webster's Collegiate Dictionary, 2008). With this sexual behavior, the anal sphincter and/or the perineum can be licked by a sexual partner's tongue or the tongue can penetrate the anus and stimulate the rectum to enhance sexual pleasure. Because the anus does not differ in sensitivity for either sex, analingus can be pleasurable for men and women, regardless of sexual orientation.

SEXUAL DIFFICULTIES AND SOLUTIONS

What if your partner wants to participate in sexual activity more often than you do? Is something wrong with you? What if you want to participate in sexual activity more often than your partner does? Is something wrong with that? How would you define high versus low levels of sexual desire? Is having a "low" level of sexual desire an area of concern? Do you consider your level of sexual desire as "too high"? What if you defined your level of sexual desire as "low," but you were with a partner who was content with the frequency of intimacy between you? Is there something wrong with both of you?

Throughout history and in different cultures, we have placed meanings on different aspects of sexual expression. For example, there was a time that a lack of sexual desire in women was considered normal, but now that is considered dysfunctional (Giraldi, 2011). Even what is considered "low" sexual desire is up for debate. There was a time that women with high sexual interest were considered nymphomaniacs, but today high levels of sexual desire in women is seen as normal and desirable (Giraldi, 2011).

The three major sex therapy paradigms in the treatment of sexual dysfunctions are the medical, psychological, and the biopyschosocial models (Winton, 2001). The *medical model* of sexual dysfunction implies that a sexual problem originates from some organic component, such as a medical condition that requires medication to alleviate the symptoms. A *psychological model* assumes the sexual problem is rooted in interpersonal and social factors. Thus, a counseling-based therapeutic approach is required to alleviate the symptoms (Winton, 2001). A *biopyschosocial* model of sexual dysfunction presumes that a sexual dysfunction is caused by both biological and psychological factors (Winton, 2000).

There does seem to be a discrepancy in the sexual difficulties that women and men report. Bancroft (2009) observed that men are more likely to complain about perceived erectile or ejaculatory problems (i.e., genital response), whereas women primarily present with perceived problems regarding the subjective quality of the sexual experience (e.g., lack of interest or pleasure). As discussed later in this chapter, depending on the sexual problem and, apparently, the sex of the person reporting the sexual complaint, the treatment options prescribed are more likely to focus on the medical rather than the biopyschosocial model.

The American Psychiatric Association's Diagnostic and Statistical Manual on Mental Disorders (DSM-IV-TR) has an entire section devoted to sexual disorders (American Psychiatric Association [*APA*], 2000). The psychosexual disorders are either linked to sexual desire, arousal/excitement, or orgasm. The DSM-IV-TR recommends clinicians consider the impact of cultural factors on sexual dysfunctions: "Clinical judgments about the presence of a sexual dysfunction should take into account the individual's ethnic, cultural, religious, and social background, which may influence sexual desire, expectations, and attitudes about performance" (APA, 2000, p. 495).

Moreover, emphasis has recently been put on the distress or interpersonal difficulties caused by a (perceived) sexual disorder (Giraldi, 2011). For example, when partners express different levels of sexual desire/need/interest, the partner who has "higher" levels of sexual desire may feel resentment while the partner with "lower" levels of sexual desire may feel guilt and shame (Rellini, Farmer, & Golden, 2011). Even so, the line between what is considered normal sexual functioning and what is perceived as a sexual disorder is not clearly defined in clinical practice and thus, precaution is warranted if a diagnosis of a sexual disorder is given (Althof, Dean, Derogatis, & Rosen, 2005).

ANTIDEPRESSANTS AND SEXUAL HEALTH

Some medications to treat depression and other psychological disorders—known as selective serotonin reuptake inhibitors (SSRIs)—are known to decrease sexual functioning. According to the American Psychiatric Association (APA, 2000), an individual experiencing sexual side effects due to medication would *not* be diagnosed with a sexual dysfunction. According to Clayton and colleagues (2006), an estimated 90 percent of men and 95 percent of women taking SSRIs experience sexual side effects in at least one area of sexual functioning (e.g., sexual desire/interest, orgasm, and vasocongestion). SSRI antidepressants, such as Prozac, Paxil, and Zoloft, work by increasing a neurotransmitter called serotonin (Gitlin, 2003). Serotonin has been found to diminish levels of dopamine. Dopamine has been found to play a role in sexual arousal/interest/desire. Thus if dopamine levels decrease, so does sexual expression (Goldstein & Silberstein, 2011). Many SSRIs do an excellent job at combating psychological disorders. It is unfortunate that they also may cause undue stress and anxiety by disrupting sexual functioning. It is recommended that individuals taking SSRIs who are experiencing sexual side effects discuss these symptoms with their doctors. A different SSRI may be used to alleviate symptoms of a psychological disorder while not adversely affecting sexual functioning.

To decrease the sexual side effects of antidepressants, Viagra has been shown in one study to improve symptoms of delayed orgasm in women (Nurnberg et al., 2008). As such, Viagra could be beneficial in alleviating symptoms experienced by men with antidepressant-associated sexual dysfunction.

MALE SEXUAL DIFFICULTIES AND SOLUTIONS

Premature Ejaculation

The most common sexual problem reported by men is *premature ejaculation* (Schuster, 2006). The American Urological Association (AUA) proposed a definition of "ejaculation that occurs sooner than desired, either before or shortly after penetration, causing distress to either one or both partners" (AUA Consensus Panel, 2004). But what constitutes "sooner than desired"? Waldinger and colleagues (1998) have suggested defining premature ejaculation (PE) as when a man reaches orgasm within one minute of (vaginal) penetration. So what if the man frequently ejaculates three minutes after penetration and leaves his partner (and as a result himself) sexually frustrated? Masters and Johnson (1970) chose not to define the disorder with a specific timeframe and instead suggested that a diagnosis be made when the man ejaculates too early for his partner's satisfaction in greater than half of sexual encounters. If a man is distressed about how soon he ejaculates after penetration, then a visit to his doctor could give him some perspective whether he is ejaculating prematurely or not, and what steps he could take to ease his anxiety.

One therapeutic approach to treating PE is called the "start-stop" method (Semans, 1956). This technique involves masturbating until the sensation of heightened arousal is met, but just prior to the emission phase of orgasm (i.e., "point of no return"). The stimulation is stopped until the sensations diminish. This is repeated (which can take days, weeks, or months) until the man can penetrate his partner without ejaculating sooner than both wish (Schuster, 2006).

Erectile Dysfunction

Erectile dysfunction (also known as *impotence*) can be defined as the "inability to attain and/or maintain a penile erection sufficient for satisfactory sexual performance" (National Institutes of Health Consensus Development Panel on Impotence, 1993). Failure to achieve an erection less than 20 percent of the time is not uncommon and in such cases treatment is rarely warranted. Experiencing erectile dysfunction (ED) more than 50 percent of the time, however, generally indicates there is a problem requiring medical attention. According to the National Institutes of Health, around 5 percent of 40-year-old men and 15–25 percent of 65-year-old men experience difficulty in achieving and/or maintaining an erection on a long-term basis.

There are various reasons why a man would experience erectile dysfunction: psychological distress, certain medications, smoking, diabetes, and recovering from prostate cancer surgery are just a few. Moreover, ED has been found to be a symptom to a serious underlying medical condition, such as cardiovascular disease (Pohjantähti-Maaroos & Palomäki, 2011). Thus, screening for cardiovascular risk factors should be considered in men with ED, because symptoms of erectile dysfunction become apparent on average three years earlier than symptoms of coronary artery disease (Heidelbaugh, 2010).

Any man, regardless of age, who experiences persistent ED needs to be seen by a doctor to rule out or confirm any underlying medical problems. According to Heidelbaugh (2010), initial diagnostic workup should include a fasting serum glucose level and lipid panel, thyroid-stimulating hormone test, and morning total testosterone level. Lifestyle changes may be necessary for the man to regain the ability to attain and maintain erections. For example, obesity, a sedentary lifestyle, and smoking greatly increase the risk of ED (Heidelbaugh, 2010).

Three conditions must occur for an erection to be achieved and maintained. First, the nerves to the penis must function properly. Second, the blood flowing into the penis must be adequate and remain within the penis when an erection is desired. Third, the man must be sexually aroused—either through indirect stimulation or direct stimulation (Pohjantähti-Maaroos & Palomäki, 2011). With indirect stimulation, a man's genitals are not being touched. Instead, his brain is being stimulated by what a man identifies as sexually arousing to him either by sight, sound, or smell. With direct stimulation, a man's genitals are being touched and he finds this physical contact sexually arousing. If any of the three conditions mentioned above are not met then a man will have difficulty attaining and/or maintaining an erection.

Nocturnal and morning erections should also be taken into account when trying to distinguish psychogenic from organic impotence (Elhanbly, Elkholy, Elbayomy, Elsaid, & Abdel-gaber, 2009). When a man wakes up with an erection he also just woke up from a dream. When we dream we are in the REM (rapid eye movement) stage of the sleep cycle. The REM stage during sleep causes an erection because, regardless of the theme of the dream (sexual or otherwise), an erection is a physiological response to the brain activity occurring during this stage of sleep (Fisher, Gorss, & Zuch., 1965). Men with physiologically based ED generally do not wake up from sleep with an erection (Karacan, Goodenough, Shapiro, & Starker, 1966), but would not necessarily have difficulty in obtaining an erection from erotic stimulation (Libman et al., 1989).

Regarding risks for the first condition (i.e., nerves to the penis function properly), certain surgical procedures to remove the prostate gland have a high risk of damaging the nerves in the perineum that assist in erections. For men with prostate cancer (discussed in chapter 5), the "gold standard" in reducing the risk of the cancer from spreading to vital organs is to remove the prostate gland (which is known as radical prostatectomy). The prostate gland is usually removed by a surgical incision in the perineum (Bella & Shamloul, 2011). Unfortunately, erectile dysfunction remains the most commonly reported problem following such a procedure (Penson et al., 2005).

Regarding the second condition (i.e., the blood flowing into the penis must be adequate and remain in the penis when an erection is desired), certain diseases, such as diabetes and cardiovascular disease, prevent the smooth muscles in the penis from relaxing. The relaxation of the smooth muscles is necessary for an erection because it allows blood to enter the erectile tissue, which then squeezes the veins nearby preventing blood from flowing away from the penis and causing an erection. However, if blood is allowed to leave the penis during an erection, the penis becomes flaccid, a condition known as a *venous leak*. For the third condition (i.e., the man must be sexually aroused either through indirect stimulation or direct stimulation), if a man is not receiving adequate stimulation to sexually arouse him, then an erection will be difficult to attain and/or maintain.

There are currently five available ED treatment options (Albaugh, 2010), not including sex therapy, even though that should always be considered a viable option. The first option includes medication taken in pill form (i.e., oral phosphodiesterase type 5 [PDE-5] inhibitors). These prescription-only drugs are more commonly known by their brand names: Viagra (sildenafil) by Pfizer, Levitra (vardenafil) by Bayer Pharmaceutical and Glaxo-Smith-Kline-Beecham/Schering Plough, and Cialis (tadalafil) by Lilly-ICOS. These drugs are taken when an erection is desired, but the medication alone does not cause the erection. The drugs help the corpora cavernosa to engorge with blood when adequate sexual stimulation is provided (Heidelbaugh, 2010).

The second option is non-invasive and involves venous and vacuum constriction devices to retain blood in the penis during intercourse. An erection is produced through a suction chamber promoting penile blood engorgement and maintaining the erection with a constriction band at the base of the penis (Heidelbaugh, 2010).

The third option is alprostadil, which is sold under the brand name Muse® (Medicated Urethral Suppository for Erection). With this prescription-only method, a man has to insert the medication (in suppository form) in the urethra at least 10 minutes before an erection is desired. Alprostadil is a prostaglandin, a chemical produced naturally by the body to help regulate the contraction and relaxation of smooth muscle tissue (Althof et al., 2006). This chemical has been manufactured for erectile dysfunction to help relax the muscle tissue in the penis to allow blood to flow to erectile tissue to attain an erection. Adequate sexual stimulation will also help maintain an erection with this approach.

The fourth option to treat ED involves penile injections (Heidelbaugh, 2010). Men using this method need to integrate the injections into their sexual relationship. Erections after an injection can last about 30–60 minutes. The goal of penile injections is to produce an erection sufficient for penetration with the least amount of untoward side effects (Albaugh & Ferrans, 2010). Side effects include pain at the injection site and *priapism* (an erection lasting three hours or more).

The fifth and final option is a penile prosthesis device or penile implant (Heidelbaugh, 2010). Penile implants have been an option available to men with ED since 1973 (Quallich, Ohl, & Dunn, 2008). This is seen as the last option if all other available approaches were unsuccessful in treating erectile dysfunction. A penile prosthesis consists of a pair of inflatable cylinders that are surgically implanted in the shaft of the penis. These cylinders are connected to a separate reservoir of fluid that has been surgically inserted under the groin muscles. A pump is also connected that allows the cylinders in the penis to fill with fluid to mimic an erection. This pump is placed in the scrotum. To obtain an erection, the man presses on the pump. The pump fills the cylinders with fluid from the reservoir causing an erection. To get rid of the erection, the man presses on a deflation valve located at the base of the pump. This returns the fluid to the reservoir and returns the penis to a normal flaccid state. This treatment is associated with permanent damage to the normal erectile cylinders. Thus,

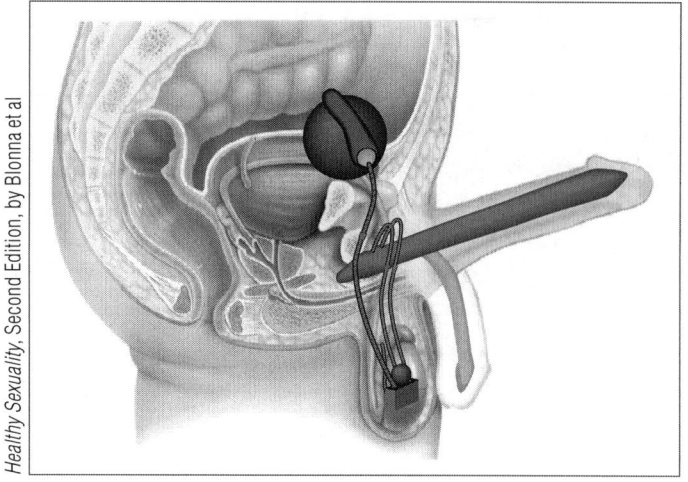

spontaneous erections are no longer possible (Heidelbaugh, 2010). Even though this method is the most invasive, it also has the highest satisfaction rate of all available treatments (Liechty & Quallich, 2008).

A new option available to men with ED or spinal cord injuries is a vibrator. In 2011, the Food and Drug Administration (FDA) approved this device specifically for men who have difficulty experiencing an erection. The vibrator is called Viberect, and it is made by the company Reflexonic. Because this vibrator is new to the market and the field of study of ED, its use and effectiveness is limited. For more information, talk to your doctor or visit the manufacturer's website at www.reflexonic.com/viberect.html.

FEMALE SEXUAL DIFFICULTIES AND SOLUTIONS

Debate continues on revising past definitions and classifications of female sexual dysfunction to decrease unnecessary distress in women and their partners when a true sexual problem does not exist (Basson, Lieblum, Brotto, & Derogatis, 2004). For example, Tiefer (2010) believes that female sexual problems should be defined as "discontent or dissatisfaction with any emotional, physical, or relational aspect of sexual experience" (p. 200). The following definitions are from the American Psychiatric Association's Diagnostic and Statistical Manual on Mental Disorders (APA, 2000). The DSM-IV-TR categorizes sexual disorders expressed in women as hypoactive sexual desire disorder, sexual arousal disorder, and orgasmic disorder (APA, 2000). Even though these sexual problems are described as complaints reported by women, men can also experience these disorders (McCarthy & McDonald, 2009).

Hypoactive Sexual Desire Disorder

Hypoactive sexual desire disorder (HSDD) can be defined as the loss or absence of any thoughts of sexual activity—an experience that causes distress in the woman (Siddall, 2010). Moreover, women are more likely to report loss of desire for sexual activity than any other sexual disorder (Clayton et al., 2009). This sexual problem is believed to affect more postmenopausal women than premenopausal women (Dennerstein & Hayes, 2005). Because HSDD has a broad definition and reasons for its existence can be complex, it remains one of the most difficult sexual problems to manage (Wylie et al., 2007). Even so, current treatment approaches that have been successful range from off-label androgen therapy to various forms of sex therapy (Davis et al., 2006; McCabe, 2001).

Sexual Arousal Disorder

Sexual arousal disorder is divided into four categories: subjective sexual arousal disorder, genital sexual arousal disorder, combined genital and subjective arousal disorder, and persistent sexual arousal disorder (Basson et al., 2003; Basson et al., 2004).

1. *Subjective sexual arousal disorder* is defined as the occurrence of vaginal lubrication despite absent or diminished feelings of sexual desire arousal, or pleasure from any type of sexual stimulation.
2. *Genital sexual arousal disorder* is defined as the absence or impaired vaginal lubrication and a considerable decrease in the intensity of genital response and orgasm.
3. *Combined subjective and genital arousal disorder* is defined as the absence or diminished sexual feelings or satisfaction from sexual stimulation and the absence or delay in vulvar swelling and vaginal lubrication.
4. *Persistent sexual arousal disorder* is defined as unexpected and unwanted genital arousal, such as tingling and pulsations in the absence of sexual desire or interest (Feldhaus-Dahir, 2009).

Orgasmic Disorder

Orgasmic disorder can be defined as absence, delay, or reduced intensity of orgasm that causes distress and interpersonal difficulty, despite the ability to experience a normal excitement phase (Graham, 2010). A woman would not fall into this category, though, if she was able to reach orgasm through cunniligus, but not coitus. As previously mentioned, there is considerable variability across women and their orgasmic ability (Meston et al., 2004). Moreover, the importance of reaching orgasm varies by woman and situation (Bancroft, 2009). Thus, each woman needs to define what is fulfilling to her.

It is well documented that some women suffer significant distress because of sexual difficulties (Johannes et al., 2009). Unfortunately, embarrassment and taboos over sexual matters mean that even when women are considerably distressed by their sexual problems, they rarely seek specific help for them (Siddall, 2010). In one study, just over a third of women with distressing sexual difficulties sought medical or psychological help, most often from their general practitioner or gynecologist (Shifren, Monz, Russo, Seggreti, & Johannes, 2008)

A woman's sexuality is complex and embedded in biological, psychological, and societal factors (Giraldi, 2011). Moreover, women are far more responsive to social, cultural, and relationship factors in determining the experience of sexual desire (Leiblum, 2002). Because of this, greater emphasis should be placed on the context of the relationship within which sexual difficulties usually occur, as well as education and support of normal variations in sexual experience (Brotto, Bitzer, Laan, Leiblum, & Luria, 2010).

Current medical therapies available for female sexual dysfunctions are limited to testosterone modalities for postmenopausal women (Siddall, 2010). These include pellets that are inserted under the skin, low-dose androgen gel, and a patch that can be worn on the skin. Medication, at times, can be enough to help women resume the frequency and enjoyment of sexual activity that they want.

However, therapy (either individual or as a couple) should always be considered a viable option.

Masters and Johnson (1970) developed a therapeutic program for couples known as sensate focus. Initially, this approach does not allow sexual contact between the couple while they work on regaining mutual trust and reducing anxiety about their sexual performance (Siddall, 2010). This program is not limited to women who have been diagnosed with a sexual problem. This method can also be used successfully with men who are experiencing sexual difficulties. Nonsexual physical intimacy, such as massaging, stroking, and touching nongenital areas, is gradually introduced through periodic tasks. More sensual contact is then allowed and finally sexual activity can be initiated (Siddall, 2010).

Reflections

Our ability to respond to sexual stimuli is multifaceted and complex. We need to take into account the biological processes that do (or do not) occur for sexual arousal, sexual desire, and orgasm to transpire. The messages we receive from our family and our social environment on sexual functioning also influence our response to sexual stimuli. Understanding and coming to terms with changing sexual functionality due to life changes can help decrease undue stress and anxiety, and also preempt relational conflicts. Satisfying sex (whatever sex means to you) is a normal and natural part of life, but only you can define what that means for you!

Critical Thinking Questions

1. Do you think our understanding of the female and male sexual response cycles has improved our ability to decrease distress and relational conflict and enhanced sexual satisfaction?

2. How does the media's portrayal of sexual functioning interfere with people's perceptions of what is normal or abnormal? How may this perception differ for males and females?

3. How do you think (female and male) gender role expectations negatively influence a woman's ability to reach orgasm?

4. How do you think life changes (i.e., puberty, pregnancy, postpartum, andropause, illness, etc.) affect sexual functioning? What are the positive and negative consequences that can be encountered in each life change?

How Much Do You Remember from the Chapter?

1. List the four phases of Masters and Johnson's sexual response cycle—order doesn't matter.

    a. _____

    b. _____

    c. _____

    d. _____

2. According to Masters and Johnson, what do men go through that women do not as part of the sexual response cycle?

    a. refractory period   b. vasocongestion

    c. myotonia   d. multiple orgasms

3. According to Masters and Johnson, what do women have the capability of experiencing that (most) men do not?

    a. refractory period   b. vasocongestion

    c. myotonia   d. multiple orgasms

(4–9) • Match the sexual behavior with its definition:

   4. Analingus   _____   a. oral stimulation of a penis
   5. Anal sex   _____   b. penile insertion in an anus
   6. Coitus   _____   c. oral stimulation of a vulva
   7. Cunniligus   _____   d. self-stimulation of the genitals
   8. Fellatio   _____   e. oral stimulation of the anus
   9. Masturbation   _____   f. penile insertion in a vagina

10. With what treatment option for ED did men typically report the highest satisfaction?

    a. penile implant   b. penile injections

    c. vacuum constriction devices d. Viagra

Challenge Yourself!

1. How can SSRIs interfere with sexual functioning?

   _____
   _____
   _____
   _____

Chapter Six **111**

2. What is the most common sexual complaint reported by men?

3. What is the most common sexual complaint reported by women?

4. Explain how hypoactive sexual desire disorder, sexual arousal disorder, and inhibited orgasm disorder differ from each other.

Websites

www.newviewcampaign.org/
A New View of Women's Sexual Problems

www.mayoclinic.com/health/premature-ejaculation/DS00578
Mayo Clinic

www.sexsmartfilms.com/
Sex Smart Films

www.sexualhealth.com/
Sexual Health Network

www.kidney.niddk.nih.gov/kudiseases/pubs/ED/
U.S. Dept. of Health and Human Services
National Kidney & Urologic Diseases Information Clearinghouse

References

Albaugh, J. (2010). Addressing and managing erectile dysfunction after prostatectomy for prostate cancer. *Urologic Nursing, 30*(3), 167–178.

Albaugh, J., & Ferrans, C. (2010). Impact of penile injections on men with erectile dysfunction after prostatectomy. *Urologic Nursing, 30*(1), 64–77.

Althof, S., Dean, J., Derogatis, L., & Rosen, R. (2005). Current perspectives on the clinical assessment and diagnosis of female sexual dysfunction and clinical studies of potential therapies: A statement of concern. *Journal of Sexual Medicine, 2*, 146–153.

Althof, S., O'Leary, M., Cappelleri, J., Crowley, A., Tseng, L., & Collins, S. (2006). Impact of erectile dysfunction on confidence, self esteem and relationship satisfaction after 9 months of sildenafil citrate treatment. *Journal of Urology, 176*(5), 2132–2137.

American Psychiatric Association (APA). (2000). *Diagnostic and statistical manual of mental disorders* (Revised 4th ed.). Washington, D.C.: Author.

American Urological Association (AUA) Consensus Panel. (2004). *Guidelines on the management of premature ejaculation*. Linthicum, MD: AUA.

Bancroft, J. (2009). *Human sexuality and its problems* (3rd ed.). Edinburgh, UK: Churchill Livingston/Elsevier.

Bancroft, J. (2010). Sexual desire and the brain revisited. *Sexual & Relationship Therapy, 25*(2), 166–171.

Basson, R. (2001). Human sexual response cycle. *Journal of Sex & Marital Therapy, 27*(1), 33–43.

Basson, R., Brotto, L., Derogatis, L., Fourcroy, J., Fugl-Meyer, K., Graziottin, A. et al. (2003). Definitions of women's sexual dysfunction reconsidered: Advocating expansion and revision. *Journal of Psychosomatic Obstetrics & Gynecology, 24*(4), 221–229.

Basson, R., Leiblum, S., Brotto, L., & Derogatis, L. (2004). Revised definitions of women's sexual dysfunction. *Journal of Sexual Medicine, 1*, 40–48.

Bella, A., & Shamloul, R. (2011). Functional anatomy of the male sex organs. In P. Mulhall, L. Incrocci, I. Goldstein,& R. Rosen (Eds.), *Cancer & sexual health* (pp. 3-12). New York, NY: Springer-Science.

Bohlen, D., Hugonnet, C., Mills, R., Weise, E., & Schmid, H. (2000). Five meters of H2O: The pressure at the urinary bladder neck during human ejaculation. *Prostate, 44*(4), 339–341.

Brotto, L., Bitzer, J., Laan, E., Leiblum, S., & Luria, M. (2010). Women's sexual desire and arousal disorders. *Journal of Sexual Medicine, 7*, 586–614.

Clayton, A., Goldfischer, E., Goldstein, I., DeRogatis, L., Lewis-D'Agostino, D. J., & Pike, R. (2009). Validation of the decreased sexual desire screener. *Journal of Sexual Medicine, 6*, 730–738.

Clayton, A., Keller, A., & McGarvey, E. (2006). Burden of phase-specific sexual dysfunction with SSRIs. *Journal of Affective Disorders, 91*, 27–32.

Clement, P., & Giuliano, F. (2011). Physiology of ejaculation. In P. Mulhall, L. Incrocci, I. Goldstein, & R. Rosen (Eds.), *Cancer & sexual health* (pp. 77–92). New York, NY: Springer-Science.

Davis, C., Black, J., Liu, H., & Bonillas, C. (1996). Characteristics of vibrator use among women. *The Journal of Sex Research, 33*, 313–320.

Davis, S., van der Mooren, M., van Lunsen, R., Lopes, P., Ribot, C., Rees, M. et al. (2006). Efficacy and safety of a testosterone patch for the treatment of hypoactive sexual desire disorder in surgically menopausal women: A randomized, placebo-controlled trial. *Menopause, 13*, 387–396.

Dennerstein, L., & Hayes, R. (2005). Confronting the challenges: Epidemiological study of female sexual dysfunction and the menopause. *Journal of Sexual Medicine, 2*(Supplemental 3), 118–132.

Dennerstein, L., Koochaki, P., Barton, I., & Graziottin, A. (2006). Hypoactive sexual desire disorder in menopausal women: A survey of Western European women. *Journal of Sex Medicine, 3*, 212–222.

Dunn, M., & Trost, J. (1989). Male multiple orgasms: A descriptive study. *Archives of Sexual Behavior, 18*, 377–388.

Elhanbly, S., Elkholy, A., Elbayomy, Y., Elsaid, M., & Abdel-gaber, S. (2009). Nocturnal penile erections: The diagnostic value of tumescence and rigidity activity units. *International Journal of Impotence Research, 21,* 376–381.

Feldhaus-Dahir, M. (2009). The physiology and causes of female sexual arousal disorder: Part I. *Urologic Nursing, 29*(6), 440–443.

Fisher, C., Gorss, J., & Zuch, J. (1965). Cycle of penile erection synchronous with dreaming (REM) sleep: Preliminary report. *Archives of General Psychiatry, 12,* 29–45.

Fugl-Meyer, K., Oberg, K., Lundberg, P., & Lewin, B. (2006). On orgasm, sexual techniques, and erotic perceptions in 18- to 74-year-old Swedish women. *Journal of Sexual Medicine, 3,* 56–68.

Giraldi, A. (2011). Classifying female sexual dysfunction. In P. Mulhall, L. Incrocci, I. Goldstein, & R. Rosen (Eds.), *Cancer & sexual health* (pp. 93–104). New York, NY: Springer-Science.

Gitlin, M. (2003). Sexual dysfunction with psychotropic drugs. *Expert Opinion on Pharmacotherapy, 4,* 2259–2269.

Goldstein, I., & Silberstein, J. (2011). Physiology of female genital sexual arousal. In P. Mulhall, L. Incrocci, I. Goldstein, & R. Rosen (Eds.), *Cancer & sexual health* (pp. 51–68). New York, NY: Springer-Science.

Graham, C. (2010). The DSM diagnostic criteria for female orgasmic disorder. *Archives of Sexual Behavior, 39,* 256–270.

Heidelbaugh, J. (2010). Management of erectile dysfunction. *American Family Physician, 81*(3), 305–312.

Hiller, J. (2004). Speculations on the links between feelings, emotions and sexual behavior: Are vasopressin and oxytocin involved? *Sexual & Relationship Therapy, 19*(4), 393–412.

Johannes, C., Clayton, A., Odom, D., Rosen, R., Russo, P., Shifren, J. et al. (2009). Distressing sexual problems in US women revisited. *Journal of Clinical Psychiatry, 70,* 1698–1706.

Jones, R., & Lopez, K. (2006). *Human reproductive biology* (3rd Ed.). Burlington, MA: Elsevier.

Kaplan, H. (1979). *Disorders of sexual desire.* New York, NY: Brunner Mazel.

Karacan, I., Goodenough, D., Shapiro, A., & Starker, S. (1966). Erection cycle during sleep in relation to dream anxiety. *Archives of General Psychiatry, 15,* 183–189.

Kinsey, A., Pomeroy, W., Martin, C., & Gebhard, P. (1953). *Sexual behavior in the human female.* Philadelphia, PA: Saunders.

Komisaruk, B., Beyer-Flores, C., & Whipple, B. (2006). *The science of orgasm.* Baltimore: The Johns Hopkins University Press.

Komisaruk, B., & Whipple, B. (1991). Physiological and perceptual correlates of orgasm produced by genital or non-genital stimulation. In P. Kothari (Ed.), *The Proceedings of the First International Conference on Orgasm* (pp. 69–73). Bombay, India: VRP Publishers.

Laan, E. (2009, June 21–25). The use of drugs and technical aids to help experiencing orgasm in women. *Paper presented at the 19th WAS World Congress for Sexual Health,* Goteborg, Sweden.

Leiblum, S. (2002). Reconsidering gender differences in sexual desire: An update. *Sexual & Relationship Therapy, 17*, 58–67.

Levin, R. (2011). Physiology of orgasm. In P. Mulhall, L. Incrocci, I. Goldstein, & R. Rosen (Eds.), *Cancer & sexual health* (pp. 35–50). New York, NY: Springer-Science.

Libman, E., Fichten, C., Creti, L., Weinstein, N., Amsel, R., & Brender, W. (1989). Sleeping and waking-state measurement of erectile function in an aging male population. *Psychological Assessment: A Journal of Consulting & Clinical Psychology, 1*(4), 284–291.

Liechty, A., & Quallich, S. (2008). Teaching a patient to successfully operate a penile prosthesis. *Urologic Nursing, 28*(2), 106–108.

Loulan, J. (1984). *Lesbian sex.* San Francisco, CA: Spinsters/Aunt Lute.

Masters, W., & Johnson, V. (1966). *Human sexual response.* Boston, MA: Little Brown.

Masters, W., & Johnson, V. (1970). *Human sexual inadequacy.* Boston, MA: Little Brown.

McCabe, M. (2001). Evaluation of a cognitive behavior therapy program for people with sexual dysfunction. *Journal of Sex & Marital Therapy, 27*, 259–271.

McCarthy, B., & McDonald, D. (2009). Assessment, treatment, and relapse prevention: Male hypoactive sexual desire disorder. *Journal of Sex & Marital Therapy, 35*, 58–67.

Merriam-Webster. (2008). *Merriam-Webster's collegiate dictionary* (11th ed.). Springfield, MA: Author.

Meston, C. (2002). The psychophysiological assessment of female sexual function. *Journal of Sex Education & Therapy, 25*(1), 6–16.

Meston, C., Levin, R., Sipski, M., Hull, E., & Heiman, J. (2004). Women's orgasm. *Annual Review of Sex Research, 15*, 173–257.

National Institutes of Health (NIH) Consensus Development Panel on Impotence. (1993). NIH consensus conference: NIH consensus development panel on impotence. *Journal of the American Medical Association, 270*(1), 83–90.

Nurnberg, G., Hensley, P., Heiman, J., Croft, H., Debattista, C., & Paine, S. (2008). Sildenafil treatment of women with antidepressant-associated sexual dysfunction: A randomized controlled trial. *JAMA, 300*(4), 395-404.

Paget, L. (2001). *The big O: Orgasms: How to have them, give them, and keep them coming.* New York, NY: Broadway Books.

Penson, D., McLerran, D., Feng, Z., Li, L., Albertsen, P., Gilliland, F. et al. (2005). 5-year urinary and sexual outcomes after radical prostatectomy: Results from the prostate cancer outcomes study. *The Journal of Urology, 173*(5), 1701–1705.

Pfaus, J. (2011). Physiology of libido. In P. Mulhall, L. Incrocci, I. Goldstein, & R. Rosen (Eds.), *Cancer & sexual health* (pp. 25–34). New York, NY: Springer-Science.

Pohjantähti-Maaroos, H., & Palomäki, A. (2011). Comparison of metabolic syndrome subjects with and without erectile dysfunction—Levels of circulating oxidised LDL and arterial elasticity. *International Journal of Clinical Practice, 65*(3), 274–280.

Quallich, S., Ohl, D., & Dunn, R. (2008). Evaluation of three penile prosthesis pump designs in a blinded survey of practitioners. *Urologic Nursing, 28*(2), 101–105.

Rellini, A., Farmer, M., & Golden, G. (2011). Hypoactive sexual desire disorder. In P. Mulhall, L. Incrocci, I. Goldstein, & R. Rosen (Eds.), *Cancer & sexual health* (pp. 105–124). New York, NY: Springer-Science.

Schuster, T. (2006). Premature ejaculation. *Urologic Nursing, 26*(4), 245–249.

Semans, J. (1956). Premature ejaculation: New approach. *South Medical Journal, 49*, 353–358.

Shifren, J., Monz, B., Russo, P., Segreti, A., & Johannes, C. (2008). Sexual problems and distress in United States women: Prevalence and correlates. *Obstetrics & Gynecology, 112*, 970–978.

Siddall, R. (2010). Diagnostic controversy: Female sexual dysfunction. *Practice Nursing, 21*(9), 450–453.

Stephenson, K., Ahrold, T., & Meston, C. (2011). The association between sexual motives and sexual satisfaction: Gender differences and categorical comparisons. *Archives of Sexual Behavior, 40*, 607–618.

Tiefer, L. (2010). Beyond the medical model of women's sexual problems: A campaign to resist the promotion of 'female sexual dysfunction.' *Sexual & Relationship Therapy, 25*(2), 197–205.

Waldinger, M., Hengeveld, M., Zwinderman, A., & Olivier, B. (1998). Effect of SSRI antidepressants on ejaculation: A double-blind, randomized, placebo-controlled study with fluoxetine, fluvoxamine, paroxetine, and sertraline. *Journal of Clinical Psychopharmacology, 18*, 274–281.

Winton, M. (2000). The medicalization of male sexual dysfunction: An analysis of sex therapy journals. *Journal of Sex Education & Therapy, 25*, 231–239.

Winton, M. (2001). Paradigm change and female sexual dysfunctions: An analysis of sexology journals. *The Canadian Journal of Human Sexuality, 10*(1–2), 19–24.

Wylie, K., Daines, B., Jannini, F., Hallam-Jones, R., Boul, L., & Wilson, L. (2007). Loss of sexual desire in the postmenopausal woman: A review of integrative therapy options. *Journal of Sex Medicine, 4*, 395–405.

chapter seven

REPRODUCTIVE TRACT INFECTIONS

CHAPTER OBJECTIVES

On completion of this chapter, students will be able to:

- recognize how RTIs can negatively impact one's reproductive health;
- distinguish between bacterial and viral sexually transmitted infections;
- list three ways to decrease the risk of exposure to sexually transmitted infections.

ABBREVIATIONS AND ACRONYMS USED IN THIS CHAPTER

AIDS	acquired immunodeficiency syndrome
BV	bacterial vaginosis
CDC	Centers for Disease Control and Prevention
ELISA	enzyme-linked immunosorbent assay
FDA	Food and Drug Administration
HIV	human immunodeficiency virus
HPV	human papillomavirus
HSV-1	herpes simplex virus-1
HSV-2	herpes simplex virus-2
IUD	intra-uterine device
PID	pelvic inflammatory disease
RTI	reproductive tract infection(s)
STD	sexually transmitted disease(s)
STI	sexually transmitted infection(s)
VD	venereal disease(s)
WHO	World Health Organization

FROM VDs TO RTIs ~ A HISTORICAL PERSPECTIVE

The adjective word *venereal* (from the Latin word *venereus*, meaning desire or love) is defined as "transmitted by sexual intercourse" in the *American Heritage Dictionary*. For hundreds of years, syphilis (which was known as the "pox") and gonorrhea (which was known as the "clap") were two of the most common venereal diseases (VDs) known to exist (McGough, 2008; Rosebury, 1971). It wasn't until the 1940s that syphilis and gonorrhea were reined in by the discovery of penicillin. During the 1960s, when 20 other diseases were recognized as being transmitted by sexual contact, public health officials in the United States introduced a new term, *sexually transmitted diseases* (STDs), to replace venereal disease in an effort to improve the clarity of their warnings to the public.

The *American Heritage Stedman's Medical Dictionary* defines the word *disease* as "a pathological condition of a body part, an organ, or a system resulting from various causes, such as infection, genetic defect, or environmental stress, and characterized by an identifiable group of signs or symptoms." Because numerous STDs were found to be asymptomatic to at least 50 percent of those infected, a new term was created in the 1990s to help clarify a long-standing misconception that everyone who has an STD is aware of their status because she/he would have the symptoms for it. With over 30 infections identified as primarily being acquired through (unprotected) sexual activity, this new term *sexually transmitted infections* (STIs) was also introduced to try to reduce the stigma attached with being diagnosed with an STD (Moore & Moore, 2005).

A new term surfaced in the mid 1990s to highlight the pathogens' role in sexual and reproductive health, as well as to move away from blaming sexual behavior and individuals. *Reproductive tract infections* (RTIs) is a relatively new term re-introduced by the editors of the 18th edition of *Contraceptive Technology* (Cates, 2004). The term RTIs is used alongside STIs in international organizations such as the World Health Organization (WHO), Engender Health, and the Population Council, to name a few. According to WHO (2005), RTIs refer to three types of infections that affect the reproductive tract: *endogenous* (en-da-ja-nas), *iatrogenic* (i-a-trə-je-nik), and *sexually transmitted infections*. The table below highlights the differences among these infections.

REPRODUCTIVE TRACT INFECTIONS

Not all sexually transmitted infections are reproductive tract infections and not all reproductive tract infections are sexually transmitted. Even so, the three types of RTIs mentioned above overlap and should be considered together. For example, some STIs, like gonorrhea or chlamydia, can be spread to the upper reproductive tract if left untreated and may lead to pelvic inflammatory disease (PID) in women, an iatrogenic infection. In addition, some endogenous infections, such as bacterial vaginosis, can also lead to PID if not properly treated. According to Hillier and colleagues (2008), BV, gonorrhea, or chlamydia can ascend

Table 7.1

RTI	Consequences
Endogenous infections	Probably the most common RTIs worldwide, they occur from an overgrowth of organisms normally present in the vagina. These infections are not usually sexually transmitted and include bacterial vaginosis and candidiasis. They are easily treated and cured.
Iatrogenic infections	These infections occur when a bacterium or other microorganism is introduced into the upper reproductive tract by a medical procedure such as endometrial biopsy, induced abortion, IUD insertion, or birth. This can happen because the infection already present in the lower reproductive tract is pushed or allowed entry through the cervix into the upper reproductive tract.
Sexually transmitted infections	Sexually transmitted infections (STIs) are caused by viruses, bacteria, or parasitic microorganisms transmitted through (unprotected) sexual activity with an infected partner. Some STIs can be easily treated, such as gonorrhea and chlamydia. Other STIs, such as the human immunodeficiency virus (HIV) and herpes simplex virus-2 (known as genital herpes), are not curable.

into the female reproductive tract during a procedure (examples are provided in Table 7.1) and, if left untreated, may cause PID.

According to Cates (2004), regardless of mode of transmission, RTIs have four serious health consequences: (1) a blockage of one or both of the fallopian tubes leading to infertility and ectopic pregnancy; (2) pregnancy loss and neonatal morbidity caused by transmission of the infection to the fetus during pregnancy and birth; (3) genital cancers, such as cervical and penile cancer; and (4) easier transmission of HIV. Any STI that produces genital lesions (such genital herpes and syphilis) or induce an inflammatory reaction places the individual at risk of acquiring HIV. Moreover, numerous infections, such as BV, chlamydia, genital herpes, and syphilis have been found to alter vaginal and cervical defenses that can lead women to increased susceptibility to HIV (Hillier, Marrazzo & Holmes, 2008).

Given the transmission dynamics of coitus, women are more likely than men to acquire an RTI from any single sexual encounter (Cates, 2004). According to Buve and colleagues (2008), when compared to men, women are also more likely to suffer from severe long-term consequences due to RTIs, such as PID, infertility, ectopic pregnancy, and cervical cancer.

RTIS DURING PREGNANCY

According to Goldenberg and colleagues (1997), some RTIs, such as genital herpes and BV, are frequently diagnosed in pregnant women in the United States. Table 7.2 shows the estimated number of women in the United States who are diagnosed during their pregnancy with specific RTIs each year (CDC, 2011).

Table 7.2

RTI	Estimated Number of Pregnant Women per Year
Bacterial vaginosis	1,080,000
Genital herpes	880,000
Chlamydia	100,000
Trichomoniasis	124,000
Gonorrhea	13,200
HIV	6,400
Syphilis	<1,000

© Centers for Disease Control and Prevention

For some women, a positive diagnosis of an RTI during pregnancy may not necessarily mean that they were infected during the pregnancy (Hitti & Watts, 2008). Many women do not routinely seek RTI screening during their lifetime. Yet many women agree to be screened during their pregnancy either to ensure a healthy pregnancy or because it is a required clinical assessment at the prenatal clinic. Moreover, because a woman's immune system is compromised during pregnancy, it is also possible that such decreased immunity provides an opportunity for symptoms to occur (Watts, 2008). For example, as shown in Table 7.2, there are a high number of pregnant women diagnosed with genital herpes during pregnancy. Yet, it is not believed that all these women were infected with HSV-2 during pregnancy.

PELVIC INFLAMMATORY DISEASE (PID)

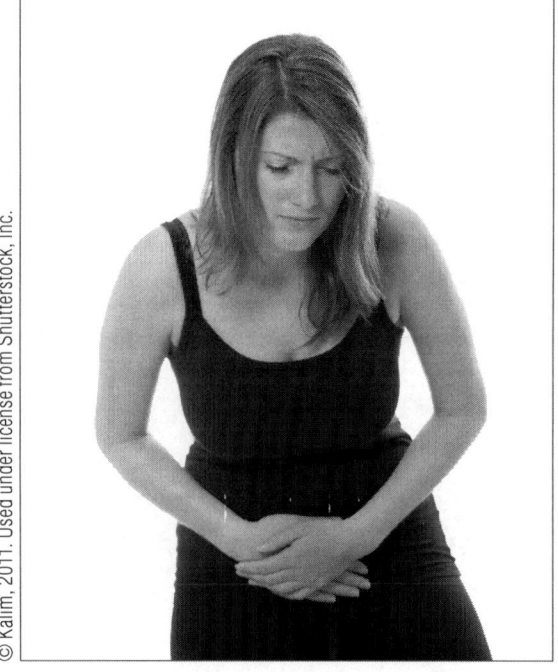

PID is an umbrella term for a variety of infections of the upper reproductive organs in females, including the ovaries, the fallopian tubes (salpingitis), the endometrial lining of the uterus (endometritis), the uterine wall, as well as the ligaments that support the uterus, and even the lining of the abdomen (Paavonen, Westrom, & Eschenbach, 2008). Because severe cellular damage of the fallopian tubes can result from PID, such a condition has also been associated with irregular bleeding, chronic pelvic pain, infertility, and ectopic pregnancy (Haggerty, Schulz, & Ness, 2003).

Infertility can be defined as having unprotected coitus for one year without becoming pregnant (this issue is discussed at length in chapter 11). An *ectopic pregnancy* occurs when the embryo grows outside of the uterus. This usually takes place in one of the fallopian tubes, but can also take place on an ovary, cervix, or somewhere else in the pelvic cavity (Jones & Lopez, 2006). An ectopic pregnancy is the leading cause of first trimester, pregnancy-related deaths in American women (Paavonen, Westrom, & Eschenbach, 2008).

Because women can be infected over and over again with chlamydia, gonorrhea, and BV, PID can occur multiple times as well. These RTIs can be cured, but that doesn't mean a person is immune from future exposure. Moreover, with every episode of PID that a woman is diagnosed with during her lifetime, she increases her risk of becoming infertile. PID is curable, but any damage done to the reproductive organs or surrounding tissues cannot be reversed (Wiesenfeld & Cates, 2008).

Every year, it is estimated that more than 1 million women experience an episode of acute PID in the United States (CDC, 2002). More than 100,000 women become infertile each year as a result of PID, and a large proportion of the ectopic pregnancies occurring every year are due to the consequences of PID. Annually, more than 150 American women die from PID or its complications (Paavonen, Westrom, & Eschenbach, 2008).

SEXUALLY TRANSMITTED INFECTIONS

The most recent national estimates, now over a decade old, estimate the total number of people living in the United States with a viral STI to be over 65 million (American Social Health Association, 1998). Every year, there are at least 19 million new cases of STIs in the United States (Weinstock, Berman, & Cates, 2004). Although young adults (15–24-year-olds) represent only one-quarter of the sexually active population, they account for nearly half of all new STIs each year (Weinstock, Berman, & Cates, 2004).

One in four women will be infected with an STI during her lifetime, with most of these infections occurring during young adulthood (Garnett, 2008). Estimates of the incidence (new cases) and prevalence (total existing cases) of most STIs are difficult to make, though, because so many people do not exhibit symptoms and thus do not seek screening or treatment.

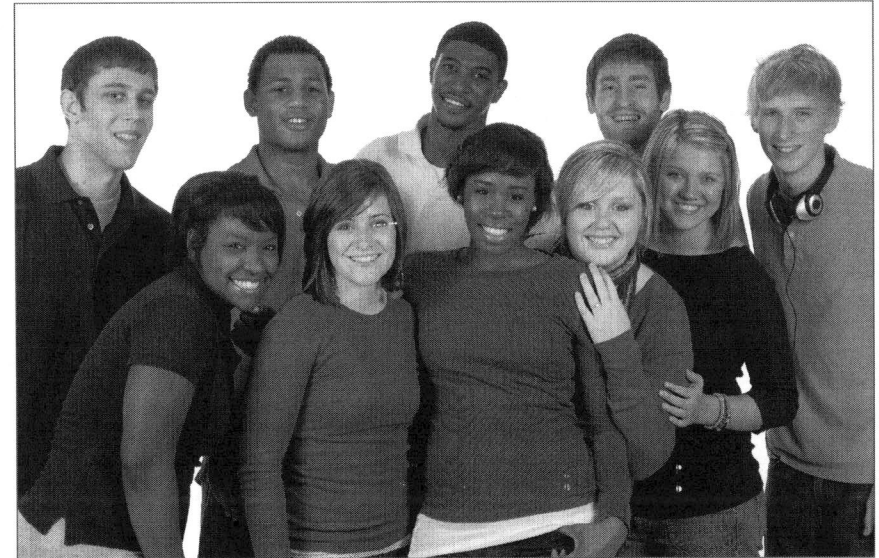

BACTERIAL INFECTIONS

Bacterial infections that are sexually transmitted are curable with antibiotics, thereby reducing any negative health consequences for an individual, as well as reducing the ability for that person to infect others. That doesn't mean, though, that the person cannot be reinfected in the future. Moreover, possible damage caused to any reproductive organs by a bacterial STI cannot be reversed even if one is cured of that infection. Prompt medical attention is needed to decrease the chances of the bacteria ascending past the vagina of females, or urethra of females and males. Unfortunately, 50–80 percent of individuals infected with an STI will not show symptoms and will probably not seek testing and treatment. Transmitting these STIs is possible with or without symptoms. It is better to get tested and find out you are not infected, than to realize you have an STI after damage has occurred to your reproductive organs, which could complicate your ability to procreate in the future. The bacterial infections discussed below are chlamydia, gonorrhea, and syphilis.

Chlamydia

Chlamydia (klu*h*-mid-ee-*uh*) is the most reported bacterial STI in the United States, with over 1 million cases documented in 2007 (CDC, 2008d). This STI is believed to be grossly underreported because 75 percent of women and 50 percent of men infected with chlamydia do not exhibit any symptoms of the infection and thus will not seek treatment (Stamm, 2008). Symptoms include abdominal pain and burning sensation when urinating in women and men, urethral discharge in men, vaginal discharge in women, and rectal pain, discharge, and bleeding in women and men participating in receptive anal intercourse (Stamm, 2008). These symptoms can present themselves anywhere from 1–3 weeks after exposure. Symptoms can disappear without treatment, which can lead to a false sense of security that your body took care of the infection or nothing was really wrong with you to begin with.

In both sexes, the urethra, mouth, throat, eyes, and anus can be infected. In women, chlamydia can infect the cervix, uterus, and fallopian tubes. Ten to 40 percent of untreated chlamydia cases will lead to PID and as many as 20 percent of women with PID will become infertile (CDC, 2009). Interestingly, chlamydial infection of the cervix can spread to the rectum. In males, chlamydia can infect the epididymis and prostate gland, which can cause discomfort, pain, and rarely, sterility.

Chlamydia can be transmitted during coitus, anal intercourse, or oral sex, as well as passed on to the fetus by an infected mother during vaginal birth. This bacterium can be inhaled by the baby during birth and cause the baby to be born with a form of pneumonia that requires antibiotics at birth to prevent further health complications (Kohlhoff & Hammerschlag, 2008). It is recommended for sexually active women 25 years and younger to be screened at least annually for chlamydia and for all pregnant women to ask to be tested for chlamydia early in their prenatal care (Stamm, 2008). Annual screening is not recommended for males even though it is in every sexually active man's best interest to be tested!

Gonorrhea

Over 350,000 cases of *gonorrhea* (gon-*uh*-ree-*uh*) were reported in the United States in 2007 (CDC, 2008d). It is believed that the actual number of cases is around 700,000. Similar to chlamydia, the majority of women (80 percent) and half of all men infected with gonorrhea do not exhibit any symptoms.

Symptoms can take as long as 30 days to appear. For men, symptoms include a burning sensation when urinating, or a white, yellow, or green discharge from the penis. Gonorrhea can cause epididymitis, a painful condition of the ducts attached to the testicles that may lead to infertility if left untreated (Geisler & Krieger, 2008). Symptoms in women include a painful or burning sensation when urinating, increased vaginal discharge, or vaginal bleeding between periods. Symptoms of rectal infection in both women and men may include discharge, anal itching, soreness, bleeding, or painful bowel movements.

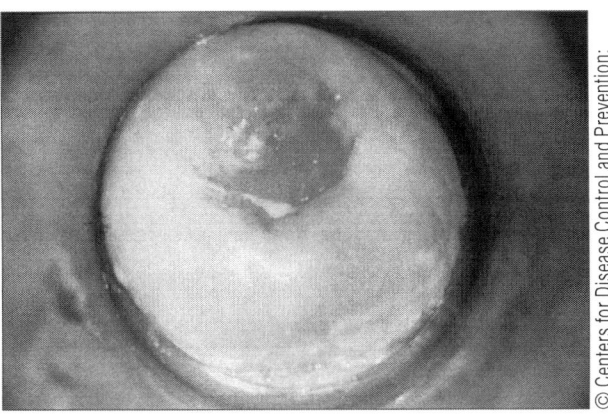
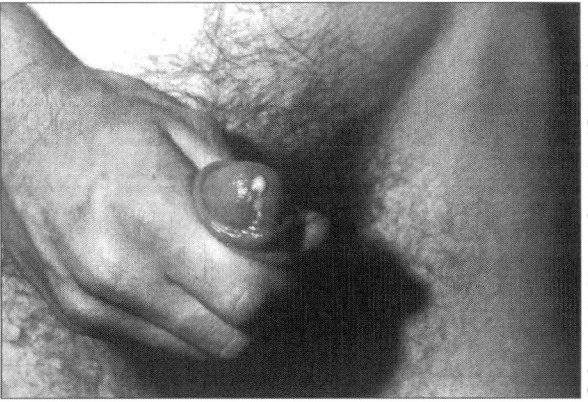

This bacterium has been found to grow and multiply easily in warm, moist areas. In the female reproductive tract, these areas include the cervix, uterus, and fallopian tubes. Gonorrhea can also grow in the mouth, throat, eyes, urethra, and anus in women and men. Interestingly, ejaculation does not have to occur to transmit or become infected with gonorrhea. This microorganism can also be spread from mother to baby during vaginal birth. This exposure can cause blindness, joint infection, or a life-threatening blood infection in the baby (Kohlhoff & Hammerschlag, 2008).

Syphilis

Over 36,000 cases of *syphilis* (sif-*uh*-lis) were reported in the United States in 2006 (CDC, 2008d). Unlike other STIs, a positive diagnosis of syphilis is required to be reported to state health departments and the Centers for Disease Control and Prevention (CDC). Incidence was highest in women 20–24 years of age and in men 35–39 years of age. The majority of cases occurred between men who have sex with men. Reported cases of congenital syphilis in newborns increased to 349 cases in 2006 from 339 cases in 2005. Because serious complications (even death) can occur to babies infected with syphilis, this is the only STI that has a federal mandate for testing during prenatal care of all women in the United

States (Shafi et al., 2008). Moreover, to help determine the cause of a stillbirth (i.e., a baby born dead), most mothers are tested for syphilis.

Transmission of the organism occurs during coitus, anal intercourse, or oral sex. Syphilis is passed from person to person through direct contact with a syphilis sore. Sores occur mainly on the vulva, penis, scrotum, vagina, anus, or in the rectum. Sores also can occur on the lips and in the mouth.

Syphilis has four stages that vary in length, symptoms, and severity of health complications. A person can only be cured during the first two stages of syphilis. A person is not curable during the third and fourth stages. In all four stages a person can infect another individual through blood or to the fetus through the placenta during pregnancy, but a person can transmit the organism sexually only during the first two stages (Sparling, Swartz, Musher, & Healy, 2008).

The primary stage is the first stage of this STI. During this stage, a sore called a *chancre* (shang-kər) appears in the area where the organism entered the body (Sparling et al., 2008). Because this sore is painless, an individual may not realize they are infected with syphilis. Moreover, if a person is unaware of the symptoms or signs associated with syphilis, she or he may not believe she or he is infected with an STI. The chancre can appear anywhere from 10–90 days after exposure. The chancre associated with primary syphilis lasts 3–6 weeks, and it can heal without treatment. However, the infection progresses to the secondary stage if treatment is not provided (Sparling et al., 2008).

During the secondary stage, a non-itchy skin rash can occur throughout the body, but it is prominent in the palms of the hands and the soles of the feet (Sparling et al., 2008). This skin rash can appear anywhere from 2–10 weeks after the disappearance of the chancre. The lesions created by the skin rash contain the syphilis bacterium and thus others can be infected by touch. The signs and symptoms of secondary syphilis resolve without treatment, and the infection progresses to the latent and possibly the tertiary (or last) stage (Sparling et al., 2008).

During the latent (or third) stage of syphilis, there are no observable signs or symptoms of infection (Sparling et al., 2008). Unfortunately, during this stage

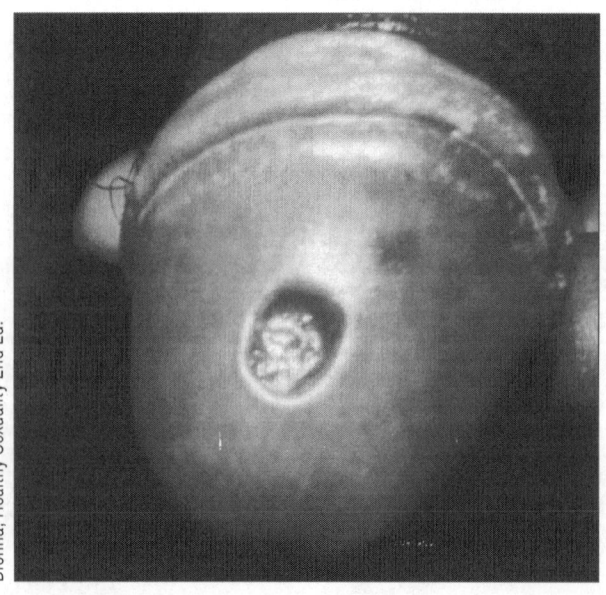

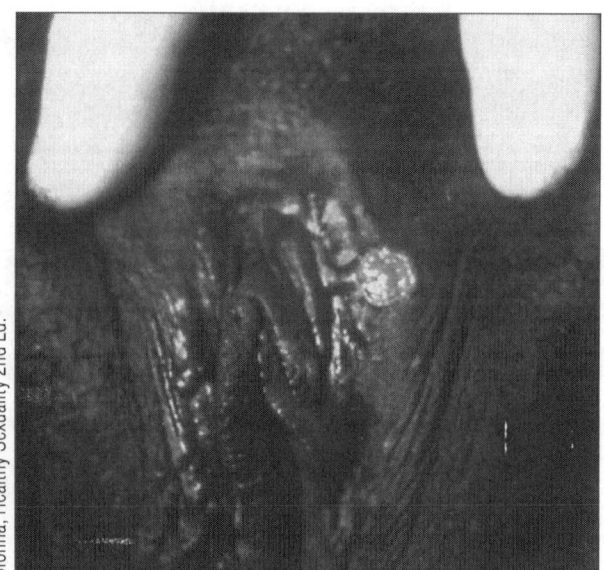

the bacterium invades the internal organs, including the brain, nerves, eyes, heart, blood vessels, liver, bones, and joints. Around 15 percent of people who have not been treated for syphilis will develop the late stages of syphilis (Sparling et al., 2008). This can occur 10–20 years after infection was first acquired.

The fourth and last stage of syphilis is called the tertiary stage. Given the irreversible damage that occurs to the internal organs during the latent stage, many in the fourth stage experience blindness, insanity, paralysis, and death (Douglas, 2009).

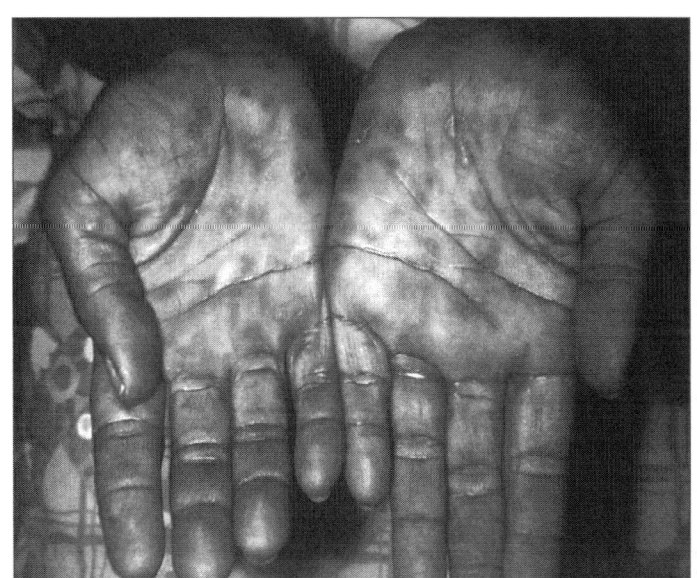

VIRAL INFECTIONS

Viral infections that are sexually transmitted are *not* curable. That means we do not have medication that can cure an individual, but we do have medication that can alleviate complications that can arise from these STIs and, for some, these medications can also reduce the risk of transmission to a sexual partner (Winer & Koutsky, 2008). Transmitting these STIs is possible, with or without symptoms. Fluid transmission, such as seminal and vaginal fluid, is not always necessary to acquire these infections (Corey & Wald, 2008; Winer & Koutsky, 2008). The viral STIs discussed below are genital herpes (Herpes Simplex Virus-2), human papillomavirus (HPV), and human immunodeficiency virus (HIV). Oral herpes (Herpes Simplex Virus-1) is also discussed, even though it is not considered an STI. As stated earlier, skin-to-skin contact can transmit certain STIs to one another. Of the STIs discussed below, only HIV cannot be transmitted through skin-to-skin contact.

Herpes Simplex Virus – 1 (Oral Herpes)

Around 80 percent of the U.S. population is believed to be infected with oral herpes. Surprised? Ever heard of "cold sores" or "fever blisters"? Well, that's oral herpes. Oral herpes belongs to the herpes family of over 100 viruses, which includes not only oral and genital herpes (discussed below), but also

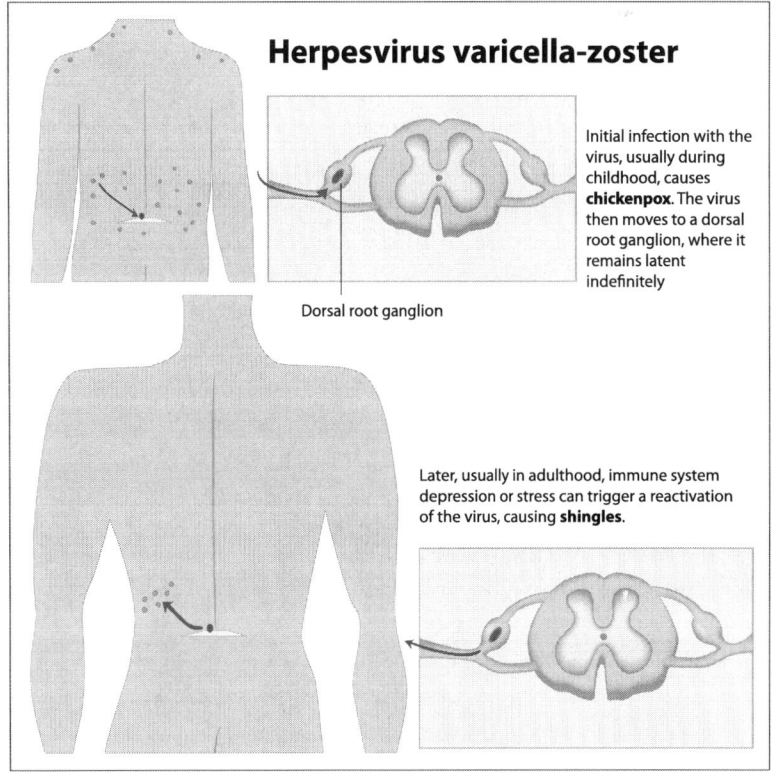

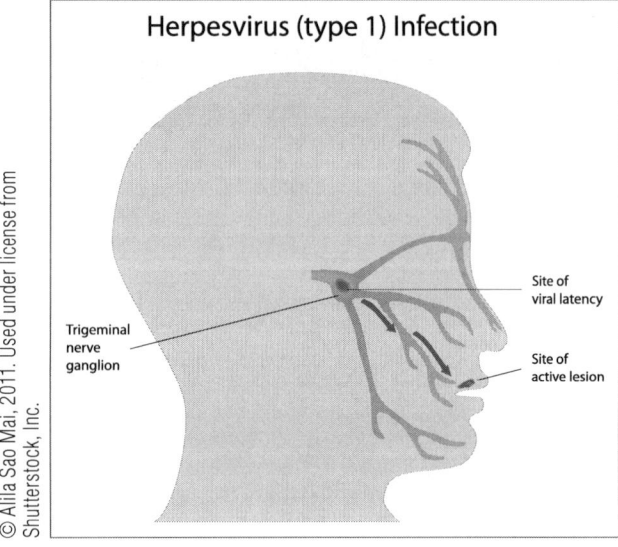

herpes varicella zoster, the virus that causes chicken pox and shingles, and Epstein-Barr, the virus that causes mononucleosis, also known as "mono" or the "kissing disease" (Pertel & Spear, 2008).

The majority of us did not acquire oral herpes by sexual transmission, and most of us weren't even sexually active when the first infamous, painful sore appeared by our lips! Many of us unknowingly became infected by a kiss from a well-meaning relative during our childhood or adolescence. This virus takes up residence in the trigeminal ganglion, a collection of nerve cells near the ear (Pertel & Spear, 2008).

Many outbreaks occur when a person has a cold or a fever, which usually means your immune system is weakened due to an illness, and this virus takes advantage to try and transmit to other "hosts." Before an outbreak, many individuals experience a tingling, burning, or itching sensation around the lips or inside the mouth (this is considered viral shedding). *Viral shedding* is a release of infectious viral particles from the affected site. Not everyone who experiences viral shedding has symptoms, yet she or he can still transmit the virus to others (Pertel & Spear, 2008), and a day or two later, a sore appears at the site. People have also been known to experience an outbreak after they've eaten spicy foods, gotten sunburn on their face, or when they are stressed. Women can also experience an outbreak during a pregnancy and along with hormonal changes during the menstrual cycle. It is unknown how those occurrences cause an outbreak.

Effective, over-the-counter medication exists for oral herpes that can shorten the duration of an outbreak and reduce viral shedding. There are some prescription drugs that can eliminate outbreaks altogether. Even though most cold sores are believed to come from Herpes Simplex Virus-1, it is possible for a person to be infected with Herpes Simplex Virus-2 (the virus that causes genital herpes) instead (Pertel & Spear, 2008). Even when an infected person is asymptomatic, she or he can pass on oral herpes through viral shedding. For those prone to regular outbreaks, oral herpes can be a downright annoying experience and cause individuals to be self-conscious. Oral herpes can be transmitted to the genitals through oral sex and this infection is much more life-altering, painful, and stressful to cope with.

Herpes Simplex Virus – 2 (Genital Herpes)

Around 16 percent of people in the United States are infected with genital herpes (CDC, 2008d). Genital herpes is more common in women (one in six) than in men (one in nine). It is believed that 25 percent of people infected with

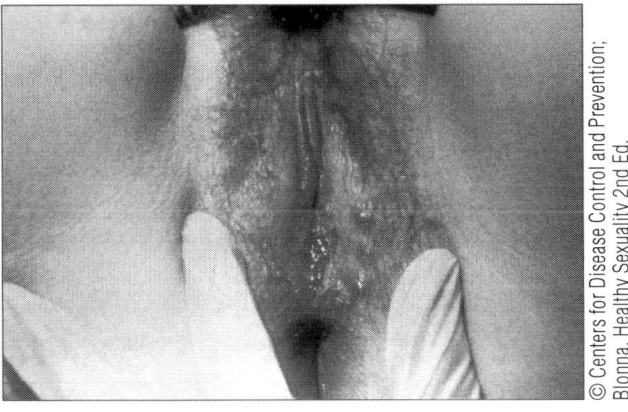
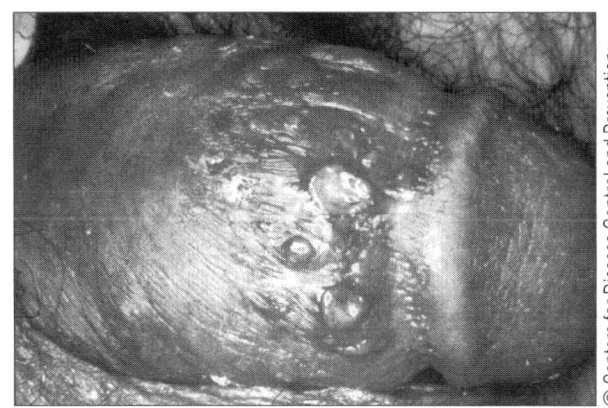

genital herpes do not know they have it because they have never had an outbreak (Corey & Wald, 2008). Within two weeks of exposure, an individual's first outbreak may occur. In genital herpes, the virus resides in the sacral ganglion at the base of the spine (Pertel & Spear, 2008). There, the virus stays dormant until a weakened immune system allows it to flare up again in the skin, usually in the genital area.

Even though there is no cure for genital herpes, three medications (available by prescription only) currently on the market, acyclovir®, famciclovir®, and valaciclovir®, are equally effective at preventing or treating outbreaks. These medications work by inhibiting an enzyme needed for the virus to replicate (Corey & Wald, 2008). Because these drugs travel through the bloodstream, they cannot eradicate the infection at its source. Thus, the only time the medications can attack the virus is when it is headed back toward the skin, which is infused by blood vessels, to cause another outbreak (Corey & Wald, 2008). Because no one really knows when another outbreak will occur, an individual has to take the medication every single day, with or without symptoms.

A pregnant woman can expose the fetus to the virus, especially if the woman is infected during the third trimester (Bradford, Whitley, & Stagno, 2008). Exposure can occur in utero or as the baby passes through the vaginal canal during birth. The health complications to the baby can be severe and can lead to death (Bradford, Whitley, & Stagno, 2008).

Human Papillomavirus (HPV)

HPV infects about 6 million people in the United States each year. The majority of these cases resolve on their own and no medical intervention is needed. Even so, the most important risk factor for cervical cancer is an HPV infection. HPV is a group of more than 100 related viruses that only infect cells on the surface of the skin, genitals, anus, mouth, and throat, but not the blood or most internal organs such as the heart or lungs (Winer & Koutsky, 2008). These viruses are called papilloma viruses because some of them cause a type of growth called a papilloma, more commonly known as warts.

Different types of HPV cause warts on different parts of the body. Some cause common warts on the hands and feet; others tend to cause warts on the lips or tongue. Still other types of HPV may cause warts on or around the female and male external genitals and in the anal area (Winer & Koutsky, 2008). These warts may barely be visible or they may be several inches across. These are known as genital warts or condyloma acuminatum. HPV 6 and HPV 11 are the two types of HPV that cause most cases of genital warts. They are called "low-risk" types of HPV because they are seldom linked to cancer.

Certain types of HPV are strongly linked to cancers and are considered "high-risk" types. As discussed in chapters 4 and 5, HPV has been linked to cancer of the cervix, vulva, and vagina, as well the penis, and anal and throat cancer in both women and men (Winer & Koutsky, 2008). High-risk types include 16, 18, 31, 33, and 45.

Although HPV can be spread during sexual activity—including coitus, anal intercourse, and oral sex—none of these behaviors have to occur for the infection to spread. All that is needed to pass HPV from one person to another is skin-to-skin contact (meaning no seminal and/or vaginal fluid transmission is needed to become infected) with an area of the body infected with HPV (Winer & Koutsky, 2008). Infection with HPV seems to be able to be spread from one part of the body to another. For example, infection may start in the vagina and then spread to the cervix. The only sure way to completely prevent anal and genital HPV infection is to never allow another person to have contact with those areas of the body. That's not very realistic for the majority of the U.S. population, though. Thus, consistent condom use is necessary to *reduce* the risk of infection.

Vaccines have been developed to prevent infection with some of the HPV types associated with cervical cancer and genital warts. Gardasil® was approved by the U.S. Food and Drug Administration (FDA) in 2006 to produce immunity to HPV types 6, 11, 16, and 18 in females between the ages of 9–26 (CDC, 2007). The first two types are known to cause around 90 percent of cases of genital warts (Winer & Koutsky, 2008). The latter two types are known to cause around 70 percent of cases of cervical cancer and cervical dysplasia (precancerous changes of cervical cells that can linger for years). HPV types 16 and 18 have also been linked to precancerous lesions and cancer of the vulva and vagina in females and the anus and throat in both females and males (Winer & Koutsky, 2008). Cervarix® was approved by the FDA in 2009 to produce immunity to HPV types 16 and 18 only. Cervarix® is approved for use in females between the ages of 10–25 years. Vaccinated women who are exposed to these viruses should not develop infections. At this time, immunity can only be guaranteed for five years with either of these vaccines.

In 2009, Gardasil® was approved by the FDA to produce immunity to HPV types 6 and 11 in males between the ages of 9–26. In late 2010, the FDA approved the use of Gardasil® to prevent anal cancer and precancerous lesions. Even though this approval is meant to decrease anal cancer in men who have sex with men, it's possible that Gardasil® can also prevent anal cancer in women who participate in this sexual behavior with men.

These vaccinations are believed to be most effective if an individual is not infected with any of the HPV types the vaccine protects a person from (even though some immunity is possible with the types that a person does not have). Both Cervarix® and Gardasil® require a series of three injections over a six-month period (first dose, then two months later, then in the sixth month after the first dose).

There are other HPV types that cause precancerous lesions, cancer, or genital warts that one is not protected against by being vaccinated (Winer & Koutsky, 2008). Thus, condoms must be used consistently with every type of sexual act to prevent fluid transmission and skin-to-skin contact to *reduce* risk. If used properly, male condoms can protect the penis and whatever the penis ends up in. This can be the vagina, the cervix, the anus, the rectum, and the mouth. If used properly, female condoms can protect the vagina, the cervix, and the penis. The vulva of a female and the scrotum of a male are not protected with female or male condoms. These areas can be infected with STIs that can be passed on through skin-to-skin contact, like HPV.

Human Immunodeficiency Virus (HIV)

In the early 1980s, a new disease infecting primarily men who had sex with men raised red flags throughout the medical community in the United States and soon after, around the world. Interestingly, the first known HIV infection was identified in a man from the Democratic Republic of Congo in 1959 (Jones & Lopez, 2006). It quickly became apparent that this disease afflicted not only men who had sex with men, but men who had sex with women, intravenous drug users, and newborns (infected by their mothers in utero, at birth, or through breastfeeding). This virus, known as HIV, is the virus known to cause Acquired Immunodeficiency Disease (AIDS). HIV can be transmitted through blood, seminal and vaginal fluids, and breast milk of an HIV+ person (American Social Health Association, 2009). Seminal fluid has the highest concentration of HIV (Jones & Lopez, 2006).

More than 1.6 million Americans have been infected with HIV since initial documentation began for this infection. More than 540,000 have already died since the first reported case in 1981. Around 56,000 new HIV infections occur each year, a number that has remained stable since 2000 (CDC, 2008a). Eighty percent of women diagnosed with HIV/AIDS in 2006 contracted the virus through heterosexual contact (CDC, 2008b). An HIV+ man is 18 times more likely to infect a woman through sexual activity than the other way around (Jones & Lopez, 2006). In 2006, as many as one in five individuals with HIV may have been unaware of their HIV+ status, down from one in four in 2003 (CDC, 2008c). HIV infection disproportionately affects the African American community, especially African American women.

Numerous drugs have been developed to delay the onset of AIDS. There are currently four classes of drugs used to prevent replication of the virus. A combination of these drugs has been found to be most effective in slowing the progression of the disease and prolonging life (Jones & Lopez, 2006). A vaccine to prevent HIV or even to cure individuals already infected has been under study for decades, yet such a development continues to elude the research community. One reason for this is that the virus is known to mutate, making development of a vaccine difficult. There are now 15 known mutations of HIV (Jones & Lopez,

2006). While AIDS doesn't kill the person, bacterial and viral infections take advantage of the person's compromised immune system and such opportunistic infections can lead to a person's death.

PREVENTION OF RTIs

What happens if you are diagnosed with chlamydia? You have been in a monogamous relationship for three months, yet both of you had sexual partners in the past. Could your recent partner have cheated on you? Did you? Or could either of you have brought this infection into the relationship? All three scenarios are possible. Screening and treatment of your partner are crucial, not only to improving your own health, but to break the cycle of reinfection that is commonly seen among patients with bacterial infections such as gonorrhea and chlamydia. Because it is often complicated to get someone's partner (or partners) to get tested and treated, many professionals in the STI field recommend that the infected partner's health care clinician provide the patient a supply of or prescription for antibiotics to the partner who was not tested.

One of three most effective ways to avoid acquiring an STI is to abstain from all sexual activity. That means no penis in a vagina, no penis in a rectum, no penis in a mouth, and no vulva on the tongue or lips! Because only skin-to-skin contact is needed to transmit some STIs, the genitals of another person should not be touching yours. What if abstinence is not an option because you want to be sexually active? Well, another way to avoid acquiring an STI is to be in a long-term, mutually monogamous relationship with a partner who does not have an STI. If that is not possible at this time, then a third way to avoid coming into contact with an STI is to use condoms. For condoms to be effective, they need to be used consistently and correctly with each and every episode of sexual activity.

PSYCHOSOCIAL RESPONSES TO STIs

People's reactions vary considerably when they find out they have an STI. Some people are nonchalant about the whole event, while others are completely horrified. How do you think you'd respond to such a diagnosis? Would it matter if you had multiple sexual partners; or were in a monogamous, long-term

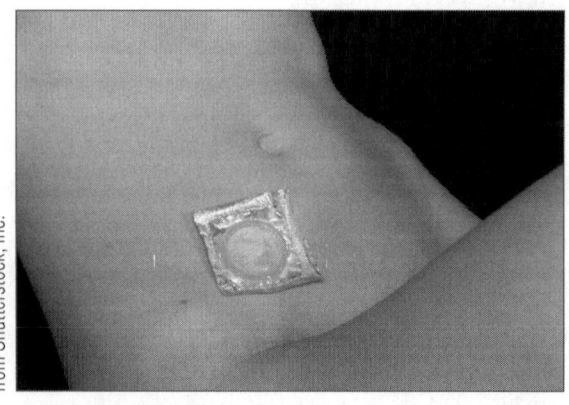
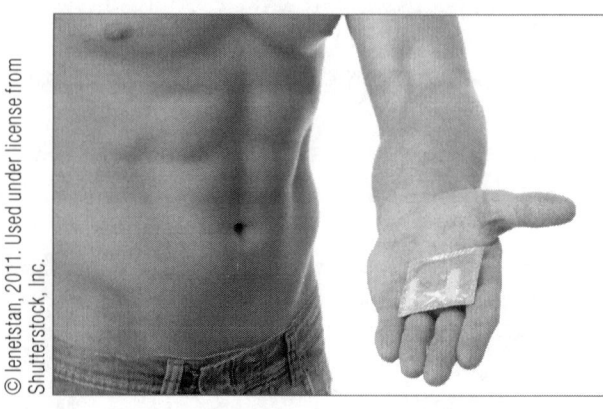

relationship; or if it happened because of a "one-night stand"? Would you respond differently if you were 15, 21, 35, or 65 years old? Ross (1986) theorized four separate meanings that individuals can place on their STI diagnosis and why it occurred. They are described in Table 7.3.

Table 7.3 Attributions Placed on an STI Diagnosis

1.	STIs are a deserved outcome of individual inadequacy that leads to sexually indiscriminate sexual sins.
2.	STIs are a consequence of individual inadequacy that leads to sexually indiscriminate behavior.
3.	STIs are a consequence of a breakdown in traditional social values and rapid social change.
4.	STIs are solely the result of an individual coming into intimate contact with a virulent pathogen.

Even though Ross' postulations are over two decades old, can you find which attribution you would mostly likely identify with if you were (or have been) diagnosed with an STI? The intention is to decrease the blame on any individual or situation and to help everyone realize that such microorganisms do not discriminate. The negative meanings we place on such a diagnosis decrease the likelihood that individuals will seek screening and treatment and will not share this information with potential sexual partners, which can lead to serious health complications and exposing others to such infections (Ross, 2008).

Reflections

The majority of STIs occur in our young adult population. One in four women will be infected with an STI during her lifetime (Garnett, 2008). Given these sobering statistics and increased openness and awareness, why haven't these infection rates decreased significantly in the past decade? The reasons why individuals have sex, with whom, and with or without protection are complex. Gender power imbalance, lack of comprehensive sexuality education, lack of access or funds to purchase protection, being under the influence of a mind-altering substance—these are just a few reasons why women and men become infected with an STI.

Critical Thinking Questions

1. What ways can you reduce your risk of being infected with an STI?
2. How would you tell a potential sexual partner you had an incurable STI, such as genital herpes?
3. Would you tell a potential sexual partner that you were once infected with a curable STI, such as chlamydia or gonorrhea? Why or why not?
4. Why do you think it is so difficult to federally mandate all children to get the HPV vaccine, even though there is strong evidence that this can greatly reduce the rate of cancers and genital warts in the cervix, vagina, vulva, penis, anus, and throat?
5. How do you think public policy has helped or hindered your generation from getting the education or access to the resources you need to protect yourselves? How has it helped?

How Much Do You Remember from the Chapter?

1. What viral STIs can be transmitted by skin-to-skin contact?
    a. chlamydia and gonorrhea
    b. genital herpes and human papillomavirus
    c. human papillomavirus and syphilis
    d. gonorrhea and HIV

2. _____ has the highest concentration of HIV.
    a. seminal fluid
    b. vaginal fluid
    c. blood
    d. breast milk

3. Men are more likely than women to acquire an RTI from any single sexual encounter.
    a. True
    b. False

4. What RTIs are women more likely to be diagnosed with during a pregnancy?
    a. HIV and chlamydia
    b. syphilis and gonorrhea
    c. human papillomavirus and HIV
    d. bacterial vaginosis and genital herpes

5. *Iatrogenic infections* can occur when:
   a. infected with herpes.
   b. an overgrowth of organisms (normally present in the vagina) occurs and *ascends* into the upper reproductive tract of a female.
   c. infected with HIV.
   d. an infection from the lower reproductive tract *ascends* into the upper reproductive tract of a female because of a medical procedure.

6. *Endogenous infections* can occur when:
   a. infected with herpes.
   b. an overgrowth of organisms (normally present in the vagina) occurs and *ascends* into the upper reproductive tract of a female.
   c. infected with HIV.
   d. an infection from the lower reproductive tract *ascends* into the upper reproductive tract of a female because of a medical procedure.

7. What RTIs can cause PID?
   a. syphilis, genital herpes, and genital warts
   b. gonorrhea, chlamydia, and bacterial vaginosis
   c. chlamydia, syphilis, and bacterial vaginosis
   d. chlamydia, genital herpes, and gonorrhea

8. The only STI testing that is currently *federally* mandated during prenatal care is for:
   a. syphilis
   b. HPV
   c. chlamydia
   d. genital herpes

9. There are now _____ known mutations that exist for HIV.
   a. 2
   b. 15
   c. 10
   d. 25

10. _____ are bacterial infections, whereas _____ are viral infections.
   a. genital herpes, HIV, and HPV / chlamydia, gonorrhea, and syphilis
   b. gonorrhea, genital herpes, and HPV / chlamydia, HIV, and syphilis
   c. chlamydia, gonorrhea, and syphilis / genital herpes, HIV, and HPV
   d. genital herpes, HPV, and syphilis / chlamydia, gonorrhea, and HIV

Challenge Yourself!

- Name the three most effective ways to avoid acquiring an STI.

- What are the four serious health consequences of RTIs?

Websites

www.ashastd.org/
American Social Health Association

www.engenderhealth.org
Engender Health

www.popcouncil.org
Population Council

www.who.int/en
World Health Organization (WHO)

References

American Social Health Association. (1998). *Sexually transmitted diseases in America: How many cases and at what cost?* Research Triangle Park, NC: Author.

American Social Health Association. (2009). *HIV and AIDS overview*. Retrieved from www.ashastd.org/learn/learn_hiv_aids_overview.cfm

Bradford, R., Whitley, R., & Stagno, S. (2008). Herpes virus infections in neonates and children: Cytomegalovirus and herpes simplex virus. In K. Holmes, P. Sparling, W. Stamm, P. Piot, J. Wasserheit, L. Corey, & M. Cohen (eds.), *Sexually transmitted diseases* (4th ed.), 1629–1658. New York, NY: McGraw-Hill.

Buve, A., Goubin, C., & Laga, M. (2008). Gender and sexually transmitted diseases. In K. Holmes, P. Sparling, W. Stamm, P. Piot, J. Wasserheit, L. Corey, & M. Cohen (Eds.), *Sexually transmitted diseases* (4th ed., pp. 151–164). New York, NY: McGraw-Hill.

Cates, W. (2004). Reproductive tract infections. In R. Hatcher, J. Trussell, F. Stewart, A. Nelson, W. Cates, F. Guest, & D. Kowal (Eds.), *Contraceptive Technology*, (18th Ed., pp. 773–845). New York, NY: Ardent Media.

Centers for Disease Control and Prevention (CDC). (2002). 2002 guidelines for treatment of sexually transmitted diseases. *Morbidity & Mortality Weekly Report, 51*, 1–80.

Centers for Disease Control and Prevention (CDC). (2007). Quadrivalent human papillomavirus vaccine: Recommendations of the Advisory Committee on Immunization Practices (ACIP). *Morbidity & Mortality Weekly Report*, Vol. 56.

Centers for Disease Control and Prevention (CDC). (2008a). *HIV/AIDS in the United States, CDC HIV/AIDS Facts*. Retrieved from www.cdc.gov/hiv/resources/factsheets/us.htm

Centers for Disease Control and Prevention (CDC). (2008b). *HIV/AIDS Surveillance Report, 2006*. Atlanta: Author.

Centers for Disease Control and Prevention (CDC). (2008c). *New estimates of U.S. HIV prevalence, CDC fact sheet, 2006*. Retrieved from www.cdc.gov/nchhstp/newsroom/docs/prevalence.pdf

Centers for Disease Control and Prevention (CDC). (2008d). *Trends in reportable sexually transmitted diseases in the United States, 2007: National surveillance data for Chlamydia, Gonorrhea, and Syphilis*. Atlanta: Author.

Centers for Disease Control and Prevention (CDC). (2009). Chlamydia screening among sexually active young female enrollees of health plans—United States, 2000–2007, *Morbidity and Mortality Weekly Report, 58*(14), 362–365.

Centers for Disease Control and Prevention (CDC). (2011). *STDs & pregnancy: CDC fact sheet*. Retrieved from www.cdc.gov/std/pregnancy/STDfact-Pregnancy.htm

Corey, L., & Wald, A. (2008). Genital herpes. In K. Holmes, P. Sparling, W. Stamm, P. Piot, J. Wasserheit, L. Corey, & M. Cohen (eds.), *Sexually transmitted diseases* (4th ed.), 399–438. New York, NY: McGraw-Hill.

Douglas, J. M., Jr. (2009). Penicillin treatment of syphilis: Clearing away the shadow on the land. *Journal of the American Medical Association, 301*(7), 769–771.

Garnett, G. (2008). The transmission dynamics of sexually transmitted infections. In K. Holmes, P. Sparling, W. Stamm, P. Piot, J. Wasserheit, L. Corey, & M. Cohen (eds.), *Sexually transmitted diseases* (4th ed.), 27–40. New York, NY: McGraw-Hill.

Geisler, W., & Krieger, J. (2008). Epididymitis. In K. Holmes, P. Sparling, W. Stamm, P. Piot, J. Wasserheit, L. Corey, & M. Cohen (Eds.), *Sexually transmitted diseases* (4th ed., pp. 1127–1146). New York, NY: McGraw-Hill.

Goldenberg, R., Andrews, W., Yuan, A., & MacKay, H. (1997). Sexually transmitted diseases and adverse outcomes of pregnancy. *Clinics in Perinatology, 24*, 23–41.

Haggerty, C. L., Schulz, R., & Ness, R. B. (2003). Lower quality of life among women with chronic pelvic pain after pelvic inflammatory disease. *Obstetrics & Gynecology, 102*, 934–939.

Hillier, S., Marrazzo, J., & Holmes, K. (2008). Bacterial vaginosis. In K. Holmes, P. Sparling, W. Stamm, P. Piot, J. Wasserheit, L. Corey, & M. Cohen (Eds.), *Sexually transmitted diseases* (4th ed., 117–127). New York, NY: McGraw-Hill.

Hitti, J., & Watts, H. (2008). Bacterial sexually transmitted infections in pregnancy. In K. Holmes, P. Sparling, W. Stamm, P. Piot, J. Wasserheit, L. Corey, & M. Cohen (Eds.), *Sexually transmitted diseases* (4th ed., pp. 1529–1562). New York, NY: McGraw-Hill.

Jones, R., & Lopez, K. (2006). *Human reproductive biology* (3rd ed.). Burlington, MA: Elsevier.

Kohlhoff, S., & Hammerschlag, M. (2008). Gonococcal and chlamydial infections in infants and children. In K. Holmes, P. Sparling, W. Stamm, P. Piot, J. Wasserheit, L. Corey, & M. Cohen (Eds.), *Sexually transmitted diseases* (4th ed., 1613–1628). New York, NY: McGraw-Hill.

McGough, L. (2008). Historical perspective on sexually transmitted diseases for prevention and control. In K. Holmes, P. Sparling, W. Stamm, P. Piot, J. Wasserheit, L. Corey, & M. Cohen (Eds.), *Sexually transmitted diseases* (4th ed., pp. 3–12). New York, NY: McGraw-Hill.

Moore, E. A., & Moore, L. M. (2005). *Encyclopedia of sexually transmitted diseases.* Jefferson, NC: McFarland & Company.

Paavonen, J., Westrom, L., & Eschenbach, D. (2008). Pelvic inflammatory disease. In K. Holmes, P. Sparling, W. Stamm, P. Piot, J. Wasserheit, L. Corey, & M. Cohen (Eds.), *Sexually transmitted diseases* (4th ed., pp. 1017–1050). New York, NY: McGraw-Hill.

Pertel, P., & Spear, P. (2008). Biology of herpesviruses. In K. Holmes, P. Sparling, W. Stamm, P. Piot, J. Wasserheit, L. Corey, & M. Cohen (Eds.), *Sexually transmitted diseases* (4th ed., pp. 381–398). New York, NY: McGraw-Hill.

Rosebury, T. (1971). *Microbes and morals: The strange story of venereal disease.* New York, NY: The Viking Press.

Ross, M. (1986). *Psychovenereology: Personality and lifestyle factors in sexually transmitted diseases in homosexual men.* New York, NY: Praeger.

Ross, M. (2008). Psychological perspectives on sexuality and sexually transmitted diseases and HIV infection. In K. Holmes, P. Sparling, W. Stamm, P. Piot, J. Wasserheit, L. Corey, & M. Cohen (Eds.), *Sexually transmitted diseases* (4th ed., pp. 137–148). New York, NY: McGraw-Hill.

Shafi, T., Radolf, J., Sanchez, P., Schulz, K., & Murphy, F. (2008). Congenital syphilis. In K. Holmes, W. Stamm, P. Piot, J. Wasserheit, L. Corey, & M. Cohen (Eds.) *Sexually transmitted diseases* (4th ed., pp. 1577-1612). New York, NY: McGraw Hill.

Sparling, P., Swartz, M., Musher, D., & Healy, B. (2008). Clinical manifestations of syphilis. In K. Holmes, P. Sparling, W. Stamm, P. Piot, J. Wasserheit, L. Corey, & M. Cohen (Eds.), *Sexually transmitted diseases* (4th ed., pp. 661–684). New York, NY: McGraw-Hill.

Stamm, W. (2008). Chlamydia trachomatis infections in the adult. In K. Holmes, P. Sparling, W. Stamm, P. Piot, J. Wasserheit, L. Corey, & M. Cohen (Eds.), *Sexually transmitted diseases* (4th ed., pp. 575–594). New York, NY: McGraw-Hill.

Watts, H. (2008). Pregnancy and viral sexually transmitted infections. In K. Holmes, P. Sparling, W. Stamm, P. Piot, J. Wasserheit, L. Corey, & M. Cohen (Eds.), *Sexually transmitted diseases* (4th ed., pp. 1563–1576). New York, NY: McGraw-Hill.

Weinstock, H., Berman, S., & Cates, W., Jr. (2004). Sexually transmitted diseases among American youth: Incidence and prevalence estimates, 2000. *Perspectives on Sexual & Reproductive Health, 36*(1), 6–10.

Wiesenfeld, H., & Cates, W. (2008). Sexually transmitted diseases and infertility. In K. Holmes, P. Sparling, W. Stamm, P. Piot, J. Wasserheit, L. Corey, & M. Cohen (Eds.), *Sexually transmitted diseases* (4th ed., pp. 1511–1528). New York, NY: McGraw-Hill.

Winer, R., & Koutsky, L. (2008). Genital human papillomavirus infection. In K. Holmes, P. Sparling, W. Stamm, P. Piot, J. Wasserheit, L. Corey, & M. Cohen (Eds.), *Sexually transmitted diseases* (4th ed., pp. 489–508). New York, NY: McGraw-Hill.

World Health Organization (WHO). (2005). *Sexually transmitted and other reproductive tract infections: A guide to essential practice.* Geneva, Switzerland: Author.

chapter eight

GENDER ISSUES

CHAPTER OBJECTIVES

On completion of this chapter, students will be able to:

- understand the differences among gender, sex, gender roles, and gender identity;
- list the cosmetic procedures performed in the United States to augment physical appearance;
- describe the steps taken for sex reassignment surgery.

ABBREVIATIONS AND ACRONYMS USED IN THIS CHAPTER

ASAPS	American Society for Aesthetic Plastic Surgery
CEO	chief executive officer
cm	centimeter
FDA	Food and Drug Administration
ISAPS	International Society of Aesthetic Plastic Surgery

DIFFERENTIATING BETWEEN SEX AND GENDER

As was discussed in chapter 1, we live in a society that uses the terms sex and gender interchangeably, even though they actually refer to two different concepts. The term *gender* encompasses the psychological and sociocultural characteristics added to our biological femaleness and maleness (Crooks & Baur, 2011). For example, in the U.S. we are more likely to expect females to be at-home moms, secretaries, or babysitters than males. We are more likely to expect males to be CEOs (chief executive officers), investment bankers, construction workers, firefighters, or soldiers than females. Fifty years ago, women and men lived in a more restricted society that frowned on "role reversal." For example, women found it difficult to be promoted to CEO of a company and men obtained little support for wanting to be an at-home dad. Progress has been made, but a gender imbalance continues to exist in certain occupations (e.g., secretarial positions, construction, and the military).

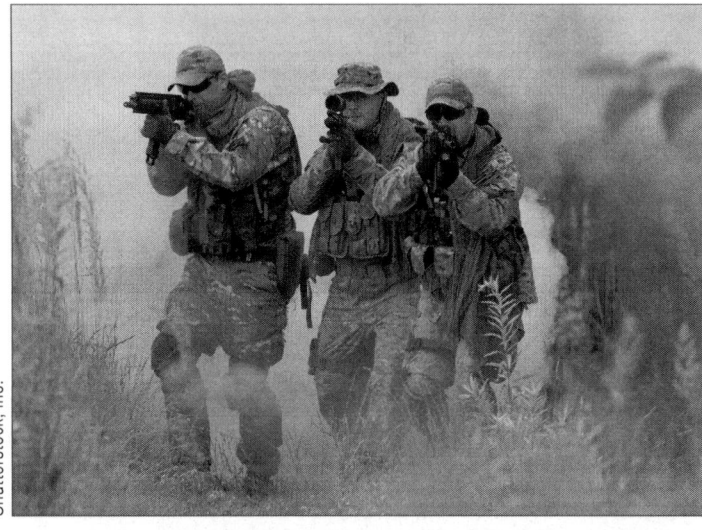

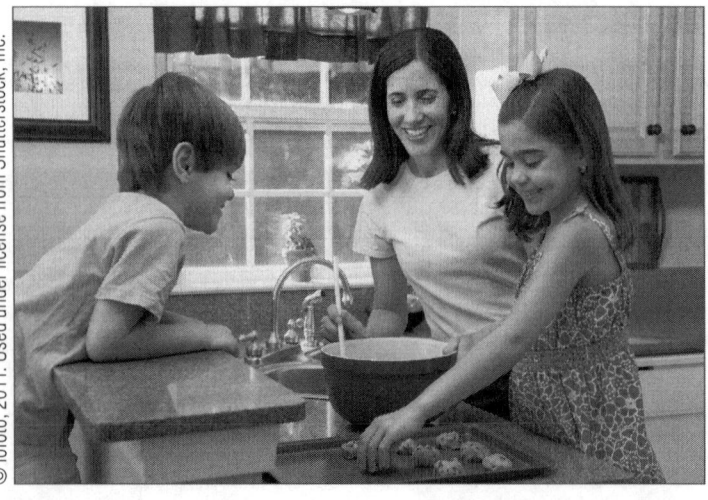

The term *sex* refers to our biological femaleness and maleness. Our biological sex is defined by three constructs: our sex chromosomes, our sex hormones, and both our external genitals and internal reproductive/sexual anatomy. The sex chromosomes for a male are XY—the X is provided by the mother and the Y is given by the father. The sex chromosomes for a female are XX—one X is provided by the mother and the other X by the father (Jones & Lopez, 2006). Thus, it is the father whose sperm decides the sex of the offspring. At birth, most of us are placed in one sex or the other ("It's a girl/boy!") by the inspection of our external genitals. For instance, it is assumed that a baby with a penis and testicles will have developed the internal reproductive organs of a male (i.e., epididymis, vas deferens, seminal vesicles, prostate gland, and Cowper's gland). At puberty, it would then be expected that this male infant's testicles (and to a lesser extent, his adrenal glands) will start producing testosterone and to a smaller degree, estrogen (Jones & Lopez, 2006). Such hormone production will then influence the development of male secondary sexual characteristics (discussed in chapter 5).

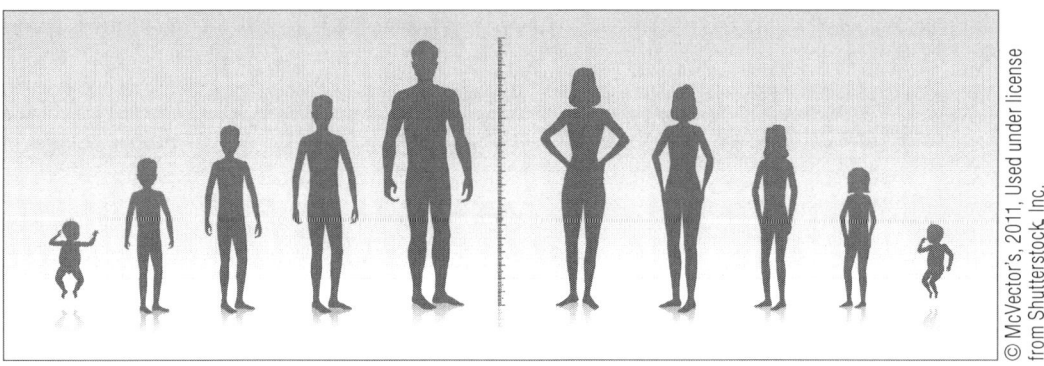

Similarly, it is assumed that a baby with a vulva will have developed the internal reproductive organs of a female (i.e., vagina, cervix, uterus, fallopian tubes, and ovaries). At puberty, it would then be expected that this female infant's ovaries (and to a lesser extent, her adrenal glands) will start producing estrogen, progesterone, and testosterone (Jones & Lopez, 2006). Such hormone production will then influence the development of female secondary sexual characteristics (discussed in chapter 4).

Intersexuality

But what if a baby is born with ambiguous external genitalia? How would that baby be identified? What if internal examinations revealed a child was born without most of the internal reproductive organs of either sex or a "mixture" of both sexes? What sex and/or gender do we place that child in? *Intersexuality* as a term was adopted by the medical community during the 20th century, and applied to humans whose biological sex cannot be classified as clearly female or male (Money & Ehrhardt, 1972). An intersex individual may have biological characteristics of both the male and the female sexes. What if a baby was born missing the sex chromosome (i.e., XO) from their father—the chromosome that dictates the body's development into a biological female or male? What if a baby was born with an extra chromosome (i.e., XXY)? What biological sex do we place this individual in? As a parent, do we explore surgical options to help our child fit more into one sex instead of "none" or do we wait until our child is old enough to make that decision? How do we then raise a child who is not considered female or male?

The prevalence of intersexuality depends on the specific condition or variation. According to the Intersex Society of North America, the prevalence of babies born either not XX or not XY is one in 1,666 births. However, including various other conditions related to sexual ambiguity (e.g., adrenal hyperplasia, vaginal agenesis, XXY), the total number of people whose internal or external reproductive/sexual anatomy differs from societal expectations is more common, with one in 100 births. For instance, in adrenal hyperplasia, individuals are born without an enzyme needed by the adrenal gland to make the hormones cortisol and aldosterone (White, 2007). Without these hormones, the body produces more androgen (i.e., testosterone) than is needed for either sex. A genetic female with this condition may be born with ambiguous external genitalia. The female's internal reproductive/sexual anatomy does not differ from a female not born with this condition, but may experience a disruption in menstruation, deeper voice, and excessive facial and hair growth (White, 2007). A genetic male born with this condition will not have obvious problems at birth, but he may enter puberty by age two or three years of age. He may start getting a deeper voice, facial and bodily hair growth, and an enlarged penis. Because his adrenal glands are producing excessive amounts of testosterone, his testes do not produce any hormones and thus, will be small (White, 2007).

Gender

Gender role refers to a collection of attitudes and behaviors that are considered normal and appropriate in a specific culture for people of a particular sex (Crooks & Baur, 2011). In many cultures, it is considered a normative behavior for women to express their emotions openly, but not for men. Moreover, various cultures not only accept, but encourage men to express themselves physically when they are angry, but do not provide such encouragement for women. More recently, various societies have been trying to reduce the restrictions placed on a particular sex to allow for the ability to experience one's full potential as a human being. For example, more men are encouraged to stay home and take care of their children. Some countries even offer generous paternity leave to motivate fathers to take a more active role in their children's lives.

However, regarding exploring one's sexuality, a double standard continues to exist between men and women. Even though women are not as restricted in their sexual attitudes and behaviors in the U.S. as they used to be, our society continues to judge women negatively if their sexual behaviors are considered "overly sexual." We continue to refer to women as "whores" and "sluts" if their number of sexual partners or appearance is deemed inappropriate for their sex. Yet, we typically do not condemn men for having numerous sexual partners, and depending on the culture, may even encourage liberal sexual expression with various sexual partners (such as in polygamous households or harems). Men are more likely to be judged positively for their sexual explorations and even possibly revered as "studs," "players," or "hustlers."

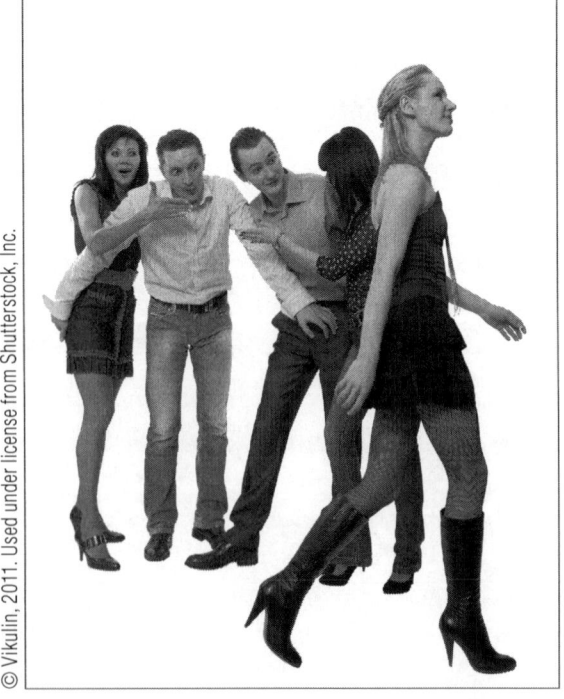

Even though it may seem that gender is irrevocably tied to our biological sex, gender is socially constructed and varies from society to society (Crooks & Baur, 2011). It may seem natural in some cultures for boys to like to play with trucks, and girls to play with dolls, but society reinforces those behaviors throughout our lives—these are not innate preferences for a particular sex. In reality, some boys like playing with dolls, and some girls like playing with trucks. Interestingly, we live in a society that allows girls greater freedom to play with toys targeted for girls or boys, but we frown on such freedom for boys. Many cultures are not comfortable with boys playing with "girl" toys. Why is that? What inferences are we making about a boy who plays with a doll, for example? Shouldn't females be insulted that toys directed at them are "not good enough" for boys?

Gender identity refers to each individual's subjective sense of being female or male or some combination of the two (Crooks & Baur, 2011). What "makes" you a woman or a man? Is it how you dress, the mannerisms you exhibit, your secondary sexual characteristics that would place you in one sex over the other (e.g., breasts for women or broader shoulders for men), or do you just *feel* like a woman or a man (whatever that means to you)? Hopefully, these questions make you realize how everyone will vary in their responses. For instance, some women never wear dresses or skirts but feel like a woman, 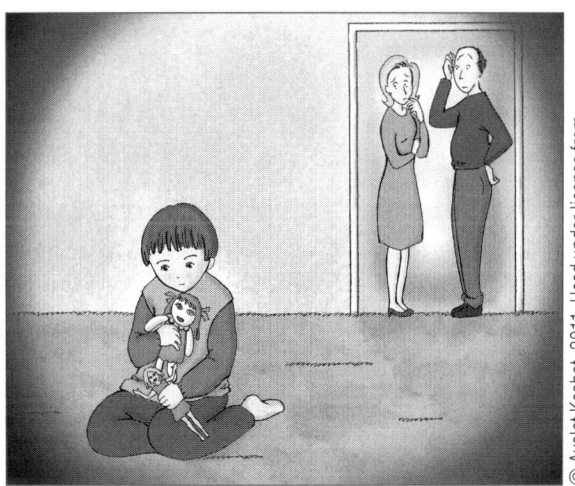 and some men are very affectionate, but feel like a man. Moreover, some men's shoulders are not very broad and some men may even accumulate more fat in the thighs than their abdomen, but they still identify as a man, and some women have very small breasts, but feel like a woman. Actually, how does someone *feel* like a particular gender? Do these feelings have more to do with the expression (or lack thereof) of emotion or the comfort in different situations? For example, some women are comfortable crying while watching a touching movie scene, whereas some men would not dare to be caught crying.

We need to also realize that even though we might identify as one gender that society has constructed for us over the other, that doesn't mean we must solely adhere to attitudes and behaviors expected for that gender. For example,

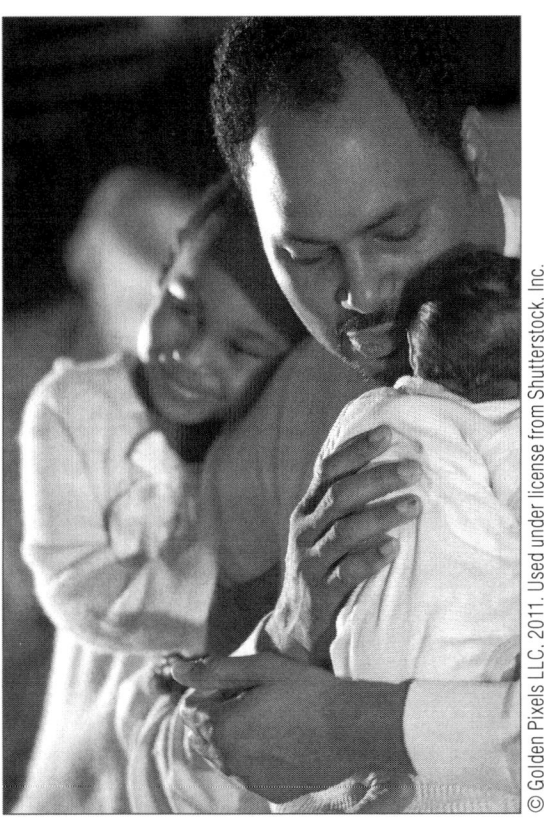

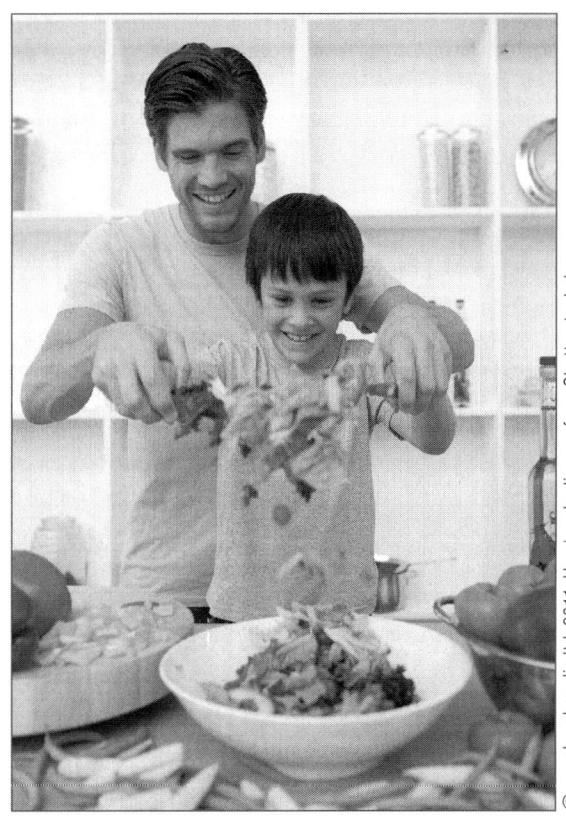

Chapter Eight **143**

throughout history, some men have undoubtedly wished that they were more involved and affectionate with their children, but were discouraged to do so, given societal expectations. Some women have also desired a life outside the home, a career, and the encouragement to explore other aspects of life, but were not allowed to, given the roles ascribed to their gender. Men can still identify as men and feel at ease in showing emotion, be nurturing to their children, and even be the main cook in their household. Women can still identify as women and feel at ease in never wearing make-up, dresses or skirts, never having children, and truly enjoying the bachelorette lifestyle.

Gender, Body Image, and Cosmetic Surgery

In many countries similar to the United States, the image of an attractive body is someone who is young, has a thin yet sculpted body, unblemished skin, and "perfect" breasts for women or "six-pack" abdominals for men (Crooks & Baur, 2011). Yet before the 20th century, Western societies preferred heavier body types, especially for women, because thinness signified poverty and poor health (Kipnis, 1996). In fact, while sporting a tan is generally considered to be fashionable, centuries ago poor servants who worked in fields would suffer the stigma of having tanned bodies, and well-to-do women would try their best to protect their fair skin from sunlight, such as with parasols. In any case, this current image of beauty is unrealistic, not only because such "perfection" is not possible for the majority of society, but because a human body varies by genes, an individual's personality, and the external environment, all of which may make it difficult to achieve such idealistic expectations. Many individuals find it difficult to reject what society deems as attractive, especially as we age and our bodies start resembling less and less the ideal body.

Cosmetic surgery has flourished as a result of the discrepancy between normal body variations and societal expectations for an attractive body. The American Society for Aesthetic Plastic Surgery (ASAPS) compiled a list of the top five cosmetic surgical procedures that occurred in the United States in 2010 (shown in Table 8.1).

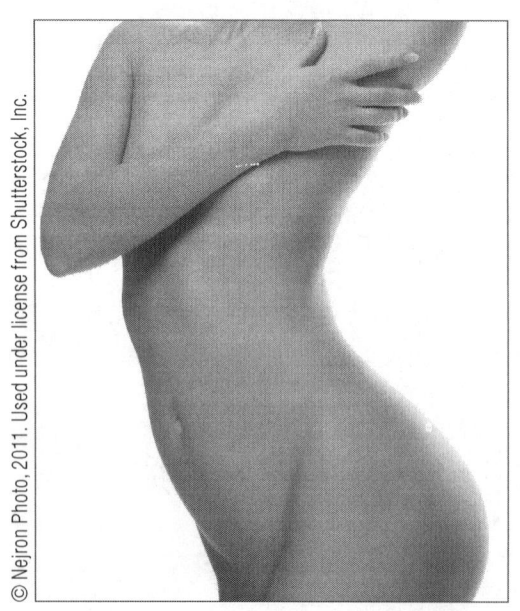
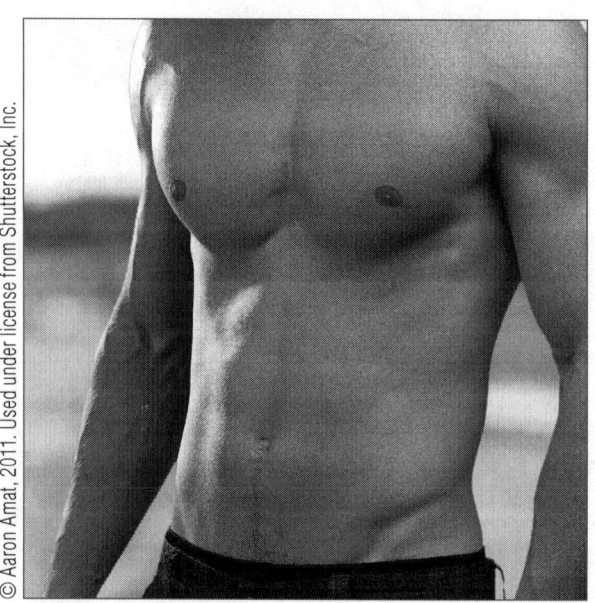

Table 8.1	TOP 5 COSMETIC SURGICAL PROCEDURES IN THE U.S. IN 2010
Procedure	**Number Performed**
Breast augmentation	318,123
Lipoplasty (liposuction)	289,016
Blepharoplasty (eyelid surgery)	152,123
Abdominoplasty (tummy tuck)	144,929
Breast reduction	138,152

Source: The American Society for Aesthetic Plastic Surgery
http://www.surgery.org/sites/default/files/2010-top5.pdf

According to the ASAPS, breast augmentation has been the most popular cosmetic surgical procedure since 2008 in the United States. Before 2008, lipoplasty was the most popular. What do you think has changed in the U.S. that can explain why there is an increase in breast augmentation and a decrease in lipoplasty in the past few years? Should we take into account the invasiveness of each procedure, the cost (most health insurance plans do not cover lipoplasty and only a small percentage cover breast augmentation), or the possibility of other means to achieve the desired results?

For example, in lipoplasty, the fat is removed for a specific area of the body. This procedure can use different means to achieve similar results. For example, plastic surgeons can use high-frequency sound waves to liquefy the fat beneath the skin's surface or they can suction out the fat with special equipment. Depending on the amount of fat removed, an individual may receive general or local anesthesia. Fat, though, can be reduced naturally if we eat healthier and exercise regularly. Even so, the timeframe to lose the desired weight through diet and exercise may vary considerably, especially

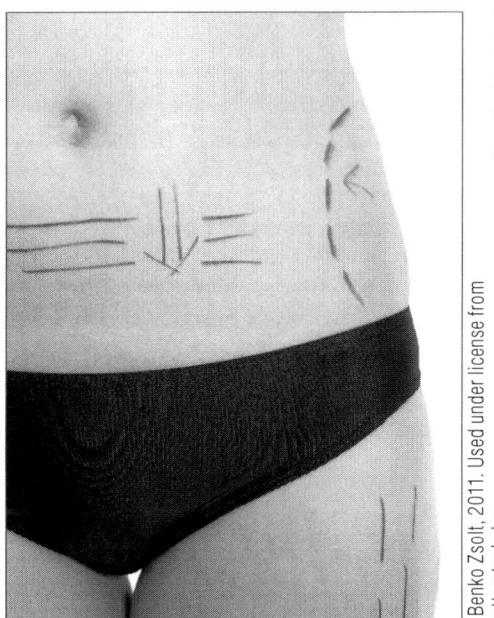

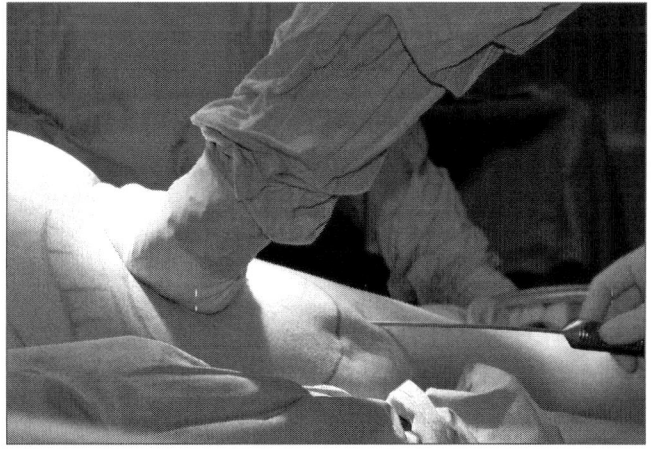

if one's metabolism is not cooperative in burning fat. Nevertheless, one reason for the decrease in lipoplasty may be that individuals are trying to find less invasive, less expensive options to have a thinner, more sculpted body.

Ironically, the breast is primarily made up of fat, and the size of a woman's breast is dictated by her weight and partly by her genes (that's why some obese women have smaller breasts and some thin women have larger breasts). There is no natural way to increase breast size without increasing fat in other parts of the body as well, even though certain bras can give the illusion of bigger breasts. Thus, women who desire bigger breasts opt for the surgical option.

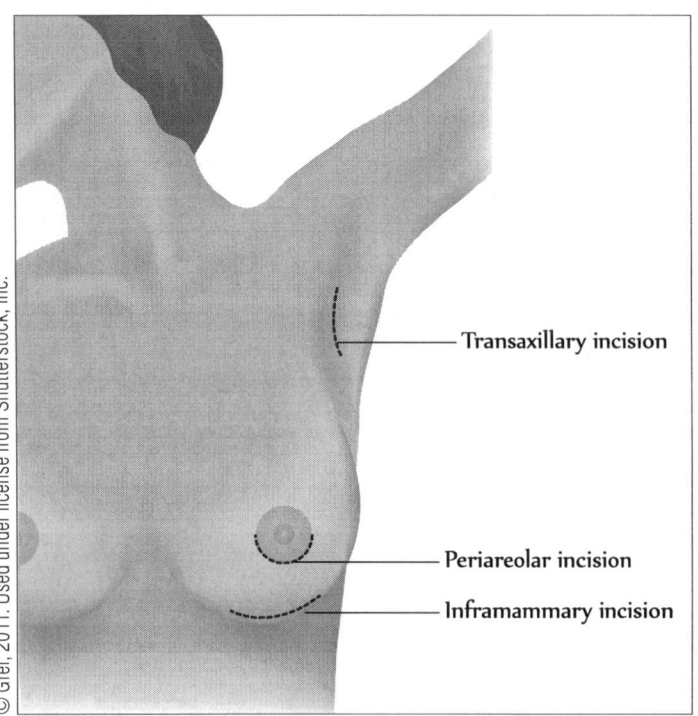

Breast implants and augmentation have been around in various forms since the late 19th century. It was not until the 1950s and 1960s that plastic surgeons started to use silicone injections in breasts, but this led to problems of breast hardening, paving the way for another device: silicone implants. Developed in 1962, silicone gel breast implants became a popular choice in breast augmentations. However the FDA removed them from the market in 1992 because of concerns that silicone leakage caused numerous autoimmune disorders in women. In fact, thousands of lawsuits against Dow Corning Corporation, a maker of silicone implants, caused it to go bankrupt in 1995. In 2006, the Food and Drug Administration (FDA) decided to make the once-popular but newly redesigned silicone gel implant available again to women. Breast implants can be inserted through the armpit (i.e., transaxillary incision), through the areola (i.e., periareolar incision), under the breast (inframammary incision), and through the navel (i.e., transumbilical breast augmentation, or TUBA).

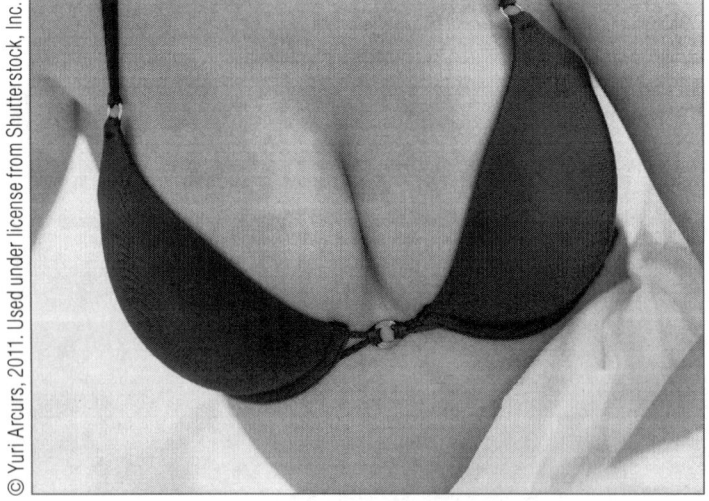

The ASAPS compiled the top five cosmetic procedures for women (Table 8.2) and the top five for men (Table 8.3) for 2010. American women and men differed in many of the cosmetic surgical procedures they requested. Did the order of popularity or any specific procedure surprise you?

Table 8.2 — TOP 5 COSMETIC SURGICAL PROCEDURES FOR AMERICAN WOMEN IN 2010

Procedure	Number Performed
Breast augmentation	318,123
Lipoplasty (liposuction)	251,834
Breast reduction	138,152
Abdominoplasty (tummy tuck)	137,925
Blepharoplasty (eyelid surgery)	131,448

Source: The American Society for Aesthetic Plastic Surgery www.surgery.org/sites/default/files/2010-top5.pdf

Women are more likely than men to undergo some types of cosmetic surgery, such as lipoplasty, abdominoplasty, and blepharoplasty. This is not surprising given societal expectations for women to strive for the ideal thin body, as well as a youthful-looking appearance. As women and men age, our skin begins to lose its elasticity and in certain areas, our skin may seem to droop. Moreover, our metabolism begins to slow down as we age and we find it harder to maintain a healthy weight, especially if we do not exercise regularly, are on medications that interfere with our metabolism or our eating habits, or we do not eat high-nutrient-dense, low-calorie meals.

Table 8.3 — TOP 5 COSMETIC SURGICAL PROCEDURES FOR AMERICAN MEN IN 2010

Procedure	Number Performed
Lipoplasty (liposuction)	37,183
Rhinoplasty (nose surgery)	30,099
Blepharoplasty (eyelid surgery)	20,675
Gynecomastia (enlarged breasts reduction)	18,256
Otoplasty (ear surgery)	10,849

Source: The American Society for Aesthetic Plastic Surgery www.surgery.org/sites/default/files/2010-gender_0.pdf

Even though the number of men who underwent some cosmetic surgical procedure is much smaller compared to women, it is interesting to note what men are choosing to modify. It is not surprising that lipoplasty was the most popular procedure, given societal expectations for men to emulate a thin, yet strong-looking body. Gynecomastia is a condition that can occur in childhood

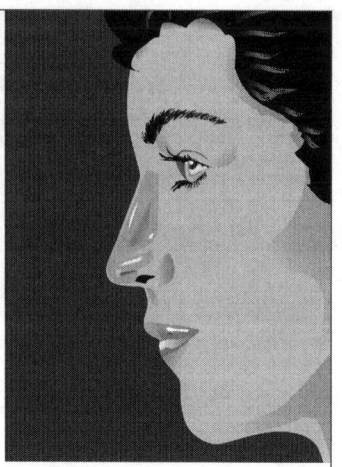 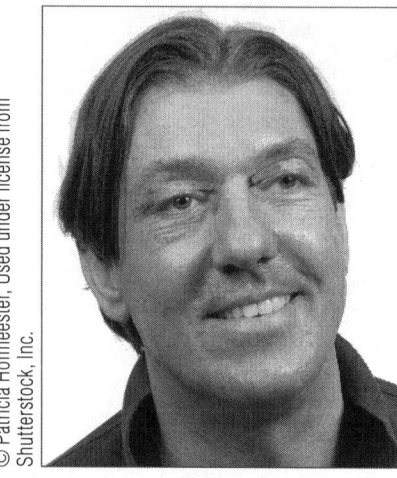

and adolescence due to hormonal imbalance. As men age, testosterone levels decrease (discussed in chapter 5) that may lead to fat accumulating in the chest and abdominal area. For some men, the breast tissue increases in fat more so than in other men. Even though many societies allow men to go shirtless in public, those men who feel the extra breast tissue on their chests is unsightly will refrain from showing their chests *even in private*, and may opt for a surgical solution to improve their body image.

The International Society of Aesthetic Plastic Surgery (ISAPS) compiled a list of the top 25 countries with the most surgical cosmetic procedures in 2009. Table 8.4 includes a list of the top 10.

Table 8.4 TOP 10 COUNTRIES FOR COSMETIC SURGICAL PROCEDURES IN 2009

- United States
- China
- Brazil
- India
- Mexico
- Japan
- South Korea
- Germany
- Turkey
- Spain

Source: The International Society of Aesthetic Plastic Surgery
http://www.isaps.org/

Do any countries on the list surprise you? Why or why not? Do you think these countries vary in what procedures are the most popular? According to ISAPS, lipoplasty was the most common surgical procedure performed around the world. There was a total of 1,607,979 liposuction surgeries performed in 2009. Breast augmentation was at #2 with 1,454,317, and blepharoplasty (eyelid surgery) came in at third with 1,153,756. China was the country with the most breast augmentations and blepharoplasty, while the United States topped the list for lipoplasty.

Gender Variance Within Papua New Guinea

Not all societies restrict their citizens' attitudes and behaviors by sex, and there are also societies in which gender restrictions are not what we would expect. Papua New Guinea is one of the most culturally diverse countries in the world, with over 850 indigenous languages and at least as many cultures, out of a population of around 7 million.

On the Vanatinai Island, near Papua New Guinea, women and men are considered equal and live in a society where their language contains no feminine or masculine pronouns (Lepowsky, 1994). Women have the same access to power and prestige as men. Moreover, both sexes appear to enjoy the same freedom to explore their sexuality (Crooks & Baur, 2011).

The people of Tchamabuli in Papua New Guinea adhere to very different gender roles than the U.S. The traditional feminine and masculine gender roles that our society dictates are reversed in this culture. It is considered the norm for men to express themselves emotionally and normal for women to show aggression (Mead, 1935). The Mundugumer of Papua New Guinea are encouraged to exhibit *only* what our society defines as masculine characteristics (i.e., aggressiveness, insensitivity) in *both* sexes (Mead, 1935). The people of this culture are hostile toward each other, regardless of their relationship (husband/wife or mother/child). This is also a culture known for headhunting (i.e., taking a person's head after killing them), cannibalism (i.e., eating human flesh), and infanticide (they strangle or throw unwanted babies into the Yuat River to drown). Unlike the Mundugumer, the Arapesh of Papua New Guinea are encouraged to exhibit *only* what our society defines as feminine characteristics (i.e., gentleness, nurturing) in *both* sexes (Mead, 1935). This culture is peaceful and loving toward each other.

Cisgender and Transgender

Even though we live in a society that makes us choose one gender and/or one sex over the other, we should strive to expand our dichotomous view of gender and biological sex. People identify with certain words. Yet, for those without words available to express one's identity—for those who find it difficult to neatly fit into our gender and sex continuum of "her/his," "female/male," "woman/man"—imagine how much more difficult it would be for their culture to show them understanding and compassion. This is why some have come to embrace such a unique, yet desperately needed, distinction for this individuality.

Since the 1960s, scholars in academia have been using a specific term that can provide recognition to an individual whose gender identity *does not* match the gender and biological sex that was assigned at birth (Burdge, 2007). That term is *transgender*. Most transgender women and men do not desire to surgically alter their external genitals. The term *trans man* refers to female-to-male transgender people and *trans woman* refers to male-to-female transgender people. They may, though, modify their physical appearance depending on their preferred gender. For example, a biological female who adheres to society's expectations of the male gender may tape her breasts so they are not apparent to others. A trans man may follow "traditional" mannerisms expected of men (i.e., how men walk, how men use their hands, and how men dress) to be identified as a man. Some trans men may also begin taking testosterone to increase muscle mass and facial and bodily hair to exhibit a more expected appearance of a man (Bolin, 1997).

The term *cisgender* is a relatively new term used to identify individuals whose gender identity *does* match the gender and biological sex they were assigned at birth (Schilt & Westbrook, 2009). We may question why we need the term cisgender since many of us use the term gender to imply the same thing. But to bring normality to gender variations that exist in society, the term cisgender is needed to refer to people who do not identify with a gender-diverse experience, without enforcing existence of a normative gender expression (Green, 2006).

An individual whose biological sex can be defined as male, but prefers to dress as a woman and wishes to be addressed with female pronouns would be considered a transgender woman in our society. For those of you unfamiliar with transgenderism, would you consider the individual described below as a "he" who's a "she," a "he" who's a "he," a "she" who's a "he," or a "she who's a "she"? Have you ever seen an individual of whose gender or biological sex you were unsure? Would you treat that person differently if you were able to place her/him in one gender over the other? Why do we need to know what a person "is"?

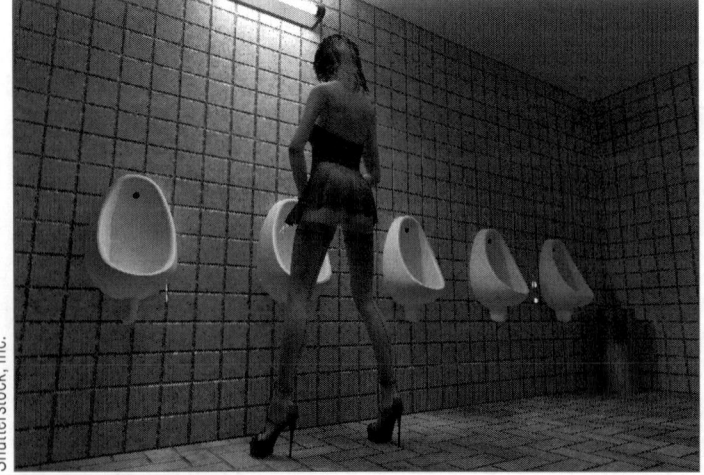

Transsexual

Transsexual is a term used to identify an individual who not only does not identify with the gender they were assigned to at birth, but also desires to modify their biological sex as much as possible to the other sex. Thus, a transsexual individual who was born a biological female would prefer not to have breasts, a vulva, and the internal female reproductive/sexual anatomy. A transsexual individual who was born a biological male would prefer not to have a penis, testicles, and the internal male reproductive/sexual anatomy (Carroll, 1999). According to Lawrence (2007), individuals who identify as male-to-female transsexual people have become common in developed countries. According to American Psychiatric Association (2000), the prevalence of roughly 1 in 30,000 biological males and 1 in 100,000 biological females seek sex reassignment surgery in the U.S.

For a transsexual individual to experience complete sex reassignment, they have to undergo extensive psychological screening, hormone therapy, and genital-altering surgery—a process that usually takes years if not decades to achieve (Crooks & Baur, 2011). Table 8.5 lists the four steps that most transsexual people follow, even though some individuals are content with completing only a few of the steps (Carroll, 1999).

Table 8.5 STEPS FOR SEX REASSIGNMENT SURGERY

Step	Procedure	Specific to Female to Male	Specific to Male to Female
1	Undergo psychological counseling	Same	Same
2	Live full-time as the other gender	Adhere to the physical appearance and mannerisms expected of the male gender; May legally change first name to match gender	Adhere to the physical appearance and mannerisms expected of the female gender; May legally change first name to match gender
3	Begin hormone therapy and/or undergo "functional procedures"	Begin taking testosterone; May undergo a radical mastectomy (remove breasts and underlying tissue)	Begin taking estrogen; May undergo breast augmentation; May undergo permanent hair removal (on the chest, arms, back, and buttocks)
4	Genital-altering surgery	May have internal reproductive/sexual anatomy surgically removed before genital-altering surgery; Undergoes a phalloplasty (a penis is created) or metoidioplasty (clitoral enlargement)	May have internal reproductive/sexual anatomy surgically removed before genital-altering surgery; Undergoes a vaginoplasty (a vulva and vagina are created)

Source: Crooks, R., & Baur, K. (2011). The World Professional Association for Transgender Health (2001).

During Step 1, transsexual individuals may be in therapy for years or even decades before they (and their therapist) feel they can proceed to other steps (The World Professional Association for Transgender Health, 2001). Some people stay in therapy throughout all the steps and even years after completing all four steps. Throughout the whole process of sex reassignment, some transsexual individuals may lose their job, their home, their family, and their friends. Supportive outlets like group or individual counseling are necessary to help them cope with the loss and rejection.

During Step 2, transsexual individuals are asked to live as the other gender full time. This means they will be seen by everyone, including their family, friends, coworkers, and acquaintances as the gender they are comfortable in. If the individuals have, after several months to a year, adjusted well to this new life, they can proceed to the next step.

During Step 3, transsexual individuals may begin hormonal therapy before undergoing specific procedures that modify their physical appearance or vice versa (The World Professional Association for Transgender Health, 2001). Hormonal therapy has to be taken for the rest of their lives. Female-to-male transsexual individuals begin taking testosterone. This ceases the production of estrogen in the ovaries and adrenal glands. The hormonal intake of testosterone (usually given as an injection every three months) increases their risk of uterine cancer. Thus, they need to have their uterus removed sooner rather than later. Testosterone also ceases a female's menstruation, but if a female-to-male transsexual person stops taking testosterone and has not undergone a *hysterectomy* (removal of the uterus), menstrual flow resumes. A *total hysterectomy* removes the uterus and the cervix. A *radical hysterectomy* removes the uterus, the cervix, fallopian tubes, and ovaries. Testosterone also lengthens the vocal chords, which in turn deepens their voice. Even if testosterone is stopped, the deeper voice remains because the vocal chords do not "shrink" back.

Male-to-female transsexual individuals begin taking estrogen. This ceases the production of testosterone in the testicles and adrenal glands. Facial and bodily hair growth is not as coarse or as full. The vocal chords do not "shrink" because of the lack of testosterone or from the influence of estrogen. Male-to-female transsexual individuals who wish for a higher-pitched voice may undergo specific surgery and speech therapy (Crooks & Baur, 2011).

During Step 4, transsexual individuals have made the decision to alter the appearance of their external genitals to be consistent with their sexual and gender identity. Months before these procedures, though, the individuals must have all their genital hair removed (electrolysis is preferred because it is permanent) to decrease the chance of the newly formed penile shaft or vagina having hair on it.

They may decide to have their internal reproductive/sexual anatomy surgically removed before or during the genital-altering surgery. For female-to-male transsexual individuals, surgical removal of their internal reproductive/sexual anatomy refers to the elimination of their vagina, cervix, uterus, fallopian tubes, and ovaries. For male-to-female transsexual individuals, surgical removal of their internal reproductive/sexual anatomy refers to the eradication of their vas deferens, seminal vesicles, ejaculatory duct, prostate gland, and Cowper's gland (The World Professional Association for Transgender Health, 2001).

For female-to-male transsexual individuals, who wish to have external genitals that appear more like a biological male, the vaginal opening is sealed and parts of the vulva are used to create the scrotum. Testicular implants are used to emulate the appearance of testicles within the newly constructed scrotum. During a metoidioplasty, the surgeon takes advantage of the fact that testosterone has enlarged the glans of the clitoris to 4–5 cm (Meyer et al., 1986). During this procedure, which takes 2–3 hours to complete and costs around $15,000, internal clitoral tissue is surgically extended externally, along with the urethra. This allows the man to urinate standing up and gives the appearance of a penis. The newly formed penis ranges in size from 4–10 cm, and because of its size it is not capable of penetration. Ejaculation is not possible because the internal male reproductive/sexual anatomy does not exist in post-operative female-to-male transsexual people (The World Professional Association for Transgender Health, 2001).

For female-to-male transsexual individuals who wish to undergo a *phalloplasty*, this surgery may take 10–15 hours to complete and may cost around $50,000. If they choose this procedure, the skin, blood vessels, and nerves are removed from an inner forearm and used to construct the shaft of the penis. The glans of the clitoris is used to create the glans of the penis. A tube is sewn onto the urethra and inserted inside the newly formed penis to allow for urination. Erection is not possible through indirect or direct stimulation, but can be achieved if an inflatable penile device is inserted (described in chapter 6). Ejaculation is not possible because the internal male reproductive/sexual anatomy does not exist in post-operative female-to-male transsexual people (The World Professional Association for Transgender Health, 2001). Because the glans of the clitoris were not removed but created into the glans of the penis and sensitive nerve endings are present on the penile shaft, sexual pleasure and orgasm are possible (Lief & Hubschman, 1993). Recovery usually takes 3–6 months.

For male-to-female transsexual individuals, a *vaginoplasty* will provide them with the external genitals that resemble a biological female vulva. The construction of a vulva and vagina costs around $30,000. The perineum and the area under it are surgically opened to create the introitus and vagina. The scrotal sac is used to construct the labia majora and labia minora. The penile shaft (and if needed skin from the abdomen) will be used to create the vagina. Vaginal dilators help the newly formed vagina retain its shape during the seven-day post-operative healing phase. Initially, the individual has to dilate the vagina 4–6 times a day for at least 45 minutes to avoid vaginal shrinkage. The time invested in dilating eventually subsides, but if vaginal penetration is expected anytime throughout their lifetime, then vaginal dilation needs to become part of their daily routine and continued for the rest of their lives. This newly formed vagina cannot lubricate when the woman is sexually aroused, thus, a water-based lubricant is needed if penetration is to occur painlessly. The glans of the penis are used to form the glans of the clitoris. The shortened urethra is sewn in place between the introitus and the location of the glans of the clitoris (The World Professional Association for Transgender Health, 2001). Complete recovery can take up to three months. Sexual pleasure and orgasm are possible after the surgery (Lawrence, 2003).

After step 4 is completed, a transsexual individual can legally change her/his birth certificate to identify her/him as their "new" sex and gender (The World Professional Association for Transgender Health, 2001). No one will ever have to know they had been born and lived as the other sex and gender. Most health insurance plans do not cover medical expenses incurred with any of the procedures for sex-reassignment surgery. Most transsexual individuals must pay for any procedure out-of-pocket. The path leading to the last step for sex reassignment surgery usually has been one filled with loss, sorrow, pain, hope, determination, and faith that it has all not been done in vain. The majority of transsexual people who undergo all four steps experience a huge wave of relief, satisfaction, and a sense of well-being (The World Professional Association for Transgender Health, 2001).

Reflections

It is difficult for many to accept that gender is a social construct and is not innate. It is also hard for some individuals to realize that they do not feel comfortable in conforming to societal expectations to their assigned gender. Pressure to conform to the roles expected for one particular sex can vary from culture to culture. Progress has been made to welcome gender variations in some cultures, but most countries continue to strongly support restricted gender roles for members of their community. You need to decide for yourself if the gender restrictions imposed on you limit your ability to live a fulfilling life. Respect and welcome gender diversity in yourself and in others and realize that humanity cannot reach its full potential without it.

Critical Thinking Questions

1. What if your child were born with ambiguous genitalia and doctors were not able to identify the child as a female or male? What would you do?

2. How do you think your parents or extended family would react to your decision to enter an occupation that is mostly associated with the other gender? Do you think most of them would be supportive?

3. A loved one confides in you that she/he wants to undergo sex reassignment surgery. She/he wants your advice on how to tell the rest of the family and asks for your support. What would you do?

How Much Do You Remember from the Chapter?

1. Define the term *sex*:
    a. refers to each individual's subjective sense of being female or male
    b. refers to our biological femaleness and maleness
    c. a collection of attitudes and behaviors considered normal and appropriate in a specific culture for people of a particular sex
    d. encompasses the psychological and sociocultural characteristics added to biological femaleness and maleness

2. Define the term *gender*:
   a. refers to each individual's subjective sense of being female or male
   b. refers to our biological femaleness and maleness
   c. a collection of attitudes and behaviors considered normal and appropriate in a specific culture for people of a particular sex
   d. encompasses the psychological and sociocultural characteristics added to biological femaleness and maleness

3. Define the term *gender identity*:
   a. refers to each individual's subjective sense of being female or male
   b. refers to our biological femaleness and maleness
   c. a collection of attitudes and behaviors considered normal and appropriate in a specific culture for people of a particular sex
   d. encompasses the psychological and sociocultural characteristics added to biological femaleness and maleness

4. Define the term *gender role*:
   a. refers to each individual's subjective sense of being female or male
   b. refers to our biological femaleness and maleness
   c. a collection of attitudes and behaviors considered normal and appropriate in a specific culture for people of a particular sex
   d. encompasses the psychological and sociocultural characteristics added to biological femaleness and maleness

Challenge Yourself!

Search online for the story of the following individuals. What happened to them? What actions could have been taken by their community, their schools, their families, and their friends to prevent the outcome?

- Victoria Carmen White, September 2010, New Jersey
- Tyler Wilson, age 11, September 2010, Ohio

Websites

www.surgery.org/media/statistics
The American Society for Aesthetic Plastic Surgery

www.isaps.org
The International Society of Aesthetic Plastic Surgery

www.isna.org/
Intersex Society of North America

www.nsrc.sfsu.edu
National Sexuality Resource Center

www.transgenderlaw.org/index.htm
Transgender Law and Policy Institute

www.wpath.org/
The World Professional Association for Transgender Health

References

American Psychiatric Association (APA). (2000). *Diagnostic and statistical manual of mental disorders* (Revised 4th ed.). Washington, DC: Author.

Bolin, A. (1997). Transforming transvestism and transsexualism: Polarity, politics, and gender. In B. Bullough, V. Bullough, & J. Elias (Eds.). *Gender blending.* New York, NY: Prometheus Books.

Burdge, B. (2007). Bending gender, ending gender: Theoretical foundations for social work practice with the transgender community. *Social Work, 52,* 243–250.

Carroll, R. (1999). Outcomes of treatment of gender dysphoria. *Journal of Sex Education & Therapy, 24,* 128–136.

Crooks, R., & Baur, K. (2011). *Our sexuality* (11th ed.). Belmont, CA: Wadsworth/Cengage.

Green, E. (2006). Debating trans inclusion in the Feminist Movement: A trans-positive analysis. *Journal of Lesbian Studies,* 10(1/2), 231–248.

Jones, R., & Lopez, K. (2006). *Human reproductive biology* (3rd ed.). Burlington, MA: Elsevier.

Kipnis, L. (1996). *Bound and gagged: Pornography and the politics of fantasy in America.* New York, NY: Grove Press.

Lawrence, A. (2003). Factors associated with satisfaction or regret following male-to-female sex reassignment surgery. *Archives of Sexual Behavior, 32,* 299–316.

Lawrence, A. (2007). Becoming what we love: Autogynephilic transsexualism conceptualized as an expression of romantic love. *Perspectives in Biology & Medicine, 50,* 506–520.

Lepowsky, M. (1994). *Fruit of the Motherland: Gender in an egalitarian society.* New York, NY: Columbia University Press.

Lief, H., & Hubschman, L. (1993). Orgasm in the postoperative transsexual. *Archives of Sexual Behavior, 22,* 145–155.

Mead, M. (1935). *Sex and temperament in three primitive societies.* New York, NY: HarperCollins Publishers.

Meyer, W., Webb, A., Stuart, C., Finkelstein, J., Lawrence, B., & Walker, P. (1986). Physical and hormonal evaluation of transsexual patients: A longitudinal study. *Archives of Sexual Behavior, 15*(2), 121–138.

Money, J., & Ehrhardt, A. (1972). *Man & woman boy & girl. Differentiation and dimorphism of gender identity from conception to maturity.* Baltimore, MD: The Johns Hopkins University Press.

Schilt, K., & Westbrook, L. (2009). Doing gender, doing heteronormativity: Gender normals, transgender people, and the social maintenance of heterosexuality. *Gender & Society,* 23(4), 440–464.

White, P (2007). Congenital adrenal hyperplasia and related disorders. In R. Kliegman, R. Behrman, H. Jenson, & B. Stanton, *Nelson textbook of pediatrics* (18th ed.). Philadelphia, PA: Saunders Elsevier.

The World Professional Association for Transgender Health. (2001). *The Harry Benjamin International Gender Dysphoria Association's standards of care for gender identity disorders* (6th Version.). Washington, DC: Author.

chapter nine

SEXUAL ORIENTATIONS

CHAPTER OBJECTIVES

On completion of this chapter, students will be able to:
- define sexual orientations, bisexuality, heterosexuality, and homosexuality;
- understand sexual fluidity;
- create a list of countries that have antidiscrimination laws based on sexual orientation;
- generate a list of countries that have criminalized homosexuality.

ABBREVIATIONS AND ACRONYMS USED IN THIS CHAPTER

AIDS	acquired immunodeficiency syndrome
CDC	Centers for Disease Control and Prevention
HIV	human immunodeficiency virus
SIECUS	Sexuality Information and Education Council of the United States
LGBT	lesbian, gay, bisexual, and transgender
MSM	men who have sex with men

SEXUAL ORIENTATIONS

Sexual orientation refers to which of the sexes we are emotionally and sexually attracted to (Crooks & Baur, 2011). For example, an individual attracted to the other sex would be referred to as a *heterosexual* person. An individual attracted to the same sex would be referred to as a *homosexual* person. Even though most societies do not have separate wording to distinguish between women and men who identify as heterosexual, many cultures have distinct wording to distinguish between women and men who identify as homosexual. For instance, in the U.S., a man attracted to another man would be referred to as a *gay* man. A woman attracted to another woman would be referred to as a *lesbian* woman. An individual attracted to both sexes would be referred to as a *bisexual* person. Findings from the National Survey of Sexual Health and Behavior indicate that in the United States about 7 percent of women and 8 percent of men identify as gay, lesbian, or bisexual. Not surprisingly, the proportion of individuals who report same-sex sexual contact at least once in their lifetimes is higher than the percentage of people who identify as lesbian, gay, or bisexual (Herbenick et al., 2010). Even though the majority of the U.S. population is assumed to identify as heterosexual, the American Psychological Association (2008), the American Psychiatric Association (2000), and the American Academy of Pediatrics (Frankowski & The Committee on Adolescence, 2004) all agree that sexual orientation is not determined by any one factor, but by a combination of genetic, hormonal, and environmental influences.

Kinsey and colleagues (1948) devised a seven-point continuum on sexual orientation from their study of men in the U.S. Table 9.1 illustrates the scale that ranges from 0 (exclusive attraction and contact with only the other sex) to 6 (exclusive attraction and contact with only the same sex):

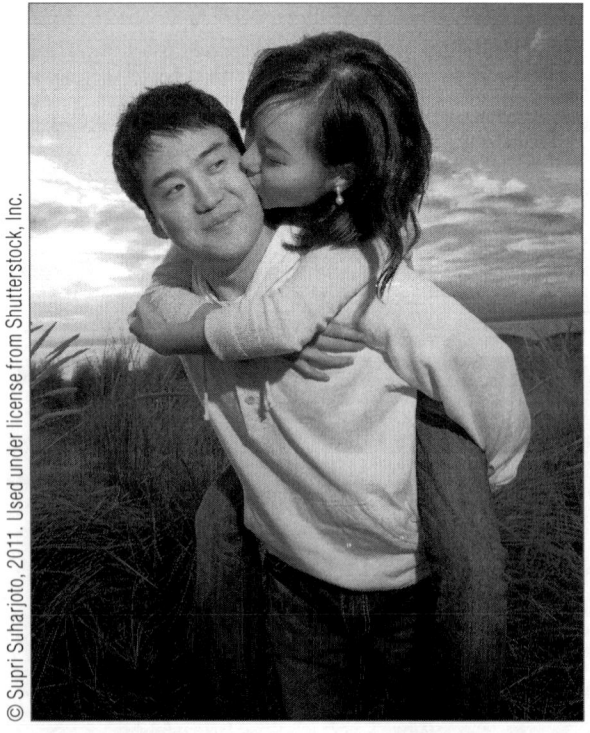
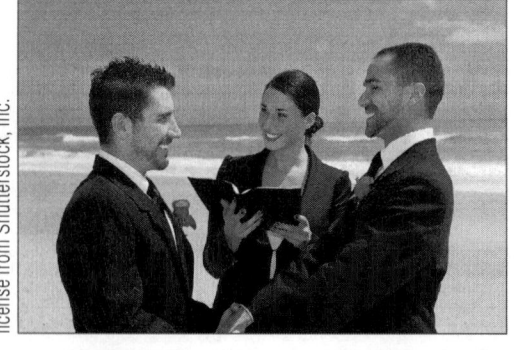
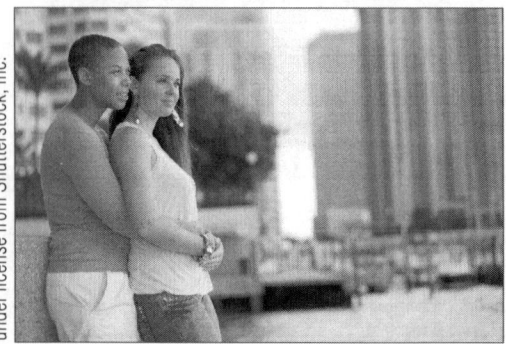

Table 9.1 KINSEY SEXUAL ORIENTATIONS CONTINUUM SCALE

0	1	2	3	4	5	6
Exclusively heterosexual with no homosexual attraction and contact	Predominantly heterosexual with only incidental homosexual attraction and contact	Predominantly heterosexual but with more than incidental homosexual attraction and contact	Equally homosexual and heterosexual attraction and contact	Predominantly homosexual but with more than incidental homosexual attraction and contact	Predominantly homosexual with only incidental heterosexual attraction and contact	Exclusively homosexual with no heterosexual attraction and contact

Source: Kinsey, A., Pomeroy, W., & Martin, C. (1948). Sexual behavior in the human male. Philadelphia, PA: Saunders; Crooks, R., & Baur, K. (2011). Our sexuality, 11th ed. Belmont, CA: Wadsworth/Cengage.

The *Kinsey Scale* was constructed using only two aspects of sexual orientation: sexual attraction and sexual behavior (Kinsey, Pomeroy, & Martin, 1948). The concept of sexual orientation, though, has been found to be more complex, with multiple variables influencing how we conceptualize our sexual identity. Klein and colleagues (1985) assert that individuals use seven aspects to shape their sexual orientation (review Table 9.2). They also rate these attributes in relation to the past (one's life since age 20), the present (one's life within the past 12 months), and the ideal (where one would like to be on the continua). If you are interested to know where you fall on the *Klein Grid*, you can take the test at www.kleingridonline.com/.

Table 9.2 KLEIN SEXUAL ORIENTATIONS GRID

	Variable
1	Sexual attraction
2	Sexual behavior
3	Sexual fantasies
4	Emotional attraction
5	Social preference
6	Heterosexual/homosexual lifestyle
7	Self-identification

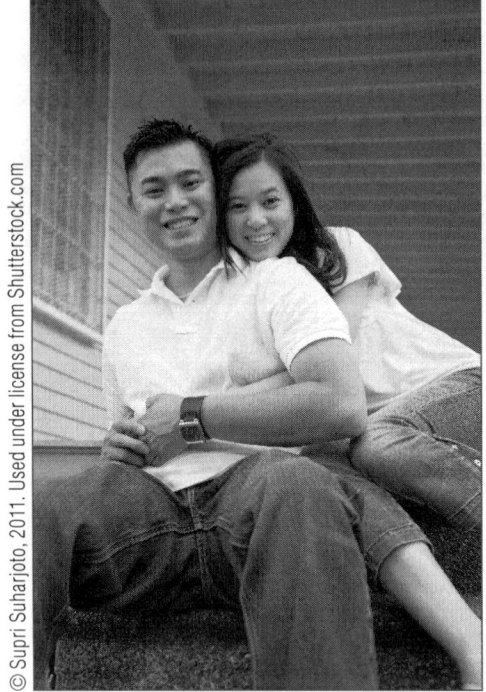
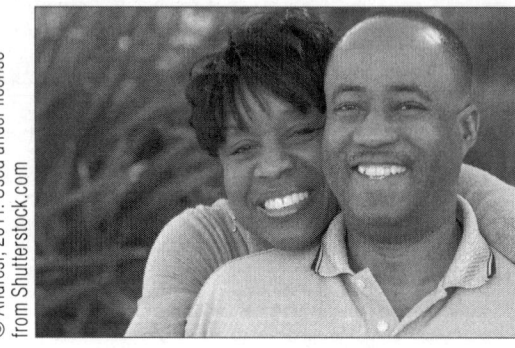
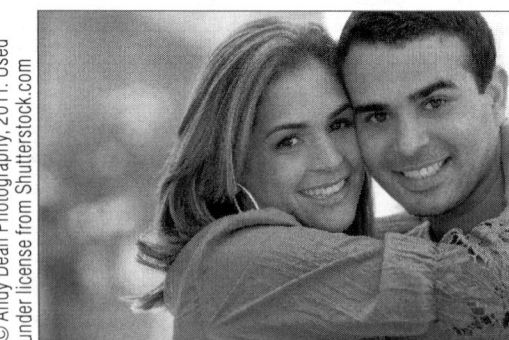

Heterosexuality

Without women and men participating in coitus, women would not become pregnant. Without women becoming pregnant, humans would not exist. Thus, the possibility of producing offspring is one of the main reasons why heterosexuality is viewed by many societies as normal, natural, and the "right" sexual orientation. Yet, attraction and desire for the other sex is not needed for reproduction. Throughout history, couples were expected to mate to produce offspring, regardless if they had romantic or sexual feelings for each other (Coontz, 2005). Most societies are generally based on the premise that most of their citizens will identify as heterosexual. Even though progress has been made to be more inclusive of other sexual orientations in the media in the U.S. for example, most advertisements, printed media, movies, and television shows continue to imply heterosexuality in some shape or form. Moreover, it is rare outside of "the Village" in New York City or San Francisco to view billboards that portray a lesbian or gay couple, unless of course the advertisement is for HIV prevention.

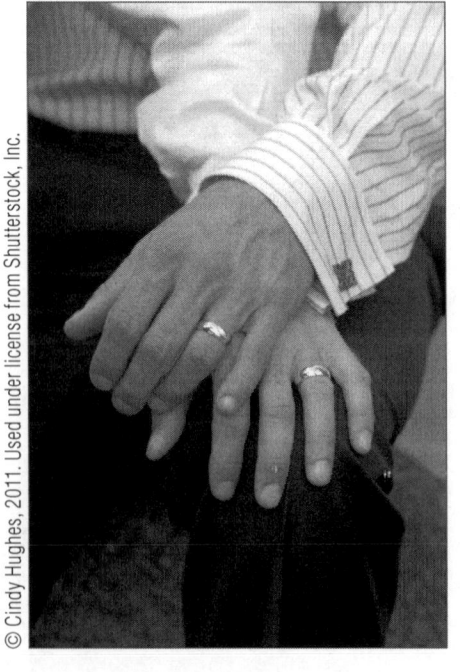

Homosexuality

Today, the world's stance on how homosexuality is perceived and accepted runs the gamut. Many countries in Europe, such as Finland, Sweden, and the Netherlands, embrace all sexual orientations and openly allow their youth to explore their sexuality. Since the 1950s, many of these countries have taught their youth about all sexual orientations, without instilling specific values of one over another (Francoeur & Noonan, 2004). Same-sex couples had legal rights in many of these countries for decades, but only recently won the right to marry in the early 21st century (this issue is discussed at length in chapter 10). In 1999, the Sexuality Information and Education Council of the United States (SIECUS, 1999) found that 14 countries around the world had antidiscrimination laws and policies based on sexual orientation. As of 2011, that number rose to 64 countries (Human Rights Campaign, 2011a)!

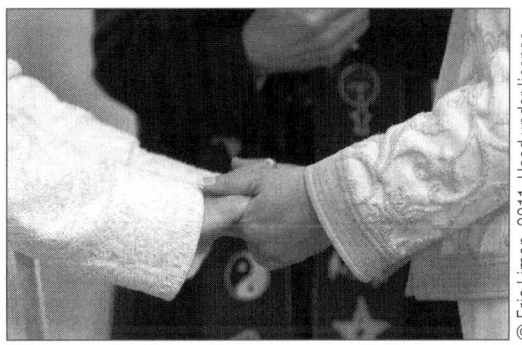

As discussed in several chapters, the U.S. has had a turbulent history in accepting homosexuality. Our own American Psychiatric Association stopped listing homosexuality as a mental disorder in the early 1970s. As of 2011, the U.S. military allows lesbian, gay, and bisexual soldiers to serve openly without threat of dishonorable discharge. Interestingly, by 2009, twenty countries, including Australia, Canada, and Great Britain had stopped discriminating on who served in the military based on sexual orientation (Quindlen, 2009). Six U.S. states legally recognize same-sex marriage and another eight allow same-sex civil unions. In 2011, San Francisco became the second city in the world (Berlin was the first) to open a GLBT museum. This museum (www.glbthistory.org/museum/index.html) provides a history of the GLBT community in San Francisco for the past 25 years.

Even so, the U.S. government does not recognize same-sex marriage at the federal level and 30 U.S. states have amended their state constitutions to outlaw same-sex marriage and/or civil unions. Religion has played a role in how a society views homosexuality. Even though some religions and denominations (such as the Catholic Church) accept bisexual, gay, and lesbian individuals openly into their congregations, on the other hand they may nonetheless condemn same-sex sexual behavior and/or refuse to bless the union between same-sex couples (The Religious Institute, 2004, 2007). Other religions (such as Mormonism and Islam) are less accepting and continue to view same-sex romantic relationships as sinful and immoral.

According to the Religious Institute on Sexuality Mortality, Justice and Healing, the following religious denominations and institutions have policies that support full inclusion of lesbian, gay, bisexual, and transgender (LGBT) persons, including ordination and marriage for same-sex couples (The Religious Institute, 2007):

1. Central Conference of American Rabbis Union for Reform Judaism
2. Reconstructionist Rabbinical Association/Jewish Reconstructionist Federation
3. Unitarian Universalist Association
4. United Church of Christ
5. Unity Fellowship Churches
6. Universal Fellowship of Metropolitan Community Churches

The following denominations ordain openly lesbian, gay, and bisexual clergy members (The Religious Institute, 2007):

1. Central Conference of American Rabbis
2. Episcopal Church U.S.

3. Evangelical Lutheran Church in America
4. Jewish Reconstructionist Federation/Reconstructionist Rabbinical Association
5. Presbyterian Church U.S.
6. Unitarian Universalist Association
7. United Church of Christ
8. United Synagogue for Conservative Judaism
9. Universal Fellowship of Metropolitan Community Churches

Bisexuality

Whereas heterosexuality has been considered natural and normal, and homosexuality has been considered immoral or sinful throughout the centuries, bisexuality has experienced indifference in the human population. Societal assumptions assert that bisexuality does not exist—either an individual is heterosexual or homosexual—and there is nothing in between (Baumgardner, 2008). Interestingly, studies have revealed that women seem to be more likely to express attraction to both sexes than men (Lippa, 2006).

Research on other species and their sexual contact has sparked great interest around the world. It is without question that bisexuality and homosexuality are widespread in the animal kingdom. It is believed that as many as 1,500 species of wild and captive animals have been observed engaging in bisexual and homosexual sexual activity (Driscoll, 2008). Giraffes, parrots, penguins, beetles, hyenas, and bonobos (a type of chimpanzee) have been observed exhibiting bisexual behavior (Crooks & Baur, 2011). For example, two male penguins native to Antarctica met in 1998 at the Central Park Zoo in New York City. Roy and Silo were a couple for six years until Silo left Roy for a female penguin, named Scrappy, who had recently arrived from SeaWorld in San Diego (Driscoll, 2008).

SEXUAL ORIENTATION AND BEHAVIOR

Contrary to societal assumptions, sexual orientation is not driven by sexual behavior. Moreover, behavior alone does not necessarily help define to whom an individual is attracted. For instance, a person who identifies as bisexual may

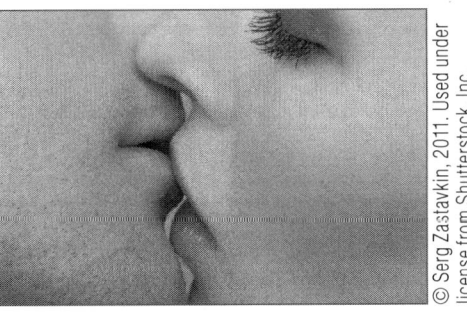 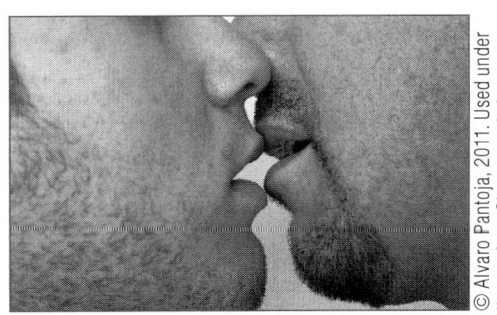 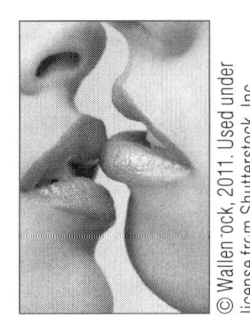

sexually prefer one sex over the other (Rosario, Schrimshaw, Hunter, & Braun, 2006). Similarly, identifying with a specific sexual orientation does not necessarily predict sexual relations with a particular sex. For instance, some people (i.e., swingers, commercial sex workers, incarcerated women and men, adult film stars, questioning youth) may define themselves as exclusively heterosexual, even though they participate in sexual activity with members of the same sex (Gilmore, Schwartz, & Civic, 1999). Also, individuals who identify as lesbian/gay may be in a sexual relationship with a person of the other sex to hide their true sexual identity from others.

Sexual identity and sexual behavior are closely related to sexual orientation. However, each attribute needs to be distinguished, with *sexual identity* referring to an individual's conception of themselves, *sexual behavior* referring to actual sexual acts performed by the individual, and *sexual orientation* referring to emotional and sexual attraction.

A Cross-Cultural Perspective in Sexual Behavior

Whereas many societies use sexual behavior to categorize an individual into a sexual orientation, the people of Sambia of Papua New Guinea do not (Herdt, 2006). Their cultural beliefs and expected roles for males may come as a surprise. From around the age of seven until between their late teens or early 20s, males are removed from their families and made to live only with other males. During this time, looking at or touching females is not allowed (Crooks & Baur, 2011). Each boy is expected to perform fellatio on a male who has already experienced puberty and has begun ejaculating. The young boys fellate the older boys to the point of ejaculation and are expected to swallow the seminal fluid (Herdt, 2006). This society believes that prepubertal boys can only become strong warriors and hunters by drinking as much semen (they call it "men's milk") as possible from postpubertal boys (Crooks & Baur, 2011). Daily fellatio and ingestion of semen occurs until the boy experiences puberty and begins ejaculating. At that time, he will no longer perform fellatio on older boys, but will have younger boys fellate him. Throughout his childhood and adolescent years, he will participate in frequent obligatory and gratifying homoeroticism (Crooks & Baur, 2011). At some point in his late teens and early 20s, the young man will marry a woman. During the first six months of marriage, the only sexual behavior allowed is fellatio. After that, the couple can participate in other sexual activities, but the man will not be allowed to participate in same-sex sexual contact again. This culture does not perceive their treatments of boys as child sexual abuse, and their language does not have a word for homosexuality (Herdt, 2006).

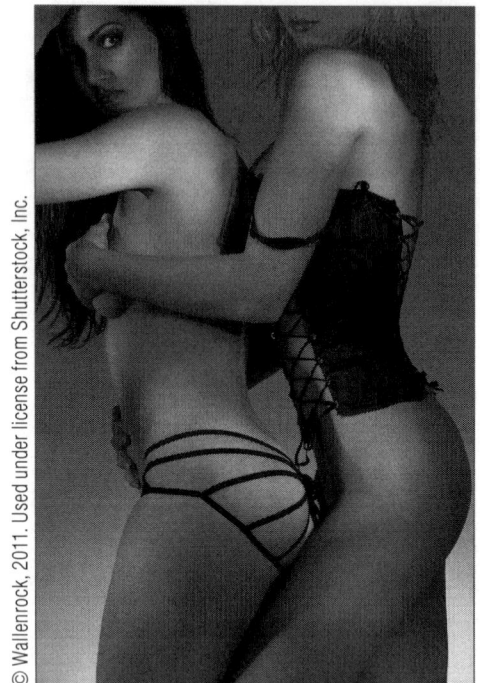
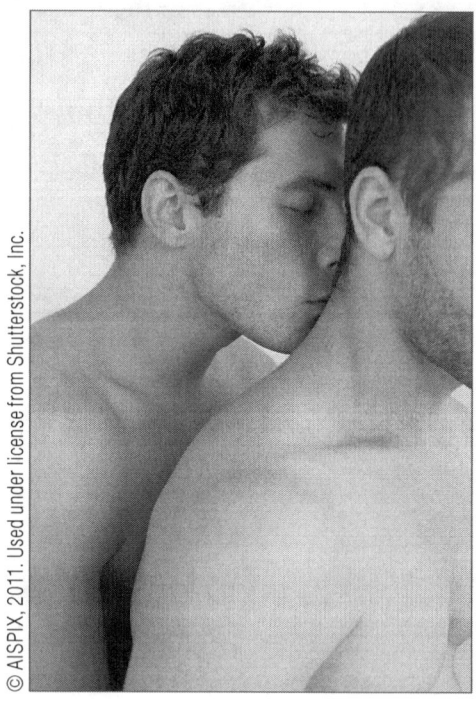

Sexual Fluidity

It has been proposed that few people identify exclusively in a specific sexual orientation or behavior with a particular sex (actual or fantasy) throughout their lives (Diamond, 2008; Kinsey et al., 1948). The concept of *sexual fluidity* helps us realize that one's sexual orientation can be broad like a continuum in which an individual can be attracted to the same sex, the other sex, or both sexes at different moments in their life rather than as a stable and fixed trait. Research has found that women have a greater likelihood of being more sexually fluid throughout their lives than men (Diamond, 2008). With the acceptance of "lesbian sex" in heterosexual pornography, it is unclear if sexual fluidity has become more acceptable—or to some extent expected—more so in women than in men. It is also unknown how much of society's social stigma of male homosexuality restricts sexual fluidity in men (Crooks & Baur, 2011).

SEXUAL ORIENTATION AND GENDER

In chapter 8, we discussed gender and defined gender identity as our own subjective sense of being female, male, or some combination of the two. Sexual orientation refers to which of the sexes we are emotionally and sexually attracted to (Crooks & Baur, 2011). Many societies, though, use appearance, mannerisms, and certain attitudes and behaviors to categorize an individual into a sexual orientation. For example, an effeminate man is more likely to be assumed to be a *gay man*. A man who controls his emotions and refrains from exhibiting behaviors stereotyped as feminine is more likely to be referred to as a *heterosexual man*.

Similar assumptions are imposed on women. A woman whose mannerisms and appearance are more characteristic of what is expected of a man is

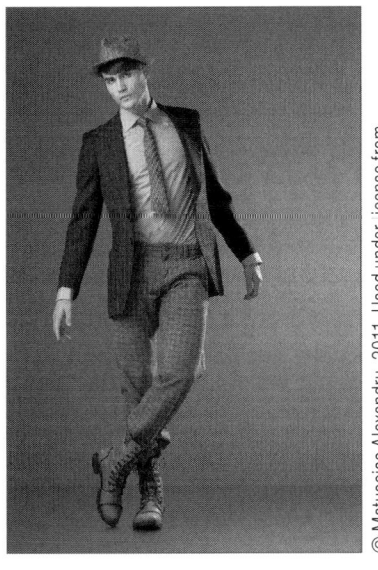
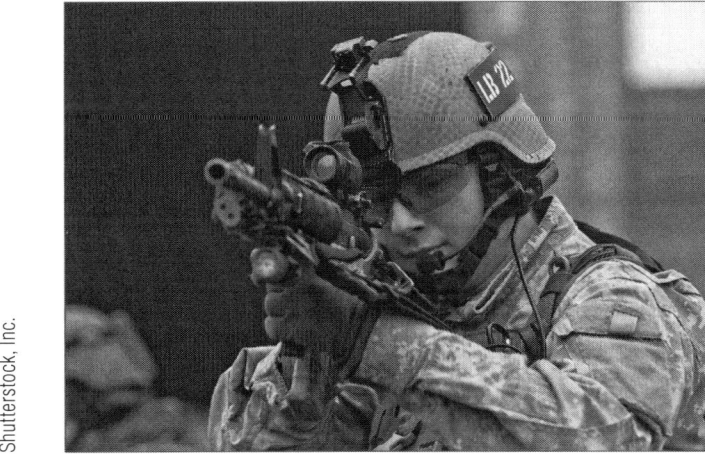

more likely to be seen as a *lesbian woman*. And a woman who exhibits attitudes and behaviors stereotyped as feminine is more likely to be referred to as a *heterosexual woman*.

DISPARITIES IN HEALTH OF LESBIAN, GAY, BISEXUAL, AND TRANSGENDER PEOPLE

Although the acronym LGBT has been used throughout this chapter as an umbrella term and certain experiences grouped together, each of these letters represents a distinct population with its own concerns. Furthermore, among bisexual women and men, gay men, lesbian women, and transgender people, there are subpopulations based on race, ethnicity, socioeconomic status, geographic location, and age (Institute of Medicine, 2011). All these factors influence sexual health. Moreover, unlike members of other minority groups (e.g., ethnic and racial minorities) in the U.S., most individuals who identify as lesbian, gay, or bisexual are not raised in a

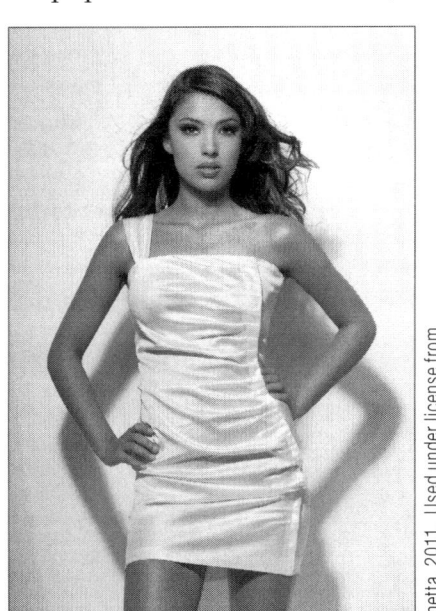
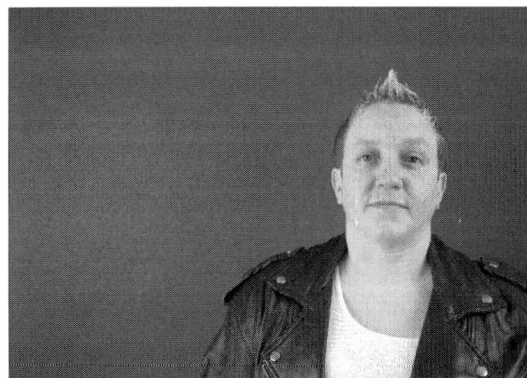

community with visible and accepted LGBT people from whom they could learn about their identity and who could reinforce and support that identity. On the contrary, most LGBT individuals are often raised in communities that are either ignorant of, or openly hostile toward, homosexuality, bisexuality, or individuals who do not conform to gender role expectations for their particular sex (Rosario et al., 2006).

HIV/AIDS remains one of the most critical health issues faced by some subgroups within LGBT populations in the United States (Institute of Medicine, 2011). Between 2006 and 2009, there was an estimated 21 percent increase in HIV incidence for all U.S. people aged 13–29. This rise was attributable to a 34 percent increase in young men who have sex with men (MSM), especially young African American MSM. According to the Centers for Disease Control and Prevention (CDC), gay and bisexual men remain the population most heavily affected by HIV in the U.S (Prejean et al., 2011). MSM represent around 2 percent of the U.S. population, but account for more than half of all new HIV infections annually from 2006 to 2009, ranging from 56 percent in 2006 to 61 percent in 2009. This increase is not fully understood, but stigma attached to HIV and same-sex sexual contact, limited access to health care, and poverty may influence the risk of HIV infection (Prejean et al., 2011). The CDC has recently increased its efforts to reach young African American and Hispanic MSM to promote sexually healthy behaviors and reduce HIV infections and transmission in this population.

According to the Institute of Medicine (2011), LGBT experience different health disparities than their heterosexual counterparts. Table 9.5 lists some of these health discrepancies:

Table 9.3 HEALTH STATUS OF LGBT POPULATIONS

LGBT individuals have an increased risk for suicidal ideation and attempts, as well as depression.

Rates of smoking, alcohol consumption, and substance use may be higher among LGB than heterosexual youth. Almost no research has examined substance use among transgender youth.

The homeless youth population comprises a disproportionate number of LGBT youth.

LGBT youth report experiencing elevated levels of violence, victimization, and harassment compared with heterosexual and nongender-variant youth.

Lesbian and bisexual women may use preventive health services less frequently than heterosexual women.

Lesbian and bisexual women may be at greater risk of obesity and have higher rates of breast cancer than heterosexual women.

LGBT people are frequently the targets of stigma, discrimination, and violence because of their sexual- and gender-minority status.

LGBT adults may have higher rates of smoking, alcohol use, and substance use than heterosexual adults.

Source: Institute of Medicine. (2011). The health of lesbian, gay, bisexual, and transgender people: Building a foundation for better understanding. Washington, DC: The National Academies Press

Reflections

Sexual orientation is a difficult concept to define. Humans are complex and complicated mammals to understand and categorize. Progress is made when we come to terms with our inability to pigeon-hole individuals into specific categories. Sexual behavior cannot be used to imply a person's sexual orientation nor can it be ignored when trying to understand the sexual health disparities in the LGBT community. In specific areas of the world, cultural beliefs and religion continue to dictate societal attitudes on homosexuality. But more liberal and progressive attitudes have taken root in other parts of the world, and given the scope of global change, common acceptance of sexual diversity is more possible in the near future than in any other time in history.

Critical Thinking Questions

1. What would you expect the sexual orientation of children of lesbian or gay parents to be? Would your answer be different if the children were raised by heterosexual parents? Why or why not?

2. Do you think children of heterosexual parents have more problems with sexual identity than do those of lesbian or gay parents or vice versa?

3. What strategies do you think are needed to decrease the rate of HIV among young African American or Hispanic MSM?

How Much Do You Remember from the Chapter?

1. What continent is more likely to include more countries with nondiscrimination laws based on sexual orientation?
    a. Africa
    b. Europe
    c. The Americas and the Caribbean
    d. Asia

2. What continent is more likely to include more countries that have laws criminalizing homosexuality?
    a. Africa
    b. Europe
    c. The Americas and the Caribbean
    d. Asia

3. LGBTs experience different health disparities than their heterosexual counterparts. List three of them.

Challenge Yourself!

Search online for the stories of the following youth. What happened to each one of them? What actions could have been taken by their community, their schools, their families, and their friends to prevent such tragedies?

- Justin Aaberg, age 15, July 2010, Minnesota
- Asher Brown, age 13, September 2010, Texas
- Tyler Clementi, age 18, September 2010, New Jersey
- Billy Lucas, age 15, September 2010, Indiana
- Seth Walsh, age 13, September 2010, California

Review the "It Gets Better Project" online. Do you think these personal stories can help youth who are struggling with bullying, emotional, mental, physical, and sexual abuse, and suicidal ideations?

Websites

www.hrc.org/
Human Rights Campaign

www.religiousinstitute.org/
The Religious Institute

References

American Psychological Association (APA). (2008). *Answers to your questions: For a better understanding of sexual orientation and homosexuality.* Washington, DC: Author. Retrieved from www.apa.org/topics/sorientation.pdf

American Psychiatric Association. (2000). *Gay, lesbian, and bisexual issues.* Retrieved from www.aglp.org/pages/cfactsheets.html#Anchor-Gay-14210

Baumgardner, J. (2008, February 26). Objects of suspicion. *Advocate*, pp. 24–27.

Coontz, S. (2005). *Marriage, a history: From obedience to intimacy, or how love conquered marriage.* New York, NY: Penguin Group.

Crooks, R., & Baur, K. (2011). *Our sexuality* (11th ed.). Belmont, CA: Wadsworth/Cengage.

Diamond, L. (2008). *Sexual fluidity: Understanding women's love and desire.* Cambridge, MA: Harvard University Press.

Driscoll, E. (2008). Bisexual species. *Scientific American.* Retrieved from www.scientificamerican.com/article.cfm?id=bisexual-species

Francoeur, R., & Noonan, R. (2004). *The continuum complete international encyclopedia of sexuality updated.* New York, NY: The Continuum International Publishing.

Frankowski, B., & The Committee on Adolescence. (2004). Sexual orientation and adolescence. *Pediatrics, 113*(6), 1827–1832.

Gilmore, M., Schwartz, P., & Civic, D. (1999). The social context of sexuality: The case of the United States. In K. Holmes, P. Sparling, P. Mardh, S. Lemon, W. Stamm, P. Piot, & J. Wasserheit (Eds.), *Sexually transmitted diseases* (3rd ed., pp. 95–105). New York, NY: McGraw-Hill.

Herbenick, D., Reece, M., Schick, V., Sanders, S., Dodge, B., & Fortenberry, J. (2010). Sexual behavior in the United States: Results from a national probability sample of men and women ages 14–94. *Journal of Sexual Medicine, 7*(supplemental 5), 255–265.

Herdt, G. (2006). *The Sambia: Ritual, sexuality, and change in Papua New Guinea*, (2nd ed.). Belmont, CA: Wadsworth Cengage Learning.

The Human Rights Campaign. (2011b). *Countries where homosexuality is criminalized*. Retrieved from www.hrc.org/issues/workplace/15677.htm

Institute of Medicine. (2011). *The health of lesbian, gay, bisexual, and transgender people: Building a foundation for better understanding*. Washington, DC: The National Academies Press.

Kinsey, A., Pomeroy, W., & Martin, C. (1948). *Sexual behavior in the human male*. Philadelphia, PA: Saunders.

Klein, F., Sepekoff, B., & Wolf, T. (1985). Sexual orientation: A multi-variable dynamic process. In F. Klein & T. Wolf (Eds.), *Two lives to live: Bisexuality in men and women* (pp. 35–49). New York, NY: Harrington Park Press.

Lippa, R. (2006). Is high sex drive associated with increased sexual attraction to both sexes? It depends on whether you're male or female. *Psychological Sciences, 17*, 46–52.

Prejean, J., Song, R., Hernandez, A., Ziebell, R., Green, T., Walker, F. et al. (2011). Estimated HIV incidence in the United States, 2006–2009. *PLoS ONE 6*(8), e17502. doi:10.1371/journal.pone.0017502

Quindlen, A. (2009, April 13). The end of an error. *Newsweek*, p. 60.

The Religious Institute. (2004). *An open letter to religious leaders on marriage equality*. Norwalk, CT: The Religious Institute on Sexual Morality, Justice, and Healing.

The Religious Institute. (2007). *An open letter to religious leaders on sexual and gender diversity*. Norwalk, CT: The Religious Institute on Sexual Morality, Justice, and Healing.

Rosario, M., Schrimshaw, E., Hunter, J., & Braun, L. (2006). Sexual identity development among lesbian, gay, and bisexual youths: Consistency and change over time. *Journal of Sex Research, 43*(1), 46–58.

SIECUS. (1999). Worldwide antidiscrimination laws and policies based on sexual orientation. *SIECUS Report, 27*, 19–22.

chapter ten

COMPANIONSHIP & MARRIAGE

CHAPTER OBJECTIVES

On completion of this chapter, students will be able to:

- discuss the varied forms of companionship;
- describe how marriage has evolved throughout the centuries;
- name the countries that legally recognize same sex marriage;
- list the U.S. states that legally recognize same-sex marriage and/or civil unions.

ABBREVIATIONS AND ACRONYMS USED IN THIS CHAPTER

ABC	American Broadcasting Company
BCE	Before the Common Era (formerly BC)
CNN	Cable News Network
DOMA	Defense of Marriage Act
ORC	Operations Research Center

COMPANIONSHIP

What motivates us to develop a relationship with another person? Do we form relationships for the support, attention, available resources, social status, pressure, intimacy, and/or affection? Companionship comes in many forms such as acquaintances, colleagues, friends, friends with benefits, lovers, and partners. All may have different meanings to different people at different points of their lives. While this chapter only focuses on human companionship, many people also enjoy companionship with their pets. Some human relationships evolve over time and others dissolve completely. Some relationships enhance our well-being, while others bring great sorrow into our lives. Sometimes we end relationships that were "good for us" and yet remain in relationships that are "unhealthy." Both endings of a healthy and unhealthy relationship are relative—what one may see as healthy, another person would not and vice versa. Even so, there are some boundaries that should not be crossed. Bringing physical, emotional, and psychological harm to another person is not a healthy aspect of any relationship.

Types of companionship vary by time period, culture, age, gender, and social status. For example, during the Victorian era, which corresponded to the reign of Queen Victoria in England from 1837 to 1901, gender roles were highly polarized and restricted, with a woman's identity centering on providing her husband a comfortable home and raising their children (Crooks & Baur, 2011). Women (especially the upper-class) in the United States and Europe were perceived as fragile, delicate, and asexual (Degler, 1980). Men were given more freedom to explore the social (and sexual) environment around them. Even though extramarital affairs were frowned upon, prostitution flourished during this period as men put morality aside and sought sexual companionship (Crooks & Baur, 2011). During this period, support and comfort were absent in most marriages and some women resorted to developing passionate friendships with other women to obtain what was lacking in their marriage, including love.

The Chemistry of Love

When we are physically intimate with another individual, our brains secrete oxytocin, a brain chemical that contributes to sexual arousal and feelings of being in love (Crooks & Baur, 2011). Oxytocin seems to help solidify certain social attachments by fostering feelings of love (Young, 2009). As we develop a deeper attachment to a particular individual, our brain starts producing a set of neurotransmitters called endorphins. Endorphins help us feel a sense of euphoria, security, tranquility, and peace (Fisher, 2004). If our "love" is taken away, these brain chemicals and neurotransmitters are lost and we experience a period of emotional pain (Crooks & Baur, 2011).

The term *love* means different things to different people (Coontz, 2006). Some individuals place a high value on the word and its meaning and others do not. Some people love only a selected group of individuals, whereas others may feel the need to spread their love (emotional, physical, psychological, and spiritual—whatever it means to them). Interestingly, love is a relatively new concept as a prerequisite to marriage, and was rare throughout world history as the main reason for marriage (Coontz, 2006). For example, in ancient India, falling in love before marriage was frowned on. In China, excessive love between the married couple was seen as a threat to the solidarity of the extended family. In Rome, the main purpose of marriage was procreation and Romans, like most of the ancient world, used marriage and inheritance as the main methods of conveying property (Coontz, 2005). For centuries, kings and noblemen married their wives to preserve bloodlines and to secure political alliances. Love, gratification, and companionship were reserved for people living at court (i.e., courtiers and courtesans) who were not their spouses.

Prior to the 17th century, Christian texts referred to the word love to feelings toward God or neighbors rather than toward a spouse (Coontz, 2005). The 1800s saw a turning point in many societies' expectations of marriage. Both North America and Western Europe began to expect marriage to include a greater importance on psychological and social needs than ever before (Coontz, 2005).

In a romantic relationship, society has constructed such attachments to include high levels of emotional and physical responsibilities and commitment. However, more causal relationships, such as "friends with benefits" may involve only sexual gratification and perhaps the responsibilities of a friendship (Puentes, Knox, & Zusman, 2008). Honest and open communication is needed in any type of relationship, but when dealing with friends with benefits, both individuals need to be aware of how this type of relationship is perceived by both parties, as well as how the relationship may intensify over time. For example, McGinty and colleagues (2007) surveyed heterosexual couples and found women were more emotionally involved and stressed the importance of the friendship, whereas men viewed the relationship as more casual and focused more on the sexual gratification.

Romantic relationships can take on many forms (Coontz, 2006). Some couples live together, while others live in separate dwellings but in close proximity (same city, for example), or live in different states and even in different countries. Some couples are sexually exclusive with each other, while others do not participate in sexual activity with each other at all, and some prefer sexual contact with someone other than their partner—either unbeknownst to the other partner or with her/his approval. All the examples provided above can occur within a marriage and none are a recent phenomenon, but have occurred throughout history (Coontz, 2005). Some couples, though, do not wish to have their union legally and/or religiously recognized. Some may only want the legal recognition of a marriage, while others would prefer only the religious recognition. Yet, others are not allowed to have their relationship legally and/or religiously recognized because their union is prohibited by the society in which they live (e.g., between two men, two women, two different races, two different religions, or one or both are already married to someone else). The rest of this chapter focuses on legally recognized unions.

THE INSTITUTION OF MARRIAGE

If you intend to marry in the future, why do you plan to do so—for the companionship, the sexual activity, to raise a family, for the social status, and/or for the money? How do you know that the person you have chosen as your future spouse is the *right* person for you? Do you feel compelled to be in love with the person in order to marry him/her? Should that person be in love with you? Do you expect the relationship to be monogamous? Or is it acceptable if one of you is monogamous, but not the other? Is premarital sexual activity acceptable to both of you? Do you or your future spouse need to be of a certain age, a certain religion, a certain sex, a certain racial/ethnic background, or have a certain job? How long should you know this person before you believe she/he is meant to be your future spouse—a week, a few months, or a couple years? Do you expect to choose your spouse or will someone (like your parents) decide for you?

Marriage has been defined differently throughout human history and in different parts of the world. Currently in the United States, marriage can be defined as an institution constructed by society in which (usually) two (genetically unrelated) individuals are legally recognized by a government and/or religion as next of kin (Coontz, 2006). This definition is simplistic and does not take into account distinctive social environments and personal expectations. For example, in some cultures, you can marry your first cousin. Many states (but not all) in the United States have laws against marrying your first cousin—namely someone who is genetically related to you because one of your biological parents and one of their biological parents are siblings. What would you add to the definition of marriage?

How does marriage benefit the individuals in a marriage? Depending on the culture, a marriage may include specific legal benefits bestowed only on a married couple, such as employer-based medical insurance, tax benefits, and inheritance to property and other wealth. Moreover, some couples get married because their parents arranged the partnership in their infancy and had no choice in the matter or welcomed their parents' involvement in picking their future spouse. Others get married for the social status that such a recognized union might bring—more money, more resources, entering adulthood, etc. For others, it's the hope of stability, love, intimacy, and support to help make their lives better and more fulfilling. And lastly, for some, it's a package deal: a little of all of the above. Yet, do we need to be married to enjoy the benefits of companionship? Is the grass necessarily greener on the other side of the marriage fence?

THE EVOLUTION OF MARRIAGE

Why do you think marriage was created? What purpose was it supposed to achieve? It is believed that marriage was constructed for a few reasons. Lombardo and Lombardo (2008) assert that the original purpose of marriage was to consolidate status, resources, and intertwine families and tribes. Other reasons they cite are for the religious sacrament and legally sanctioned contract, and most recently, is to expect love and devotion from a spouse (Lombardo and Lombardo, 2008). These evolutions vary by country, religion, and period in history. For instance, some societies (e.g., most of India) still expect the parents to choose an offspring's future spouse while others do not place much social significance on the institution of marriage.

The union of two individuals was not always consensual between the pair but was considered necessary for the greater good of the community. With time and depending on the culture, a marriage was also seen to allow the couple to acknowledge their bond with each other and to society (Shlain, 2003). Depending on the culture, polygamist men could be married to more than one woman, but most cultures have not allowed women to have more than one husband (at the same time or ever again if the husband died or dissolved the marriage). Thus, depending on the culture and time period, a married couple would either need to stay monogamous (because that was the social norm) or could be in a polygamous relationship where the man could marry other women (Coontz, 2005).

Another reason for marriage was to determine who the father was if a woman became pregnant (Watson, 2005). It is assumed that when a woman becomes pregnant within a marriage that the husband is the father. The need to establish paternity could be a pressing matter if the husband has wealth or property to pass onto his children. He would like to make sure (and supposedly being married gave him that assurance) that the children who inherit his wealth and property are his biological children and—before DNA testing—the only way to be sure is if his wife had the baby.

By 1000 BCE (Before the Common Era), many societies had established a double standard, which perceived men as dominant and superior to women. Any rights women had before this time diminished considerably, especially as patriarchy solidified with the rise of Christianity and Judaism (Lombardo & Lombardo, 2008).

THE MEANING PLACED ON FAMILY/LAST NAMES

Many naming systems exist throughout the world. The term *surname* comes from the medieval French word *surnom*, which means above or over name. The surname was initially used to distinguish people with the same given or first name. Surnames were drawn from a number of sources and were not initially passed down from generation to generation (Hook, 1982). According to Dodgson Bowman (1931), most surnames were drawn from places (Hill), occupations (Brewer), physical descriptions (Little), moral characteristics (Good), and relationships (Williamson).

Over time, however, surnames became hereditary and were used to facilitate the inheritance of property. The custom of passing the father's surname on to the children was further developed in response to England's legal system and social practices in which the ownership and management of all marital property was vested in the husband (Seng, 1984). Under this doctrine, the wife's legal identity was considered the husband's. The husband had all legal rights, duties, and powers with respect to the children of the marriage and the children born of the marriage were given the surname of their father (Kelly, 1996). In ancient Rome, though, power in the relationship was tied to property rather than to gender. Thus, a man would assume the surname of his wife if she came to the marriage with more property than he did (Kelly, 1996). This also occurred in England in order for husbands to align themselves with their wife's estate. This practice ceased around the 11th and 12th century when property inheritance was restricted only to the eldest son in the family (Mahoney Frandina, 2009).

According to Seng (2008), in China, patrilineal (father-line) family names started with Emperor Fu Xi in 2852 BCE to facilitate census taking and as a symbol of a man's pride and honor. Toward the 8th century, the Catholic Church began to have a stronger influence over marriage in Europe and helped contribute to patrilineal naming customs (Coontz, 2006). Ireland started using surnames around the year 900, but these surnames were not hereditary, and were created with the influence of the Catholic Church. For example, modern Irish surnames, in particular those beginning with *Gil-* or *Kil-*, originate from the Irish word *giolla*, meaning follower or devotee. Even though Britain began to adopt surnames around the 13th and 14th century (mostly among the aristocracy), it wasn't until 400 years later that King Henry VIII (1491–1547) ordered marital births to be recorded under the surname of the father (Doll, 1992). Family names were uncommon in Japan except among the aristocracy up until the 19th century.

As families started to emigrate to other parts of the world, names started to represent one's sense of self and an expression of one's social identity. Families also started to associate last name with identity through ethnic and familial history. In the United States, a patrilineal naming tradition continues to be followed by the majority of married heterosexual couples. For most of America's history, women were forced to take their husband's last name when married. During the 20th century, though, women in Western countries gained the right to choose to take their husband's last name, hyphenate his last name with her last name, keep her last name, or create a whole new last name with her husband. The United Nations (2003) reaffirms women's equality around the world and endorses the same personal rights as husband and wife, including the right to choose a family name. Most women, though, continue to change their last name to her husband's. Interestingly, legal authority for a man to change his surname to his wife's upon marriage only exists in 7 of the 50 U.S. states (Mahoney Frandina, 2009). The seven states are Georgia, Hawaii, Iowa, Louisiana, Massachusetts, New York, and North Dakota.

A child's last name is not required by law to be that of the father's, whether or not the couple is married. Most couples, though, pass the father's last name to the children, regardless of marital status. American citizens have the legal right to change any part of their name (first, middle, and/or last) through the court system (Mahoney Frandina, 2009). The naming system continues to be redefined as more same-sex couples marry in the United States and around the world, as more men choose to take their wife's last name, or as more couples choose to create a new surname to uniquely identify their family unit.

Marriage Statistics in the U.S.

For the first time since the U.S. Census Bureau began collecting data on marriage, less than half (45 percent) of all households in this country included a heterosexual married couple in 2010. Married couples are more likely to have a college education and be affluent (heterosexual or lesbian/gay). In 1960, the heterosexual marriage gap between college and high school graduates was minimal—76 percent versus 72 percent, respectively. According to the Pew Research Center, this gap has widened to 16 percentage points. Marriage has become for many a luxury instead of a rite of passage for heterosexual couples. Moreover, a woman with a high school diploma is more likely to raise her children out of wedlock than a woman with a college education. Forty-four percent of babies born to mothers whose education ended with high school were raised outside of marriage, versus only 6 percent of children born to college-educated mothers. Single-parent households are more likely to live in poverty than married couples (regardless of sexual orientation).

The Williams Institute at the UCLA School of Law estimates that around 165,000 same-sex couples have gotten married, entered into a civil union, or entered into a domestic partnership in the U.S. Even though there is no data on the dissolution of marriage for same-sex couples, around 2 percent of same-sex couples who had entered a civil union or a domestic partnership have ended that relationship. Moreover, U.S. states that legally recognize same-sex couples in the name of marriage or civil unions had the lowest number of divorces in the nation in 2009. For example, Massachusetts, the first state to legalize same-sex marriages, had a rate of 1.8 divorces per 1,000 residents. The nation's highest divorce rate, at 6.6 per 1,000 residents was in Nevada.

MARRIAGE EQUALITY FOR SAME-SEX COUPLES AROUND THE WORLD

Below is a list of the first 10 countries that legally recognized two women or two men as a married couple. None of them occurred during the 20th century. Do any of the countries on the list surprise you? Why or why not?

Table 10.1 COUNTRIES THAT LEGALLY RECOGNIZE SAME-SEX MARRIAGE

Country	Year Enacted
The Netherlands	2001
Belgium	2003
Spain	2005
Canada	2005
South Africa	2006
Norway	2009
Sweden	2009

Portugal	2010
Iceland	2010
Argentina	2010

Civil Union vs. Marriage

What *is* a civil union and how does it differ from marriage? A civil union allows a couple to take advantage of all the benefits available to married couples in that state. Thus, a civil-unionized couple has the legal right to be considered next of kin which would give them the right to each other's employer-based medical insurance; inheriting a partner's social security benefits, wealth, and property; and be able to make medical decisions if one of them is incapable of doing so for themselves. Yet, even though the only difference between a civil union and a marriage is the words used to separate same sex couples from heterosexual couples, the difference is huge! Some states in the United States have made great strides in recognizing the rights of lesbian and gay individuals (and the Obama administration has been the most gay-friendly in America's history), and younger generations are more likely to accept marriage equality for same-sex couples. Even so, we still have a long way to go to stop marginalizing a group of people because of their sexual orientation. Why do we need separate words to refer to same-sex relationships that are legally recognized instead of the term legally used to recognize heterosexual couples?

Technically, a civil union can only be legally recognized in another state that offers it as well. However, it is unclear if a civil union performed in one state is considered a marriage in a different state that only offers same-sex marriage but not same-sex civil unions. The uncertainty even exists for heterosexual couples. For instance, it is possible for heterosexual couples to obtain a civil union

Table 10.2 U.S. STATES WITH CIVIL UNIONS

State	Branch of Government	Date Enacted
Vermont	State Supreme Court	July 1, 2000
Connecticut	State Legislature	October 1, 2005
New Jersey	State Supreme Court & Legislature	February 19, 2007
New Hampshire	State Legislature	January 1, 2008
Illinois	State Legislature	June 1, 2011
Rhode Island	State Legislature	July 2, 2011
Hawaii	State Legislature	January 1, 2012
Delaware	State Legislature	January 1, 2012

instead of a marriage license (in states that offer civil unions), but it is unclear if that civil union is then considered a marriage in another state that offers only marriage—not civil unions—for heterosexual couples.

Table 10.2 lists eight states that have passed civil unions in the United States through January 1, 2012. Even though each civil union law was passed to provide a path for legal recognition of same-sex couples, a heterosexual couple could choose to obtain a civil union over a marriage license, but they cannot do both. Depending on the state, a same-sex couple may only have the option of a civil union.

MARRIAGE EQUALITY FOR SAME-SEX COUPLES IN THE UNITED STATES

In 2011, several national polls showed a slight majority of Americans supporting legal recognition of same-sex marriage. Gallup and ABC/*Washington Post* surveys reported that 53 percent of Americans polled support marriage equality for same-sex couples, whereas CNN/ORC and the Public Religion Research Institute surveys found 51 percent of Americans support legal same-sex marriage in the United States (*U.S. News and World Report*, 2011). Since the 1990s, over half of the U.S. states, though, have amended their state constitution to *not* legally recognize same-sex civil unions and/or same-sex marriage in their state. If history is any indication, it is unlikely that many of these states would amend their state constitution to allow the legal recognition of same-sex civil unions and/or same-sex marriage. For example, interracial marriage was not legally recognized in this country until the U.S. Supreme Court ruling of Loving *v.* Virginia in 1967 (388 U.S. 1). Before this, only a handful of states legally recognized a heterosexual marriage between a white person and a nonwhite person. Moreover, several states had laws making such unions illegal (with the possibility of going to jail). It took Congress to propose amending the U.S. constitution, followed by the states' ratification of the amendment, for the United States to prohibit any U.S. citizen to be denied the right to vote based on sex. In 1920 the Nineteenth Amendment gave American women the right to vote. Thus, it will be up to the U.S. Supreme Court to decide if marriage equality is a right that should be offered to same-sex couples or a right that should remain available only to heterosexual couples in this country.

In the United States, the top five states with the strongest support for marriage equality for same-sex couples in 2009 were New York, Rhode Island, Connecticut, Massachusetts, and California. How many of these states do you think legally recognize same-sex civil unions or marriage? Do you think any of them have amended their state constitution to *not* legally recognize same sex couples? The top five U.S. states with the strongest opposition to same-sex marriage in 2009 were Utah, Oklahoma, Alabama, Mississippi, and Arkansas. How many of these states do you think legally recognize same-sex civil unions or marriage? Do you think any of them have amended their state constitution to *not* legally recognize same-sex couples?

The six states that currently provide legal recognition in the name of marriage to same-sex couples in the United States are listed in Table 10.3. Washington, D.C. began to legally recognize and perform marriage for same-sex couples in early 2010. For states where the law to allow same-sex marriage was created by the state legislature, either the governor signed the bill into law or the legislature had enough votes to override a gubernatorial veto (as was the case in Vermont).

Table 10.3 U.S. STATES THAT LEGALLY RECOGNIZE SAME-SEX MARRIAGE		
State	**Branch of Government**	**Date Enacted**
Massachusetts	State Supreme Court	May 17, 2004
Connecticut	State Supreme Court	November 12, 2008
Iowa	State Supreme Court	April 24, 2009
Vermont	State Legislature	September 1, 2009
New Hampshire	State Legislature	January 1, 2010
New York	State Legislature	July 24, 2011

Voting Against the Right to Marry

California's State Supreme Court granted same-sex couples full marriage rights in May 2008. It became legal on June 16, 2008. Over 20,000 same-sex couples from California got married. On November 3, 2008, that right was subsequently taken away from California residents with the passage of Proposition 8. Adoption of Proposition 8 changed the state constitution to recognize marriage only between one man and one woman. When this constitutional amendment passed, marriage for same-sex couples was no longer a right in California. The California Supreme Court upheld Proposition 8, but interestingly did not nullify the 20,000 same-sex marriages that had been previously performed. The state of California has to legally recognize all of those marriages even though California can no longer perform same-sex marriages nor legally recognize same-sex marriages from other U.S. states or countries.

The Maine legislature approved a bill legally recognizing same-sex couples in the name of marriage in May 2009. The governor signed the bill into law and it took effect September 15, 2009. However, on November 4, 2009 the residents of Maine overturned this law by passing Question 1. Passing Question 1 amended the state constitution to recognize marriage only between one man and one woman. When this amendment passed, marriage for same-sex couples was no longer a right in Maine.

Changing the State Constitution

Thirty states have laws that make it virtually impossible to legally recognize same-sex couples. Table 10.4 lists the 14 states that ban marriage for same-sex couples. Table 10.5 lists the states that ban both marriage and civil unions for same-sex couples. Across both lists, 23 states (denoted with an asterisk) were more likely to vote Republican in the 2008 Presidential election. Is this a coincidence? Would you expect to see more states that voted Republican than Democratic in either list? Why or why not?

Table 10.4 — STATES BANNING MARRIAGE ONLY FOR SAME-SEX COUPLES

Arizona*	Alaska*	California
Colorado	Florida	Idaho*
Kansas*	Mississippi*	Missouri*
Montana*	Nevada	Oregon
South Carolina*	Wisconsin*	

* States that were more likely to vote Republican in the 2008 Presidential election

Table 10.5 — STATES BANNING MARRIAGE AND CIVIL UNIONS FOR SAME-SEX COUPLES

Alabama*	Arkansas*	Georgia*
Kentucky*	Louisiana*	Maine
Michigan	Nebraska*	North Dakota*
Ohio	Oklahoma*	South Dakota*
Tennessee*	Texas*	Utah*
Virginia		

* States that were more likely to vote Republican in the 2008 Presidential election

Most of these states have laws that were approved by the voters to change the state constitution by specifically defining marriage as between "one man and one woman." These revisions to state constitutions served not only to derail any chance of legally recognizing same-sex couples (either by civil unions, marriage, or both), but also to condemn polygamous marriages. Both Islam and Mormonism condone a man having more than one wife at the same time, even though not everyone who follows either religion adheres to this proclamation. Polygamous religions and cultures rarely allow a woman to have more than one husband at the same time.

In Table 10.4, of the 14 states that revised their state constitution to ban marriage for same-sex couples (and polygamy), 9 of them were more likely to vote Republican in the 2008 presidential election. In Table 10.5, of the 16 states that revised their state constitution to ban marriage and civil unions for same-sex couples (and polygamy), 12 of them were more likely to vote Republican in the 2008 Presidential election.

Even though conservative voters are more likely to vote against legally recognizing same-sex couples, not everyone in favor of marriage equality for same sex-couples is liberal. Moreover, it was a Democratic president (President Bill Clinton) who signed the Defense of Marriage Act (DOMA) into law in 1996 (Public Law 104-199, 110 Stat. 2419). This federal law defines marriage as a legal union between one woman and one man, and ensures that no state is obligated to recognize another state's legal recognition of same-sex couples. Moreover, the federal government does not recognize civil unions or marriage for same-sex couples deemed legal in a particular U.S. state or another country. Thus, when a same-sex married couple in Massachusetts completes their taxes, they are married on their state tax return, but they need to identify as single on their federal tax returns because of DOMA. There is strong vocal support in the federal government for this to change. For example, in 2011, the Justice Department announced it would no longer defend the constitutionality of DOMA in court.

Reflections

Companionship encompasses a variety of meanings to an individual. Some societies continue to restrict certain types of companionships, while others allow their citizens to expand their perceptions of such relationships. Marriage is a social construct that has evolved throughout the centuries. The last century has seen a rise in acceptance to such concepts as divorce, remarriage, interracial marriage, same sex marriage and the right *not* to marry. Yet, marriage means different things to different people. Thus, meanings placed on these differences have created a new "cultural war" in which you have one side fighting for specific rights to marriage and another side fighting to keep marriage as traditionally defined.

Critical Thinking Questions

1. Do you believe recent changes in marriage laws have strengthened or weakened the institution of marriage?

2. If civil unions were offered to all heterosexual couples, do you think they would choose that option over marriage? Why or why not?

3. In the future, will marriage continue to be relevant?

4. Do you think marriage provides certain benefits to society? If so, what?

5. If you are married or intend to marry in the future, how do you think your marriage will be different from your parents' or grandparents' marriage (if they were married)?

How Much Do You Remember from the Chapter?

1. Which *eight* states in the U.S. have legal civil unions for lesbian and gay couples?
    a. New Jersey, California, Vermont, Connecticut, Illinois, Delaware, Hawaii, Texas
    b. Connecticut, Hawaii, Vermont, Rhode Island, New York, Maine, Nevada, Arizona
    c. New York, Vermont, New Jersey, Hawaii, Iowa, Minnesota, Colorado, Alabama
    d. Vermont, New Jersey, New Hampshire, Connecticut, Hawaii, Rhode Island, Illinois, Delaware

2. What U.S. state offers civil unions because of their state's Supreme Court decision?
    a. California
    b. Vermont
    c. New Jersey
    d. Connecticut

3. What U.S. state offers civil unions because of their state's Supreme Court decision *and* their legislature?
    a. Delaware
    b. Vermont
    c. Connecticut
    d. New Jersey

4. What *six* U.S. states have legal same-sex marriage?
    a. Massachusetts, California, Iowa, Connecticut, Maine, Nevada
    b. California, Connecticut, Maine, Vermont, Iowa, Mississippi
    c. Vermont, New Jersey, Connecticut, New Hampshire, Iowa, South Dakota
    d. Connecticut, Massachusetts, Vermont, Iowa, New Hampshire, New York

5. What *two* U.S. states had same-sex marriage by their state's Supreme Court or legislature, but then the voters took it away?
    a. Colorado, Texas
    b. Florida, Oregon
    c. California, Maine
    d. Arizona, Kansas

Challenge Yourself!

Name the 10 countries that have same-sex marriage.

1. _____   2. _____
3. _____   4. _____
5. _____   6. _____
7. _____   8. _____
9. _____   10. _____

Websites

www.hrc.org/
Human Rights Campaign

www.pewresearch.org/
Pew Research Center

http://www.pollingreport.com/civil.htm
Polling Report, Inc.

www.religiousinstitute.org/
The Religious Institute-Faithful Voices on Sexuality and Religion

www3.law.ucla.edu/williamsinstitute/
Williams Institute - UCLA Law School

References

Coontz, S. (2005). *Marriage, a history: From obedience to intimacy, or how love conquered marriage.* New York, NY: Penguin Group.

Coontz, S. (2006). *Marriage, a history: How love conquered marriage.* New York, NY: Penguin Group.

Crooks, R., & Baur, K. (2011). *Our sexuality.* Belmont, CA: Wadsworth/Cengage.

Defense of Marriage Act. (1996). *To define and protect the institution of marriage.* Retrieved from www.gpo.gov/fdsys/pkg/PLAW-104publ199/pdf/PLAW-104publ199.pdf

Degler, C. (1980). *At odds: Women and the family in America from the Revolution to the present.* Oxford, UK: Oxford University Press.

Dodgson Bowman, W. (1931). *The story of surnames.* London, England: George Routledge & Sons.

Doll, C. (1992). Harmonizing filial and parental rights in names: Progress, pitfalls, and constitutional problems. *Howard Law Journal, 35,* 227–234.

Fisher, H. (2004). *Why we love: The nature and chemistry of romantic love.* New York, NY: Henry Holt and Company.

Hook, J. (1982). *Family names: How our surnames came to America*. New York, NY: Macmillan.

Kelly, L. (1996). Divining the deep and inscrutable: Toward a gender-neutral, child-centered approach to child name change proceedings. *West Virginia Law Review, 99*, 1–80.

Lombardo, T., & Lombardo, J. (2008). The evolution and future direction of marriage. In C. Wagner (Ed.). *Seeing the future through new eyes*. Bethesda, MD: World Future Society.

Mahoney Frandina, M. (2009). A man's right to choose his surname in marriage: A proposal. *Duke Journal of Gender Law & Policy, 16*, 155–168.

McGinty, K., Knox, D., & Zusman, M. (2007). Friends with benefits: Women want 'friends,' men want 'benefits.' *College Student Journal, 41*, 1128–1131.

Puentes, J., Knox, D., & Zusman, M. (2008). Participants in 'friends with benefits' relationships. *College Student Journal, 42*, 176–180.

Seng, B. (1984). Like father, like child: The rights of parents in their children's surnames. *Virginia Law Review, 70*, 1303–1355.

Seng, S. (2008). *Origin of Chinese surnames*. Retrieved from www.genealogy.about.com/library/authors/ucboey2a.htm

Shlain, L. (2003). *Sex, time, and power: How women's sexuality shaped human evolution*. New York, NY: Viking.

United Nations. (2003). *Convention on the elimination of all forms of discrimination against women*. Retrieved from www.un.org/womenwatch/daw/cedaw/text/econvention.htm#article16

U.S. News & World Report. (2011). New study: Support for gay marriage grew faster in past two years. Retrieved from www.usnews.com/news/articles/2011/07/27/new-study-support-for-gay-marriage-grew-faster-in-past-two-years

Watson, P. (2005). *Ideas: A history of thought and invention from fire to Freud*. New York, NY: HarperCollins Publishers.

Young, L. (2009). Being human: Love-neuroscience reveals all. *Nature, 457*, 148–149.

chapter eleven

CONCEPTION, PREGNANCY, & OUTCOMES

CHAPTER OBJECTIVES

On completion of this chapter, students will be able to:

- identify the possible outcomes of a pregnancy;
- recognize the hormones necessary to sustain a pregnancy;
- describe the three trimesters of pregnancy;
- list the causes of maternal and infant deaths.

ABBREVIATIONS AND ACRONYMS USED IN THIS CHAPTER

ACOG	American Congress of Obstetricians and Gynecologists
BMI	body mass index
cm	centimeters
GDM	gestational diabetes mellitus
hCG	human chorionic gonadotropin
hPL	human placental lactogen
IOM	Institute of Medicine

PREGNANCY OUTCOMES

In the United States, an estimated 6 million women become pregnant annually (Martin et al., 2009). In any given year, around 10 percent of reproductive age women experience a pregnancy (Mosher & Jones, 2010). According to Ventura and colleagues (2009), of the 6.4 million pregnancies in the United States in 2006, 4 million resulted in births, 1.3 million in abortions, and 1.1 million in miscarriages and stillbirths. The proportions of pregnancies that were intended (51%) and unintended (49%) were almost identical.

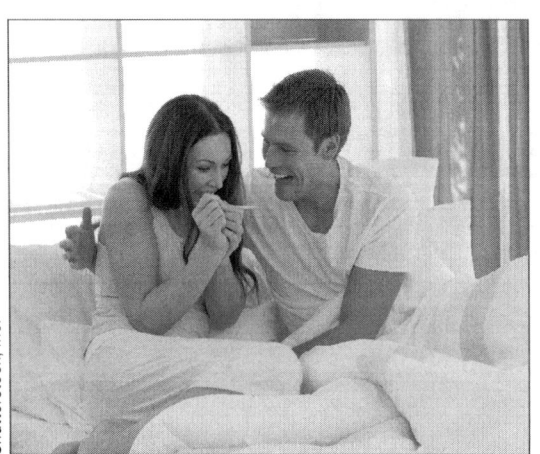
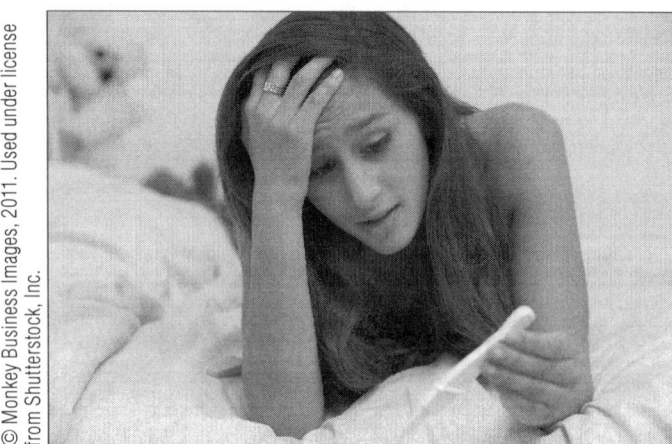

PREGNANCY OUTCOME • BIRTH

Of the 3.3 million intended pregnancies in the United States in 2006, 80 percent resulted in births. Of the 3.1 million unintended pregnancies, 44 percent ended in births (Ventura, Abma, Mosher, & Henshaw, 2009). A baby can be born through the vagina or through the abdomen via a cesarean section. Cesarean delivery involves major abdominal surgery and is associated with higher rates of surgical complications. In 2007, nearly one-third (32%) of all births were cesarean deliveries—the highest rate ever reported in the United States (Menacker & Hamilton, 2010). New Jersey had the highest rate at 38 percent, whereas Utah had the lowest rate at 22 percent.

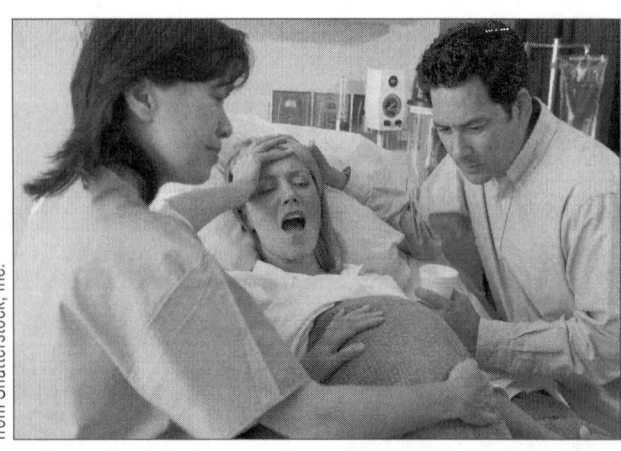
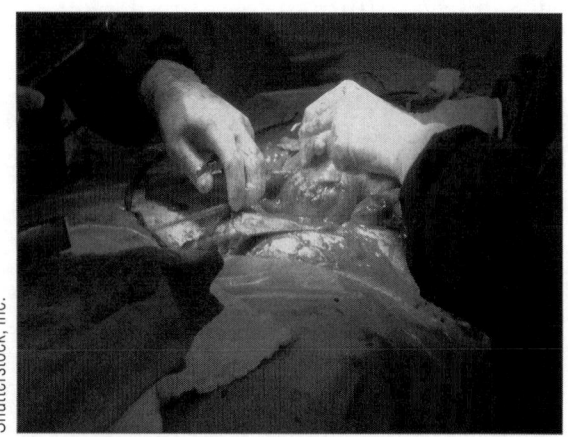

Even though women can request a c-section even if it's not medically necessary, most women have this procedure because of a prior c-section (especially if it occurred less than five years prior), the fetus is not in a head-down position in the uterus during labor, the woman is experiencing a medical emergency, and/or the baby is under fetal distress. Moreover, pregnant women between 40–54 years old are more likely to have a c-section than any other age group (Menacker & Hamilton, 2010).

Age at First Birth

The average age women are giving birth in this country is 25 years old (Martin et al., 2009). In 1970, the average age was 21 years old. In 2006, Asian/Pacific Islander women had the oldest average age at first birth (28.5 years), and American Indian/Alaska Native women had the youngest (21.9 years). Women postpone parenthood for various reasons and more and more women are choosing to give birth for the first time later in life. With the advancements of assisted reproductive technology, many couples are able to begin a family in their 30s, 40s, and even 50s! Keep in mind, though, that any pregnant woman 35 years or older is considered carrying a "high risk" pregnancy due to her age and the increased risk of pregnancy complications and negative outcomes (Brown, 2007).

PREGNANCY OUTCOME • ABORTION

Women do terminate a planned pregnancy, but the number is low and cannot be represented in percentage terms. Of the 3.1 million unintended pregnancies in the United States in 2006, though, 42 percent resulted in abortions (Ventura et al., 2009). The national average rate of abortion is 19.6 per 1,000 women. In 2008, Delaware had the highest rate of abortion (40 per 1,000 women) and Wyoming had the lowest abortion rate, less than 1 per 1,000 women (Jones & Kooistra, 2011). Abortion levels also differed widely by racial or ethnic group. In 2000, the abortion rate was 12 among Caucasian women, 31 among Hispanic women, and 57 among African American women (Jones, Darroch, & Henshaw, 2002). In the United States, 88 percent of abortions occur in the first 12 weeks of pregnancy (Jones & Kooistra, 2011). The remaining 12 percent break down as follows: 6.6 percent of abortions occur during 13–15 weeks of pregnancy, 3.8 percent during weeks 16–20, and 1.5 percent occur at 21 weeks or more (The Alan Guttmacher Institute, 2011).

Medical Abortion

In 2000, the FDA approved mifepristone (also known by the trade name Mifeprex or its original French name, RU-486) for use along with a prostaglandin (a hormone that causes uterine contractions and softens the cervix) for terminating pregnancies up to 49 days from the onset of a woman's last menstrual period (Jones & Henshaw, 2002). These early medication (nonsurgical) abortions accounted for 11 percent of all abortions in 2006 (Pazol et al., 2009). With a medical abortion (meaning a woman ingests and/or a suppository containing the medication is inserted in her vagina), the contents of the pregnancy are expelled

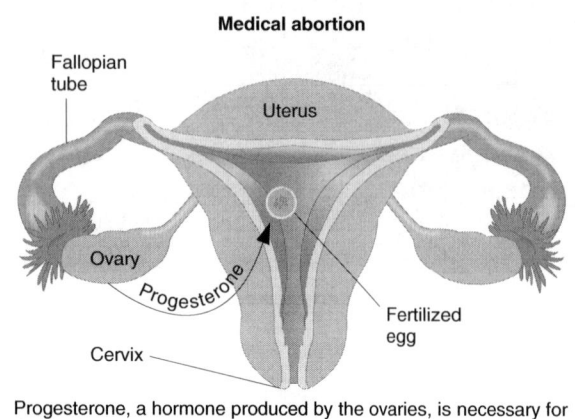

Progesterone, a hormone produced by the ovaries, is necessary for the implantation and development of a fertilized egg.

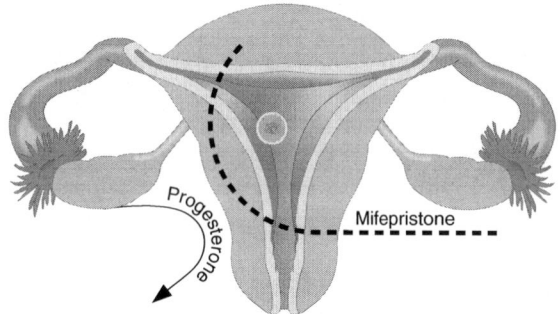

Taken early in pregnancy mifepristone blocks the action of progesterone and makes the body react as if it isn't pregnant.

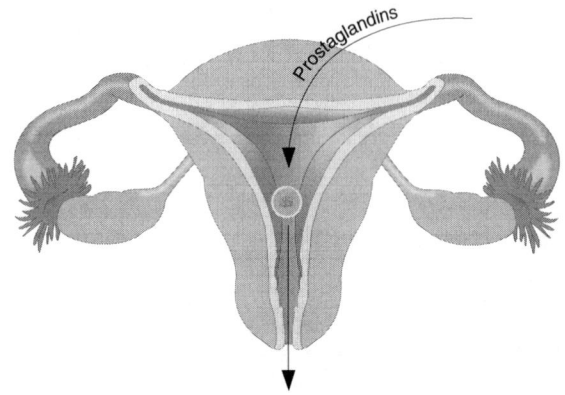

Prostaglandins, taken two days later, cause the uterus to contract and the cervix to soften and dilate. As a result, the fertilized egg is expelled in 97% of the cases.

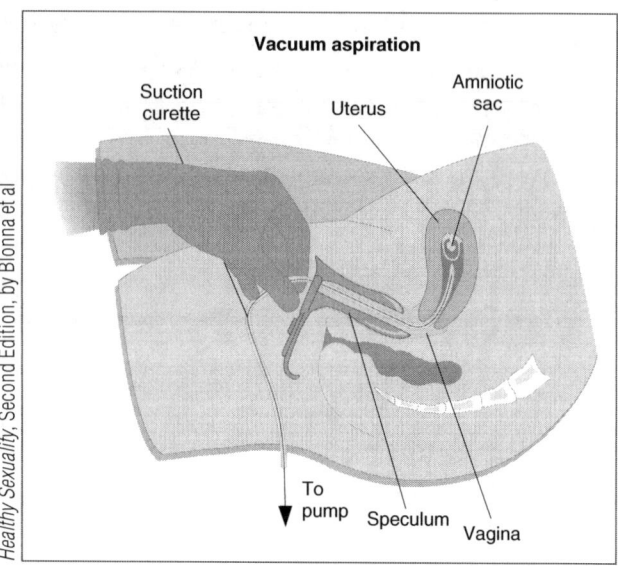

through the vagina two days to two weeks after the ingestion or insertion of the medication.

Surgical Abortion

According to Pazol and colleagues (2009), around 88 percent of abortions were surgically performed by *curettage* (i.e., dilating the cervix and scraping the endometrial lining), along with vacuum or suction aspiration (i.e., removing uterine contents during the first trimester), or dilation and evacuation procedures (i.e., removing uterine contents during the second trimester).

Around the world, Cuba and the Russian Federation have more abortions than births annually (Sedgh, Henshaw, Singh, Bankole, & Drescher, 2007). At current rates, the average Cuban or Russian woman will have more than one abortion in her lifetime. These countries do not have the highest rates of abortion in the world, though. Azerbaijan (AZ-ər-by-JAHN), a former state of the Soviet Union, has the highest rate recently reported for any country at 116 per 100 live births. According to Sedgh and colleagues (2007), women in this country will have an average of three abortions each if current levels prevail throughout their reproductive lives.

The United States has one of the highest rates of abortions when compared to other developed countries (The Alan Guttmacher Institute, 2011). If reducing the number of abortions in this country is a goal, then society needs to concentrate on reducing the number of unintended pregnancies experienced every year. Studies have demonstrated that abortion levels are strongly linked to contraceptive use patterns (Marston & Cleland, 2003).

For example, Brown and colleagues (2008) compiled a list of interrelated factors that contribute to the high rates of unintended pregnancies in the United States. Identified factors were: (1) lack of adequate sex education; (2) general discomfort with sexuality; (3) insidious effects of poverty; (4) improper use of specific contraceptive methods; (5) poor communication between sexual partners; (6) ambivalence about pregnancy; (7) difficulties obtaining access to the most effective contraceptive methods; (8) increased public acceptance of nonmarital childbearing; (9) exaggerated fears about the side effects of certain contraceptive methods; and (10) a culture that glamorizes sex yet rarely portrays it in responsible ways. Thus, increasing access to comprehensive, evidence-based, medically accurate family planning education and contraceptive services can prevent unintended pregnancies. Reducing access to and increasing barriers to abortion services and providers does not prevent the termination of pregnancies, but helping couples get pregnant only when they want to get pregnant will (Cohen, 2006).

PREGNANCY OUTCOME • FETAL LOSS

According to Ventura and colleagues (2009), of the 3.3 million intended pregnancies in the United States in 2006, 20 percent resulted in fetal losses (miscarriage or stillbirth). Of the 3.1 million unintended pregnancies, 14 percent ended in fetal losses.

Miscarriage

A miscarriage is defined as a spontaneous abortion that occurs before the 20th week of pregnancy. Approximately one in four clinically recognized pregnancies ends in miscarriage. It is considered the most common disorder of pregnancy. If miscarriages include a loss that occurs before a positive pregnancy test, then some estimate that 40 percent of all conceptions end in a miscarriage. The risk of miscarriage increases with a woman's age. For example, 30–50 percent of women over the age of 40 will miscarry whereas 7–15 percent of women under the age of 30 will experience such a loss.

Even though there is a variety of reasons (biological and environmental) why a miscarriage occurs, more than one half of all miscarriages that happen during the first trimester are a result of chromosomal abnormalities affecting the fetus (Jones & Lopez, 2006). Miscarriages that transpire during the second trimester result from an incompetent (i.e., weak) cervix that cannot hold the weight of the pregnancy. To decrease the chance of a miscarriage due to an incompetent cervix, the American Pregnancy Association recommends women consider having their cervix sewn during the pregnancy. This is called a *cervical cerclage* (sir-klahj). A doctor stitches a band of strong thread around the cervix, and the thread will be tightened to hold the cervix firmly closed for the remainder of the pregnancy. The thread is removed at the 37th week of pregnancy, but it can be removed earlier in the pregnancy if a woman's water breaks or contractions start. Moreover, most women who need a cerclage in one pregnancy will need to have one in future pregnancies. Unfortunately, it is difficult to detect a weak cervix without knowledge of prior trauma (such as procedures to eliminate cervical dysplasia, cervical cancer, or previous second-trimester miscarriages).

Stillbirth

A *stillbirth* is defined as a fetal death occurring after 20 weeks of pregnancy. Unlike miscarriage, which is more common, a stillbirth occurs in 1 out of 160 pregnancies (ACOG, 2009). The most prevalent risk factors in women associated with this tragic event is being African American, being over the age of 35, no previous births, and having a body mass index (BMI) over 30. Other risk factors related to those listed above include chromosomal abnormalities affecting the fetus, multiple pregnancies, diabetes, hypertension, preeclampsia, syphilis, and smoking (McClure, Nalubamba-Phiri, & Goldenberg, 2006).

A SPERM'S JOURNEY FOR THAT "GOLDEN" EGG!

Given the amount of unintended pregnancies experienced in the United States every year, one might think that getting pregnant is an easy task. After ejaculation, it can take 75 minutes for the sperm to reach the outer portion of the fallopian tubes (Gilbert & Harmon, 2002). That's pretty impressive, but many factors have to be in line for that one sperm to be successful in its mission. Any sperm making the journey into a woman's reproductive tract has a difficult road ahead!

When a man ejaculates into a woman's vagina (and remember that an average ejaculation can carry around 200 million sperm), the sperm have to make it through the acidic environment of the vagina to the cervix (Jones & Lopez, 2006). Over 99 percent of sperm *do not* survive their journey through the vagina. Around 1 million sperm make it to the cervix from the vagina. At the cervix, the sperm can only hope a woman is close to ovulating or recently has, thus ensuring that their journey through the cervix is not blocked by cervical mucus. When ovulation occurs, the cervical mucus becomes more hospitable to sperm to improve chances of survival and ease of passage. Yet, the cervix has numerous crevasses that sperm find it difficult to escape. From there, the 1,000 sperm that survive the cervix now have to swim their way through the uterus. When the sperm reach the uterus, the uterus activates an upsurge of white blood cells (cells of the immune system involved in defending the body against both infectious disease and foreign materials). These cells begin to engulf any sperm that have not made their way to the fallopian tubes. Approximately 200–500 sperm make it to the fallopian tubes from the uterus. Some swim to the fallopian tube that does not contain an oocyte, while around 20–200 make it to the egg (Jones & Lopez, 2006). So from a starting point of almost 200 million sperm, less than 1 percent will actually have a chance of fertilizing an egg—against all odds, though, only one is needed!

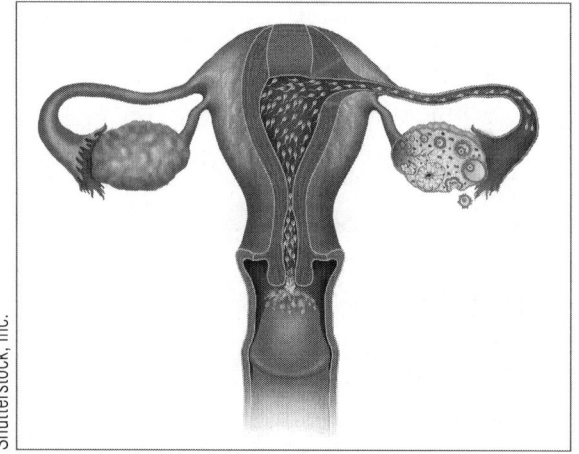

The sperm and egg unite in one of the fallopian tubes to form a one-celled entity called a *zygote*. Fertilization (or conception) must take place near the fimbriae of the fallopian tube. The process of fertilization can take 1–2 days to occur. If fertilization is successful, the zygote is pushed toward the uterus by the cilia of the fallopian tube. The zygote has 46 chromosomes—23 from the mother and 23 from the father. These chromosomes determine the fetus' sex and traits, such as eye and hair color. The zygote begins to divide rapidly, forming a cluster of cells resembling a tiny raspberry as it journeys through the fallopian tube to the uterus (Jones & Lopez, 2006).

Six to seven days after fertilization, this new cell mass is around 100 cells and is called a *blastocyst*. The inner cell mass becomes the embryo and the outer portion of cells becomes the placenta, umbilical cord, and amniotic sac. Implantation in the endometrial lining can only occur at this stage of development (Heffner & Schust, 2006). Time is of the essence! Depending on the length of a woman's menstrual cycle, she may only have days from menstruating. If the blastocyst does not burrow in the endometrial lining and "hijack" the woman's menstrual cycle, the fertilized egg is sloughed off with the rest of the endometrium (Wilcox, Baird, & Weinberg, 1999). The woman will never know that a pregnancy was imminent.

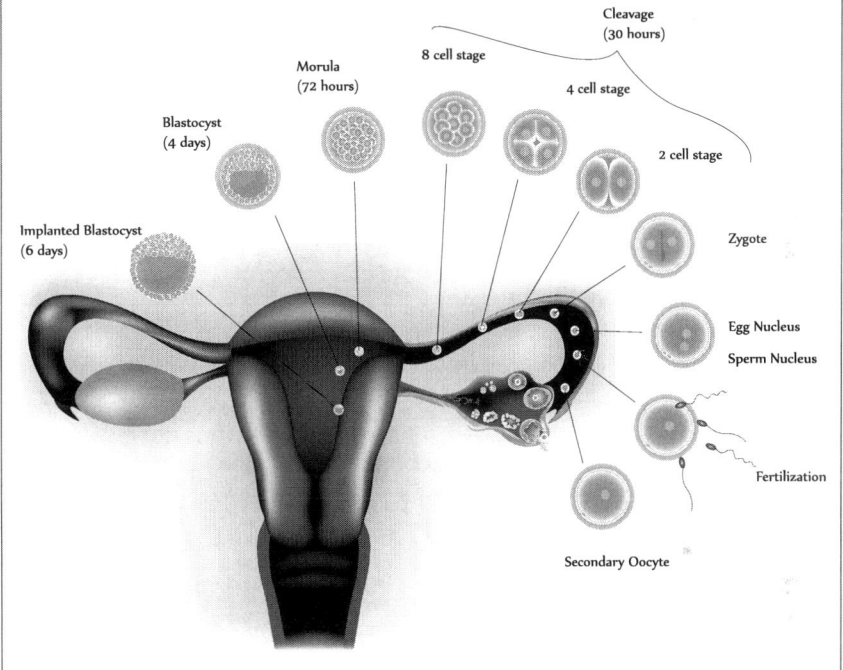

PLANNING A PREGNANCY

There is no reason why couples who want to get pregnant cannot plan the pregnancy to improve their chances of a healthy pregnancy and birth outcome. If a couple is seriously contemplating becoming parents, then what can they do besides participate in unprotected coitus? First of all, the couple should discuss when they want to have

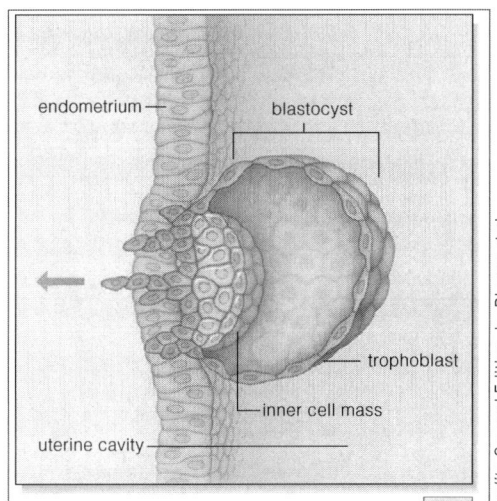

f DAYS 6–7. The blastocyst attaches to the endometrium and starts burrowing into it. Implantation is under way.

actual size

Chapter Eleven **195**

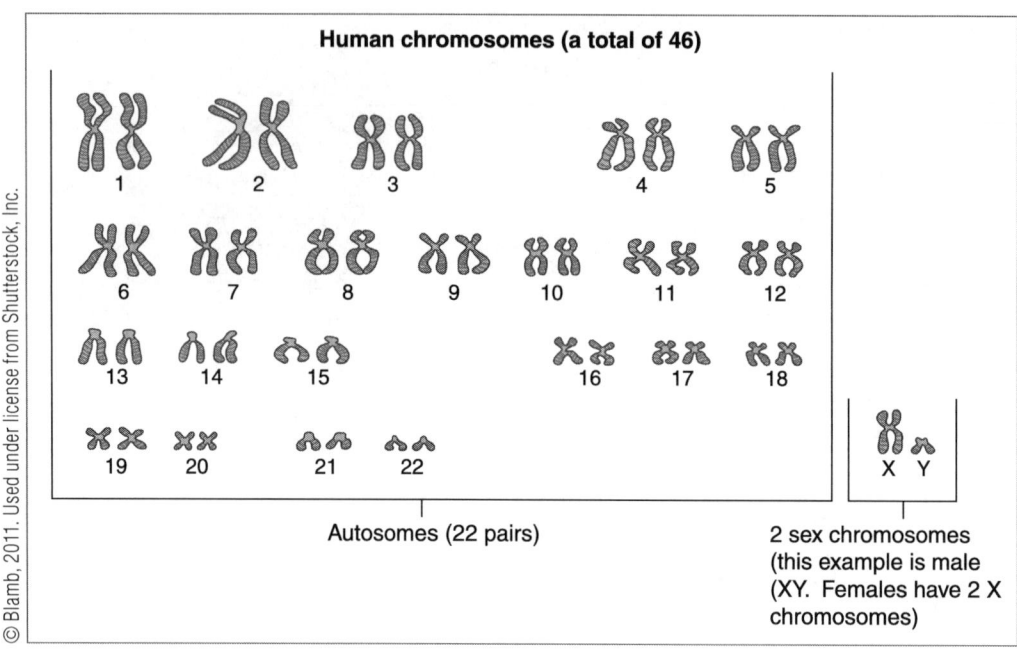

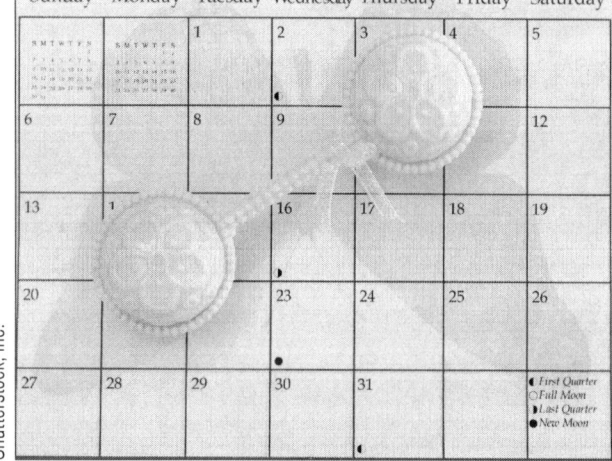

the baby born. If it is September and they were hoping for a May baby, well, that's not going to happen. A couple should begin planning a pregnancy a year *before* the planned birth.

A woman needs to stop any hormonal method that was preventing her from getting pregnant at least three months before initiating unprotected coitus. One reason is to give her body enough time to orchestrate a menstrual cycle of its own to help determine the days a woman is close to ovulating.

Also, women need to consider taking a prenatal vitamin daily at least three months before participating in unprotected coitus. Why? Well, when do women usually find out they are pregnant? If they were planning the pregnancy, it might be weeks into it, if it was unintended, they might not realize (or be in denial) that they are pregnant until months into it.

Taking prenatal vitamins before a pregnancy helps ensure that when a woman does find out she is pregnant, the embryo or fetus has been receiving the nutrients needed from the mother. Moreover, folic acid taken before pregnancy and for the first three months of pregnancy can reduce the risk of neural tube defects (Mosley et al., 2009).

196 Conception, Pregnancy, & Outcomes

HORMONAL SURGE

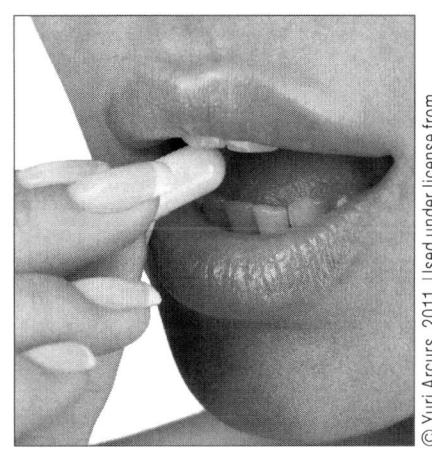

After ovulation, the *corpus luteum* (the disintegrating follicle that contained the ovum) increases the production of estrogen and progesterone to maintain a receptive uterine lining for the expected blastocyst (Gilbert & Harmon, 2002). When a pregnancy is established (meaning the blastocyst has burrowed into the uterine lining), the woman's body begins producing large quantities of estrogen, progesterone, and human chorionic gonadotropin (hCG) to help the pregnancy continue. Pregnant women will make more estrogen in nine months than a woman who never is pregnant will make in her entire lifetime! Pregnant women will also produce eight times the amount of progesterone that nonpregnant women produce (Bonillas & Feehan, 2008). Review Table 11.1 for changes that can occur during a pregnancy because of these hormones.

Table 11.1 INTERNAL AND EXTERNAL PHYSICAL CHANGES DURING PREGNANCY

First Trimester Weeks 1–13	Explanation for Change
Missed period	Hormones secreted by the blastocyst (after burrowing into the endometrial lining) take control of the menstrual cycle.
Nausea and vomiting	Due to rapidly increasing levels of the hormone human chorionic gonadotropin (hCG). Nausea tends to peak around the same time as levels of hCG rise.
Sensitivity to odors	Due to high levels of the hormone estrogen.
Fatigue	Due to higher levels of the hormone progesterone so the body can focus its energy on sustaining the pregnancy.
Breast enlargement	Due to increased levels of estrogen, the mammary glands begin to enlarge in preparation for breastfeeding.
Breast tenderness	The enlargement of the mammary glands make the breasts become tender.
Areola darkening	The pigmented areas around each breast darkens due to the increased levels of progesterone and estrogen (and believed to help the newborn find the breast at birth).
Areola size increase	Due to increased hormone levels (and believed to help the newborn find the breast at birth).
Mood swings	Partly due to surges in hormones—characterized by change in emotional stability and irritability.
Expanding uterus	The placenta produces progesterone, which relaxes the muscles of the uterus so they can stretch as the pregnancy progresses.

Table 11.1   INTERNAL AND EXTERNAL PHYSICAL CHANGES DURING PREGNANCY (CONTINUED)

Second Trimester Weeks 14–27	Explanation for Change
Slower digestion	High levels of progesterone slow down the contractions of the esophagus and intestines, thus slowing down digestion.
Constipation	Due to slower digestion.
Hemorrhoids	Due to constipation.
Heartburn	The placenta produces progesterone, which relaxes the valve that separates the esophagus from the stomach, allowing gastric acids to seep back up and cause an unpleasant burning sensation.
Backaches	Due to the expanding uterus affecting posture.
Pinching of sciatic nerve	Nerve in the hip/buttock area gets pinched because of pressure exerted on it by the expanding uterus.
Facial skin darkening	Due to hormonal changes.
Increased urination frequency	Due to increased blood flow to the kidneys and pressure from the weight of the pregnancy on the bladder.
Edema	Swelling of the ankles, hands, and face due to fluid retention.
Expanding uterus	Due to progesterone, which in turn relaxes the muscles of the uterus so they can stretch as the pregnancy progresses.
Abdominal enlargement	Due to the progression of the pregnancy, the uterus expands into the abdominal cavity.
Blood volume increase	Due to the need for extra blood to flow to the uterus.
Heart growth	Due to the body needing to supply more blood for the growing fetus and placenta.
Quickening	Feeling fetal movements for the first time.
Stretch marks	Due to the expanding abdomen, breasts, legs, buttocks. Stretch marks occur when the dermis, the middle layer of skin, is stretched to a point where its elasticity begins to break down.
Sweating	Due to hormonal changes, increased effort of physical activities due to the expanding uterus, and the fetus causes the body to radiate heat.
Sleeping difficulties	Due to fetal movements or frequent urination at night.
Leukorrhea	Higher levels of estrogen increase blood flow to the vagina, which increases the release of a white-colored odorless vaginal discharge (sign of a healthy vagina).

Table 11.1 INTERNAL AND EXTERNAL PHYSICAL CHANGES DURING PREGNANCY (CONTINUED)

Second Trimester Weeks 14–27	Explanation for Change
Hair growth	Due to hormone stimulation of hair follicles on the head, arms, legs, and face.
Dry, itchy skin	Particularly on the abdomen as the skin continues to grow and stretch due to the expanding uterus.
Linea nigra	A dark line running from the pubic bone up the center of the abdomen to the ribs which is caused by the increase in hormones.

Third Trimester Weeks 28–40	Explanation for Change
Heart turns on its side	Creates room for expanding uterus, which pushes other organs up.
Varicose veins	Swollen/bluish veins may bulge near the surface of the skin, usually behind the legs. As the uterus grows, it puts pressure on the large vein on the right side of the body, which increases pressure on the veins in the legs, making the veins swell from the extra pressure to return the blood from the extremities to the heart (as they work against gravity).
Heartburn	The growing fetus crowds the abdominal cavity, pushing the stomach acids back up into the esophagus.
Hemorrhoids	Due to constipation.
Leg cramps	Believed to be due to lack of calcium in the body.
Shortness of breath	Due to the expanding uterus pushing up against the diaphragm.
Braxton-Hicks contractions	Usually painless uterine contractions that help the uterus prepare for labor.
Increased urination frequency	Due to increased blood flow to the kidneys and pressure from the weight of the pregnancy on the bladder.
Stretch marks	Due to the expanding abdomen, breasts, thighs, and buttocks.
Dry, itchy skin	Particularly on the abdomen as the skin continues to grow and stretch due to the expanding uterus.
Navel protrusion	Due to the expanding abdominal cavity.
Colostrum	Yellow, watery fluid produced by the mammary glands. Colostrum contains large amounts of antibodies that protect the mucous membranes in the throat, lungs, and intestines of the infant. White blood cells are also present in large numbers and protect infant from harmful bacteria and viruses. Beneficial bacteria are also established in the digestive tract of an infant when colostrum is ingested.

Table 11.1	INTERNAL AND EXTERNAL PHYSICAL CHANGES DURING PREGNANCY (CONTINUED)
Third Trimester Weeks 28–40	**Explanation for Change**
Increased estrogen	A pregnant woman will have more estrogen in her body during the nine months of pregnancy than a woman who never gets pregnant will have in her entire lifetime.
Increased progesterone	By the end of the pregnancy, levels of this hormone will increase to 7 times its normal levels.

Source: Republished with permission of Lamaze International from "Tools for Teaching: Normalizing the Changes Experienced During Each Trimester of Pregnancy" by C. Bonillas and R. Feehan, in *Journal of Perinatal Education*, 2008, 17, 39-43. Permission conveyed through Copyright Clearance Center, Inc.

CALCULATING A DUE DATE

The medical community counts the duration of a pregnancy beginning from the first day of the last menstrual period to 40 weeks in the future. At that last menstrual period, the woman hadn't even participated in coitus that resulted in fertilization. Depending on the length of a woman's menstrual cycle, the dating of a pregnancy is measured beginning 1–3 weeks before ovulation. This practice, though, is convenient because it is easy to determine when the last menstrual period was, while both fertilization and implantation can only be hypothesized.

TRIMESTERS

According to the American Congress of Obstetricians and Gynecologists (ACOG, 2010), the 40 weeks (around 280 days) of pregnancy are divided into three trimesters. Each trimester lasts about 12–13 weeks each (or about three months). The first trimester is considered weeks 0–13 (or months 1–3), the second trimester is weeks 14–27 (months 4–6), and the third trimester is deemed to be weeks 28–40 (months 7–9).

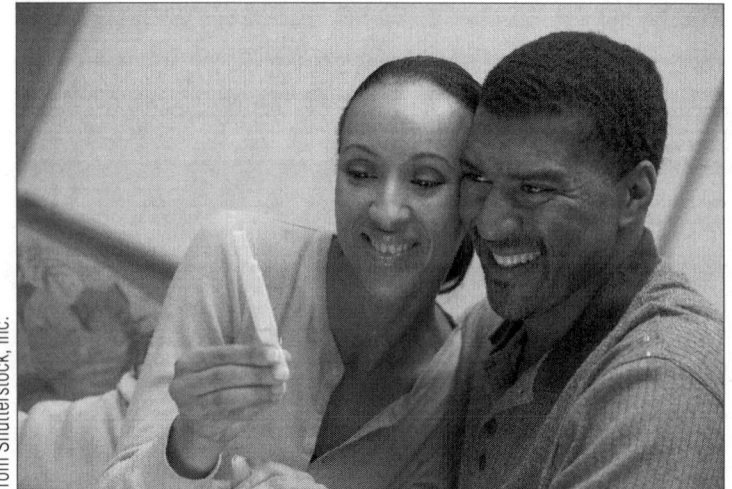

First Trimester

Finding out you or your partner is pregnant is always a surprise even if the pregnancy was planned! As exciting as being pregnant (or having a partner who's pregnant) is, it is strongly recommended that a pregnancy be kept a secret during the first trimester. Losing a pregnancy during the first three months of pregnancy is likely, regardless of the health of the woman (Gilbert & Harmon, 2002). Because of this, it is best to wait until the 14th week of pregnancy to let everyone in on the wonderful surprise.

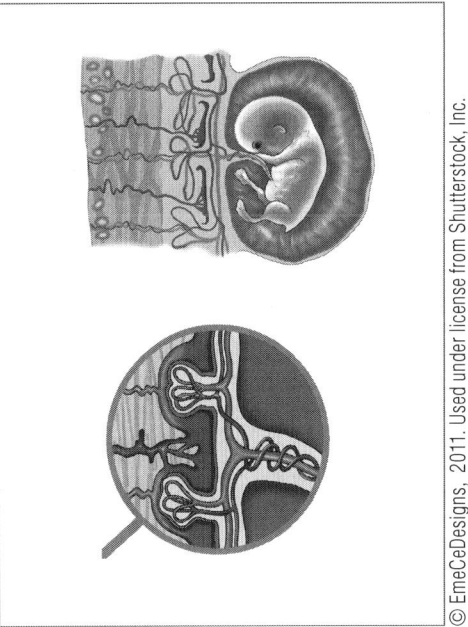

Most women will not see a difference in the size of their abdomen at this time, but they might with their breast size! Many women experience certain symptoms that imply a pregnancy has occurred. Most obvious is that every pregnant woman stops menstruating. Hormonal changes during pregnancy cease the endometrial lining from growing. Moreover, the cervix creates a mucous plug that prevents passage to the uterus. Thus, withdrawal bleeding similar to menstruation is not possible during pregnancy. If a woman is bleeding, that might indicate bleeding from the vagina or cervix, but endometrial bleeding is rare (Gilbert & Harmon, 2002). Around 80 percent of women experience nausea and/or vomiting. This is a good thing! For most women, the nausea and/or vomiting are side effects to the upsurge in certain hormones that help sustain the pregnancy. Table 11.1 also lists the internal and external physical changes women may experience during pregnancy (compiled by Bonillas and Feehan [2008]).

When a pregnancy occurs, a woman's body is no longer her own. She has now become the "host" to this pregnancy. If the fetus is in need of calcium, for example, and the mother is not providing sufficient nutrients via the placenta, fetal cells travel through the placenta to a woman's calcium supply (i.e., her bones) to obtain what they need! Thus, establishing healthy eating habits before and during pregnancy is of utmost importance to ensure optimal nutrition is provided to the fetus and the mother.

Embryo Development

According to ACOG (2010), the embryonic period begins around three weeks after conception occurred and lasts until the end of the eighth week of gestation. The placenta has not fully developed during this stage. The embryo creates a yolk sac that provides nourishment until the placenta is capable of that responsibility. The embryo's brain, spinal cord, heart, and other organs begin to form during the first trimester. At the gestational age of three weeks, the embryo is around the size of the tip of a pen! Five weeks after conception the embryo is a

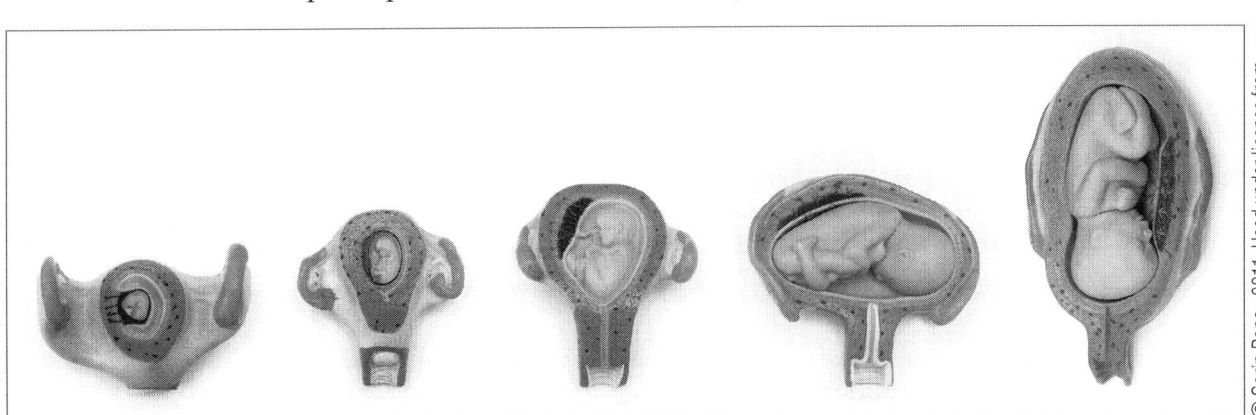

little bigger than the top of a pencil eraser. By the end of this stage, the embryo is now a whopping one-half inch long!

Second Trimester

Don't be shy about sharing the great news with anyone and everyone! Of course, some people probably have suspected something, especially if the woman was running to the bathroom all the time (to vomit or to urinate) or craving uncommon foods, such as liver (which probably means she is low in iron). Most women's abdomens start to protrude during this trimester. That means most of her clothes will feel tight. By 14–16 weeks into the pregnancy, the placenta assumes the responsibility for maintenance of the pregnancy by delivering oxygen and nutrients and producing the necessary hormones (Gilbert & Harmon, 2002). Along with estrogen, progesterone, and hCG, the placenta produces human placental lactogen (hPL). This hormone helps break down fats in the pregnant woman to provide fuel to the developing fetus. Elevated levels of this hormone may lead to insulin resistance and carbohydrate intolerance in the pregnant woman, which increases the risk of gestational diabetes mellitus (GDM). As discussed later in this chapter, healthy eating habits (i.e., eating nutrient-dense foods over calorie-dense/low-nutrient-dense foods) throughout the pregnancy provide the fetus and the mother with the needed nutrients.

Fetal Development

According to ACOG (2010), the fetal period begins around the ninth week of gestation and lasts until birth. At this stage, the fetus has functioning organs, nerves, and muscles. Tissue that becomes bone develops around the fetal head and within the arms and legs. Fat begins to accumulate under the skin around the 17th week. Around the 24th week, the uterus and ovaries are in place in a female fetus. The ovaries are filled with 5 million immature ovarian follicles (Jones & Lopez, 2006). For a male fetus, the testes are beginning to descend from the abdomen to the outside of the body. By the end of the second trimester, the fetus will be around nine inches long and weigh nearly two pounds.

Third Trimester

During the last three months of the pregnancy it is hard to deny that a woman is pregnant! There are women, though, especially if they are obese, who do not "show" at all. By the end of the pregnancy, the uterus has expanded to around 40 inches! As it expands, it moves a woman's organs out of the way to make room for itself. The uterus does not actually grow. The uterus stretches to accommodate the growing fetus, placenta, and amniotic fluid. For many women, their breasts increase at least one cup size during the pregnancy. Their shoe size also increases, as does the width of their feet. Fluid retention is normal in the hands and feet, but if it is felt suddenly (instead of a gradual increase over days or weeks), this warrants a call to the doctor to confirm it is not *preeclampsia* (a medical condition in which high blood pressure rises in pregnancy).

Many couples prepare for the upcoming arrival of their baby by participating in birthing classes, touring the hospital or birthing center where they will deliver, packing a bag for the mother and baby, having an infant car seat if leaving the hospital or birthing center by car (the medical staff does not allow a newborn in a car without an infant car seat), and having at least a crib waiting for the baby's homecoming.

Fetal Development

At this stage, the fetus is busy gaining weight—about one-half pound a week during the last month. The lungs are the last organ to develop. From 38–40 weeks gestation, the fetus is around 14 inches long and weighs about 7½ pounds.

Sexual Activity During Pregnancy

For most couples, sexual activity can continue as it did before the pregnancy was established. During the first trimester, a woman does not have to feel constrained in any way in regard to coital position or experiencing an orgasm. Women can feel free to engage in sexual activities they are comfortable with. Many times their sexual partners find the pregnant body sensual and amazing to experience during sexual activity. A woman cannot lie on her back during any sexual activity after her fourth month of pregnancy. As the uterus expands, the creativity in sexual activities also needs to progress to find positions comfortable for the woman. Experimenting with different coital positions after the fourth month of pregnancy, such as "woman on top" or "rear-entry," helps continue sexual activity. Remember that the fetus is surrounded by water and thus protected from movements or thrusting that may occur. Of course, coitus is not the only type of sexual activity that is possible and the couple needs to think outside the box during this time.

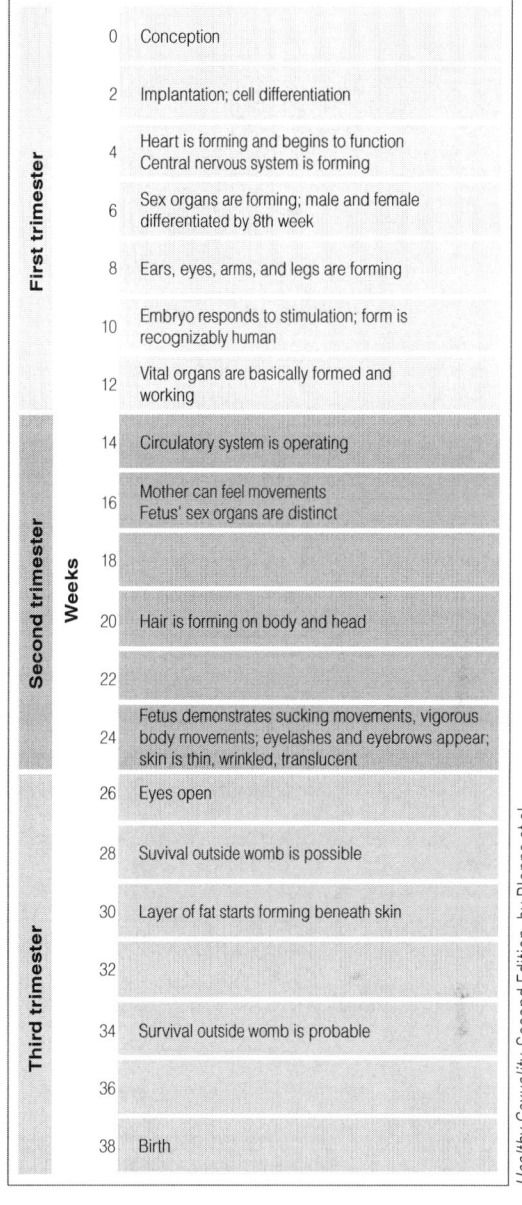

	Weeks	Fetal development
First trimester	0	Conception
	2	Implantation; cell differentiation
	4	Heart is forming and begins to function. Central nervous system is forming
	6	Sex organs are forming; male and female differentiated by 8th week
	8	Ears, eyes, arms, and legs are forming
	10	Embryo responds to stimulation; form is recognizably human
	12	Vital organs are basically formed and working
Second trimester	14	Circulatory system is operating
	16	Mother can feel movements. Fetus' sex organs are distinct
	18	
	20	Hair is forming on body and head
	22	
	24	Fetus demonstrates sucking movements, vigorous body movements; eyelashes and eyebrows appear; skin is thin, wrinkled, translucent
	26	Eyes open
Third trimester	28	Survival outside womb is possible
	30	Layer of fat starts forming beneath skin
	32	
	34	Survival outside womb is probable
	36	
	38	Birth

Healthy Sexuality, Second Edition, by Blonna et al

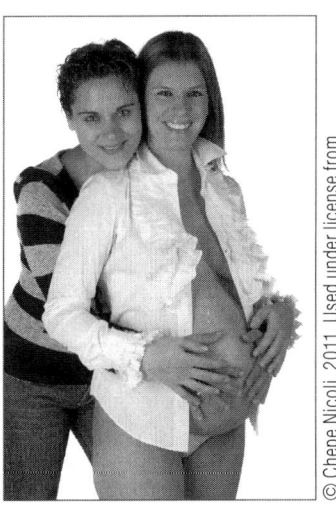
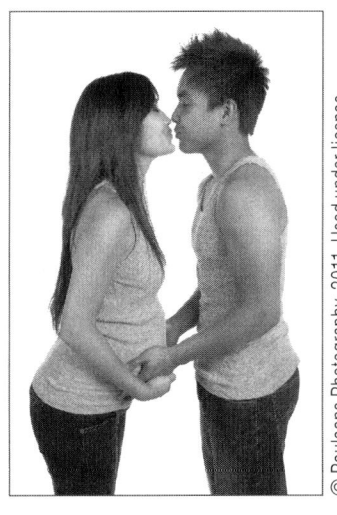
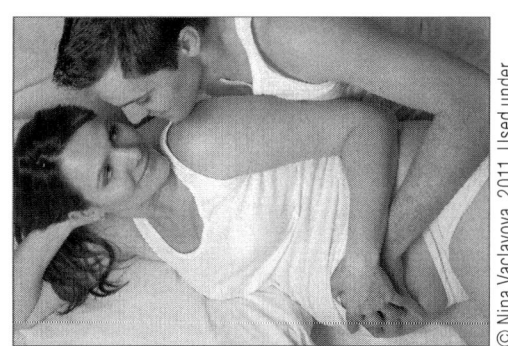

As discussed in chapter 6, oxytocin, our antistress hormone, is produced in humans when we are physically close to each other and it is made in abundance when we orgasm. Unless otherwise recommended by her doctor, there is no reason why a woman should not indulge in experiencing orgasm throughout her pregnancy! Moreover, remember that in chapter 4, it was explained that the middle layer of the uterus, the myometrium, contracts during orgasm. Imagine a woman having an orgasm with a uterus that has expanded to 40 inches. Now *that's* an orgasm!

Reasons to Abstain from Sexual Activity During Pregnancy

If bleeding is an issue during pregnancy, then a woman needs to see her doctor to identify the cause and solution and discontinue participating in any sexual activity (alone or with a partner). Moreover, if a woman has experienced a first trimester miscarriage, she may also be advised against sexual activity (and orgasm) during the first trimester. For women who have experienced premature labor in the past (or during the current pregnancy), sexual abstinence (and orgasm) may be necessary during the whole pregnancy. If a woman is starting a new sexual relationship during her pregnancy, then consistent condom use is strongly recommended to reduce the risk of exposing herself and the pregnancy to STIs (discussed in chapter 7).

LABOR AND BIRTH

The majority of women do not deliver on their due date (only around 10 percent do). If labor is not induced for any reason, most women give birth between two weeks before or two weeks after their due date. A woman delivering "at term" is defined giving birth between 37–42 weeks gestation. Most women are not allowed to carry a pregnancy past 42 weeks because the placenta starts to disintegrate, which places the fetus at risk of death (ACOG, 2010). A premature delivery is giving birth before 37 weeks' gestation.

First Stage of Labor

This stage begins when uterine contractions are consistent and can be timed every 5–20 minutes. The purpose of these contractions is not to push the baby out but to open the cervix to allow the woman to push the baby out during the second stage of labor. Levels of oxytocin and prostaglandins increase in women during labor. Oxytocin has been found to improve the uterus' ability to contract during labor and prostaglandins help the cervix become softer and shorter (Gilbert & Harmon, 2002). Many women describe the contractions as menstrual cramps that progressively increase in intensity and duration. This stage ends when the cervix is completely *effaced* (i.e., thinned out) and *dilated* (i.e., opened up) to 10 cm (around 4 inches).

This is the longest stage and is broken into three phases. The early labor phase begins at the onset of labor until the cervix is effaced and dilated to 3 cm. The active labor phase continues until the cervix is 100 percent effaced (completely thinned out) and 7 cm dilated. It is during the active labor phase that women can request pain relievers, such as an epidural. During this stage, the mucous plug dislodges and the amniotic sac may rupture. On average, the first stage of labor lasts around 10–16 hours. Just as every pregnancy can be experienced differently, so can every labor. Some women end this stage after 3 hours, other women take 24 hours or longer. Many women experience a shorter first stage of labor in subsequent pregnancies. The transition phase continues until the cervix is fully dilated to 10 cm.

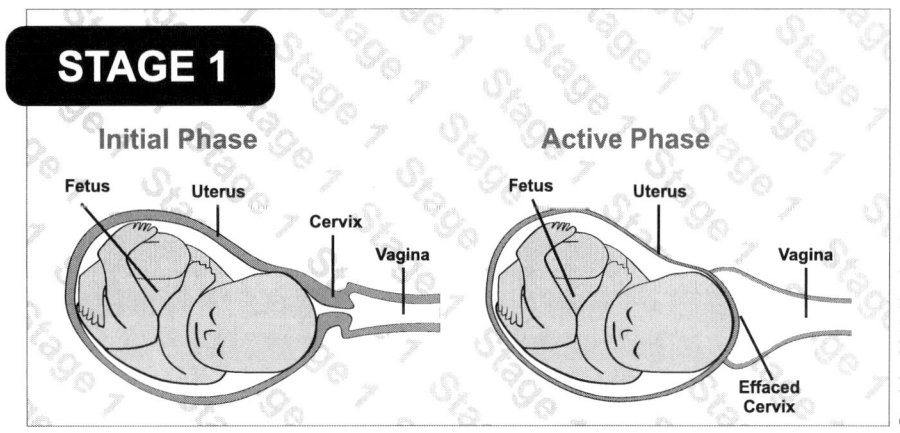

Second Stage of Labor

This stage begins when the cervix has dilated to 10 cm and it is time for the mother to push. On average, the second stage of labor lasts around 30 minutes to two hours. This stage ends at the delivery of the baby.

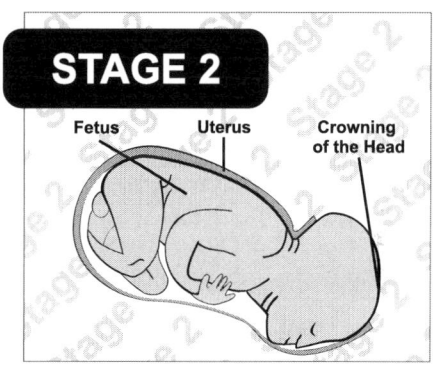

Third Stage of Labor

This stage begins when the baby has been delivered. On average, the third and final stage of labor occurs up to 30 minutes after birth. This stage ends at the delivery of the placenta.

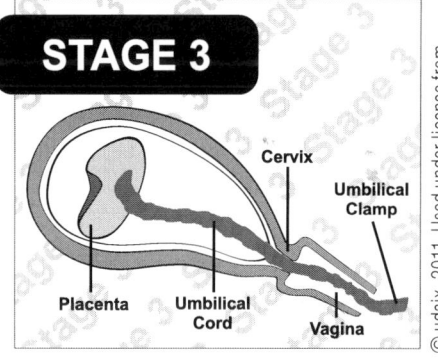

CAN PARTICIPATING IN COITUS TRIGGER LABOR?

Some of you may have heard that doctors (or well-read family and friends) sometimes tell pregnant women to participate in coitus to stimulate the uterus to start the labor process. How can coitus possibly cause labor? According to Jones and Lopez (2006), two gynecologists discovered in 1930 that seminal fluid contains a substance that causes the uterus to contract. This substance was later named prostaglandin because it was believed to be secreted by the prostate gland into the semen. It is now known that the seminal vesicles, not the prostate gland, are the major sources of prostaglandins in

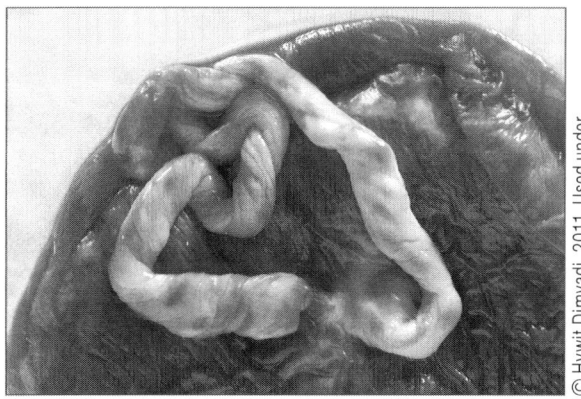

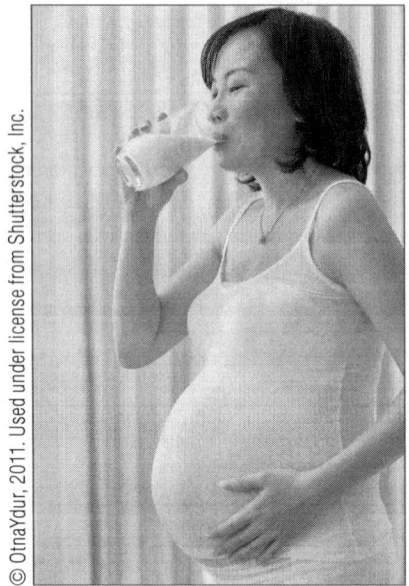
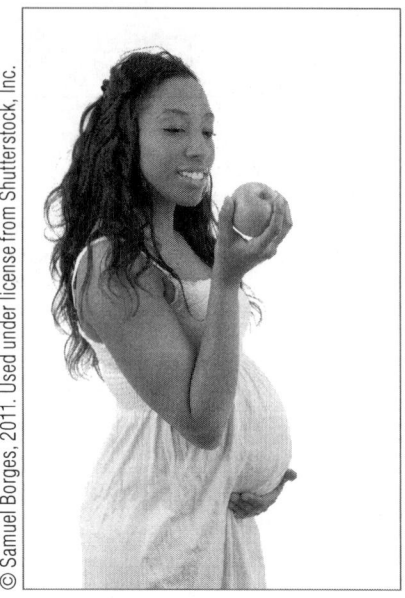

semen. Remember that the seminal vesicles produce around 70 percent of the seminal fluid. So if you ever meet a pregnant woman who is at least 38 weeks pregnant and can't wait to give birth (and has a male partner), tell her to participate in coitus to help her go into labor!

HAVING A HEALTHY PREGNANCY

Prenatal Nutrition

One of the few times that a woman purposely gains weight is during pregnancy (O'Toole, Sawicki, & Artal, 2003). Extra energy is required during pregnancy for the growth and maintenance of the fetus, placenta, and maternal tissues (IOM, 1990; Rasmussen & Yaktine, 2009). The fetus is a continuous feeder, whereas the mother is a periodic feeder (Gilbert & Harmon, 2002). A woman's dietary intake during pregnancy affects fetal growth and development. But just because a woman is gaining gestational weight does not mean she is providing the nutrients needed by her body and the fetus to achieve an optimal birth weight and pregnancy outcome (Stotland et al., 2005).

Seiga-Riz and colleagues (2002) found that pregnant women were more likely to compromise their nutrient intake by drinking soft drinks over more nutrient-dense beverages, such as milk. High-fat diets, specifically high-fat animal products, were also common. These findings follow the trend in the expansion of fast food restaurants, both in number and in nontraditional locations, such as gasoline stations, department stores, and even hospitals (Morland, Wing, & Diez, 2002). The traditional menus (e.g., soft drink, French fries, and hamburger) are high in fat and low in nutrient density, which increase the risk of obesity, particularly with the trend in supersizing these low-cost meals. Diets high in fat and empty calories need to be of concern for pregnant women given a tendency to gain weight above the weight gain recommendation and lack of nutrient-dense foods needed to achieve a healthy pregnancy (Davis, Zysanski, Olson, Stange, & Horowitz, 2009).

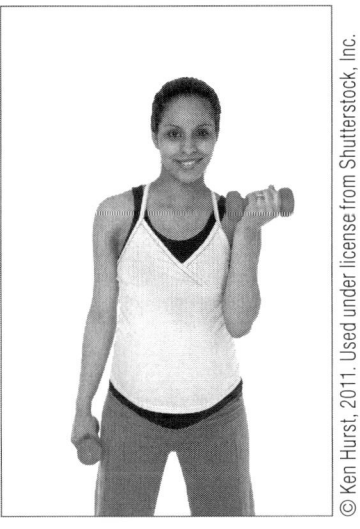
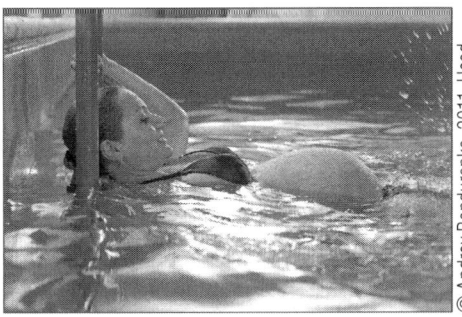
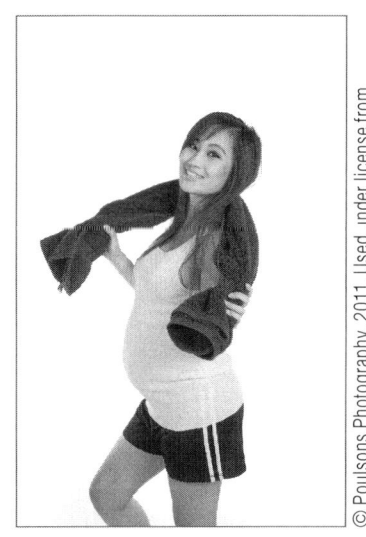

Physical Activity During Pregnancy

In 2002, ACOG concluded that exercise during pregnancy may provide additional health benefits to women (ACOG, 2002). The ACOG guidelines for exercise during pregnancy state that "in the absence of either medical or obstetric complications, 30 minutes or more of moderate exercise a day on most, if not all, days of the week is recommended for pregnant women" (p. 171). Recommended prenatal exercises include swimming, walking, and yoga (American College of Sports Medicine, 2000).

Weight Gain During Pregnancy

In 1990, the Institute of Medicine (IOM) issued guidelines for weight gain during pregnancy (IOM, 1990). These guidelines have recently been revised because of changing weight patterns among women in the United States and because the 1990 pregnancy guidelines did not offer specific advice for obese women (Rasmussen & Yaktine, 2009). A woman with a normal body mass index (BMI) of 18.5–24.9 is advised to gain between 25–35 pounds during a pregnancy. A woman considered overweight (BMI of 25.0–29.9) is advised to gain between 15–25 pounds during a pregnancy. An obese woman (BMI ≥30.0) is counseled to limit her gestational weight gain to 11–20 pounds (Expert Panel on the Identification, Evaluation, and Treatment of Overweight in Adults, 1998; Rasmussen & Yaktine, 2009).

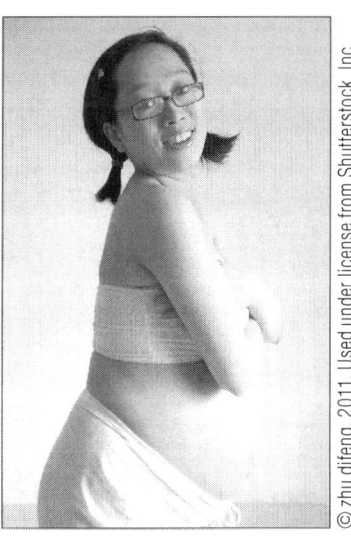

Where is this extra weight going? The March of Dimes created a list, provided in Table 11.2, that describes how the weight is distributed. Women vary, though, in how much they gain and where that extra weight ends up, especially with the size of the baby and how much extra fat they have gained during the pregnancy.

Where You Gain the Weight

The average BMI is increasing among all age categories, and women are entering pregnancy at higher weights (Ogden et al., 2006; Siega-Riz, Siega-Riz, & Laraia, 2006). Currently one in five women is obese

Table 11.2 GESTATIONAL WEIGHT GAIN

Baby	7½ lbs
Fat and proteins	7 lbs
Retained water	4 lbs
Blood	3 lbs
Amniotic fluid	2 lbs
Breasts	2 lbs
Uterus	2 lbs
Placenta	1½ lbs
TOTAL	**29 lbs**

at the beginning of pregnancy (Kim, Dietz, England, Morrow, & Callaghan., 2007). Moreover, overweight and obese women are more likely to gain excessive weight during their pregnancy and are less likely to lose it after delivery (Olson, Strawderman, Hinton, & Pearson, 2003).

Maternal obesity during pregnancy has been connected to such complications as cesarean delivery (Myles, Gooch, & Santolaya, 2002), gestational hypertension (Yogev & Visser, 2009), preeclampsia (Robinson, O'Connell, Joseph, & McLeod, 2005), GDM (Rosenn, 2008), and macrosomia (Murphy et al., 2008). Obesity during pregnancy is also associated with greater use of health care services and longer hospital stay (Chu et al., 2008). Interestingly, a recent study found that more than half of all obstetricians consider their training on weight management as "inadequate" or "non-existent" (Power, Cogswell, & Schulkin, 2006).

PREGNANCY COMPLICATIONS

Infertility

Infertility can be defined as having unprotected coitus for one year without becoming pregnant. Thirty-five percent of fertility problems reside with the woman, 35 percent with the man, 20 percent with both partners, and 10 percent of the time, the cause is unknown (Jones & Lopez, 2006). The leading cause of infertility in females is the failure to ovulate. The leading cause of infertility in males is a low sperm count. According to Jones and Lopez (2006), sperm count has to be lower than 20 million per ejaculate to be considered low.

Even though the majority of births (99.8 percent) occur to women under 45 years of age (Martin et al., 2009), age is known to affect fertility for both women and men. A woman's fertility peaks around age 20–24 (Crooks & Baur, 2011). Fecundity begins to wane around the age of 30 with a dramatic fall for women over the age of 35 (Spandorfer, Avrech, Colombero, Palermo, &

Rosenwaks, 1998). A woman in her late 20s does not produce as much progesterone as she did when she was younger. The number and quality of ovarian follicles also diminish. This causes a decline in estrogen production, and ovulation does not occur on a monthly basis, making conception more difficult (Harvard Medical School, 2005).

According to the American Society for Reproductive Medicine, cigarette smoking is harmful to a woman's ovaries, and the degree of harm depends on how much and how long a woman smokes. Smoking appears to accelerate the loss of oocytes and may advance the time of menopause by several years. Moreover, components in cigarette smoke have been shown to interfere with the ability of cells in the ovary to make estrogen and to cause a woman's eggs to be more prone to genetic abnormalities.

Men's fertility can also be affected by smoking. Smoking can decrease sperm motility and increase the number of structurally abnormal sperm in ejaculated semen. If realizing the dangers of smoking to one's heart or lungs isn't enough to help people stop smoking, maybe acknowledging the link between infertility and smoking will!

Ectopic Pregnancy

An ectopic pregnancy occurs when the embryo grows outside of the uterus. This usually takes place in one of the fallopian tubes, but can also take place on an ovary, cervix, or somewhere else in the pelvic cavity (Jones & Lopez, 2006). This is a life-threatening situation and immediate medical attention is needed. Women at risk for an ectopic pregnancy have a history of reproductive tract infections (Cottrell, 2010; Honey & Templeton, 2002), are smokers (Roelands, Jamison, Lyerly, & James, 2009), or have undergone fertility treatment (Chang & Suh, 2010).

Multiple Pregnancies

Carrying twins occurs in 1 of every 85 pregnancies. Carrying a multiple pregnancy is considered a high-risk pregnancy. *Dizygotic* (or fraternal) twins occur when two ova are released and each is fertilized by a different sperm (Jones & Lopez, 2006). The incidence of fraternal twins is genetic and influenced by race and inherited factors from the mother, but not the father. Around the world, African American women have the highest rate of fraternal twins, whereas Japanese women have the lowest rate. *Monozygotic* (or identical) twins are rarer than

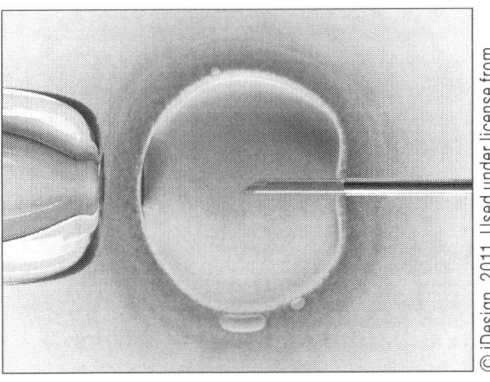
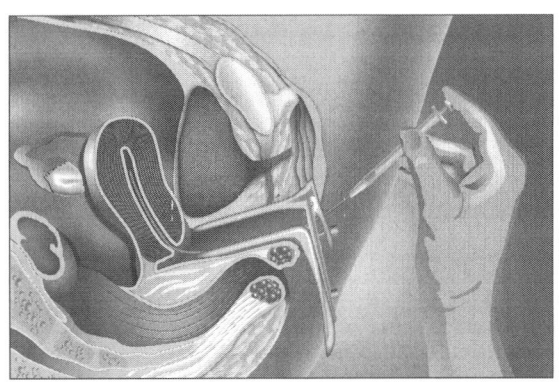

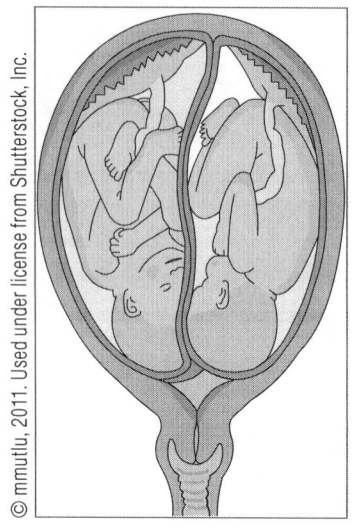
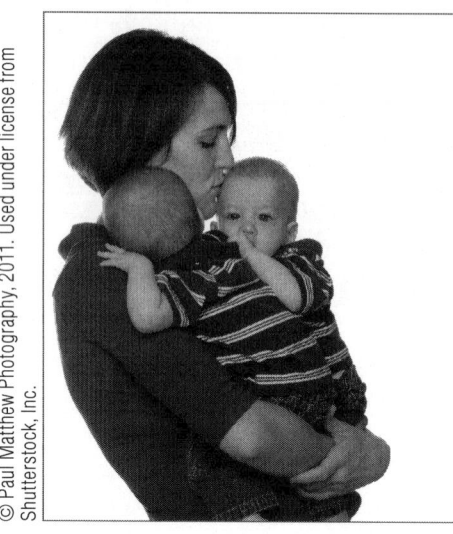

fraternal twins and occur when a zygote divides into two. Carrying a pregnancy with identical twins is not genetic and, thus, is not influenced by race, inheritance, or the mother's age.

Women who use assisted reproductive technology to get pregnant increase their chances of carrying multiple pregnancies (Jones & Lopez, 2006). Given the recent publicized accounts of women carrying sextuplets or more, the Society for Assisted Reproductive Technology has reported that multiple pregnancies carrying triplets has decreased to almost 2 percent of women under the age of 35 in 2007. In 2003, that number was 6.4 percent. As more clinicians transfer no more than two embryos into a woman's uterus, the likelihood that a woman will carry a pregnancy with more than one fetus decreases. Multiple pregnancies and pregnancies assisted by reproductive technology are more likely to end before term and have babies born at low or very low birth weight (Kogan et al., 2000).

Gestational Diabetes Mellitus (GDM)

GDM is considered the most common medical complication of pregnancy (Baptiste-Roberts et al., 2009). GDM can be defined as glucose intolerance with an onset or first recognition occurring during pregnancy (American Diabetes Association, 2004). The risk of developing GDM is about 2–4 times higher among overweight and obese women, respectively, when compared with normal weight pregnant women (Chu et al., 2007). In a recent study, Zhang and colleagues (2006) found that women who lived a sedentary lifestyle had a higher risk of GDM than women who were physically active before and during their pregnancy. GDM increases the risk of developing type-2 diabetes not only for the mother, but for the baby as well (Baptiste-Roberts et al., 2009).

POSTPARTUM HEALTH

Postpartum Bleeding

After a birth, a woman will bleed anywhere from 4–6 weeks. This is not the time to wear tampons, but a time to make sure she has a good supply of menstrual pads for many heavy days. This should not be considered a normal menstrual period. This postpartum bleeding and discharge is called *lochia*. The bleeding occurs for so long because the detached placenta has left a wound on the uterine lining. This area has to heal, and part of that healing is bleeding.

The bleeding is not an indication that a woman cannot become pregnant at this time. It is recommended that women with male sexual partners wait at least six weeks postpartum to participate in coitus. But that timeframe should also adhere to when the woman is ready to resume vaginal-penile intercourse (which could be longer than six weeks). As the uterus heals, the vaginal discharge will change from a bright red, to a pink, to a yellow. By the time a woman attends her six-week postpartum visit, the lochia should be yellow or ceased completely. This postpartum visit is needed so the obstetrician or midwife can check on the woman's physical recovery from pregnancy and delivery, see how she's doing emotionally, and address any needs. This is also a good time to speak with the clinician about contraceptive options so an unplanned pregnancy doesn't occur, especially so soon after giving birth. The World Health Organization (2009) recommends spacing pregnancies at least two years apart. This can help ensure the mother's body has recovered from the previous pregnancy and birth and that the infant has received the nutrients and attention needed during this time.

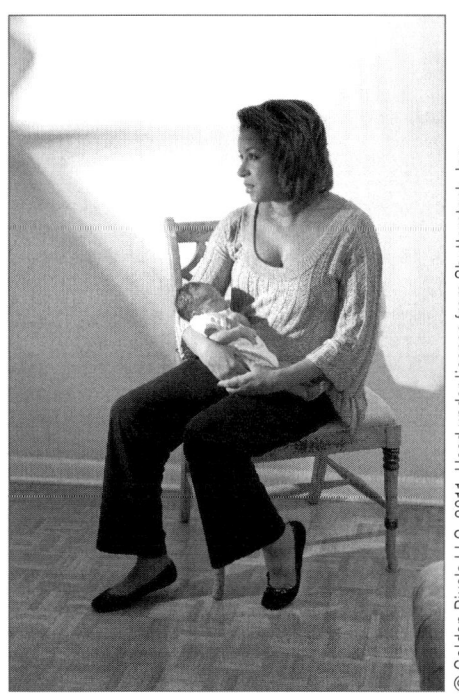

Postpartum Depression (PPD)

According to Postpartum Support International, while many women experience some mild mood changes during or after the birth of a child, 15–20 percent of women experience more significant symptoms of depression or anxiety. One cause for this is the sharp and rapid drop in estrogen and progesterone soon after giving birth. A number of hormones, including estrogen and progesterone, directly affect the brain chemistry that controls emotions and mood (Bloch, 2003).

A woman with PPD might experience feelings of anger, sadness, irritability, guilt, lack of interest in the baby, changes in eating and sleeping habits, trouble concentrating, thoughts of hopelessness, and sometimes even thoughts of harming the baby or herself. This is a serious condition that should not be taken lightly. With medication and/or therapy, the majority of women recover from PPD.

"Breast Is Best"

Breastfeeding is the preferred method of infant feeding for the first year of life or longer and exclusive breastfeeding is recommended for the first six months of life (Gartner et al., 2005). Figure 11.1 illustrates the percentage of infants that are breastfed at six months of age in the United States. How does your state measure up? The majority of American infants are breastfed at birth (over 70 percent in 2007), but we lag behind in breastfeeding our infants at three or six months of age. Why do you think that is the case? And why do European countries have better breastfeeding rates than the United States? According to the National Centers for Health Statistics (McDowell, Wang, & Kennedy-Stephenson, 2008), Mexican American women, regardless of income and age are more likely

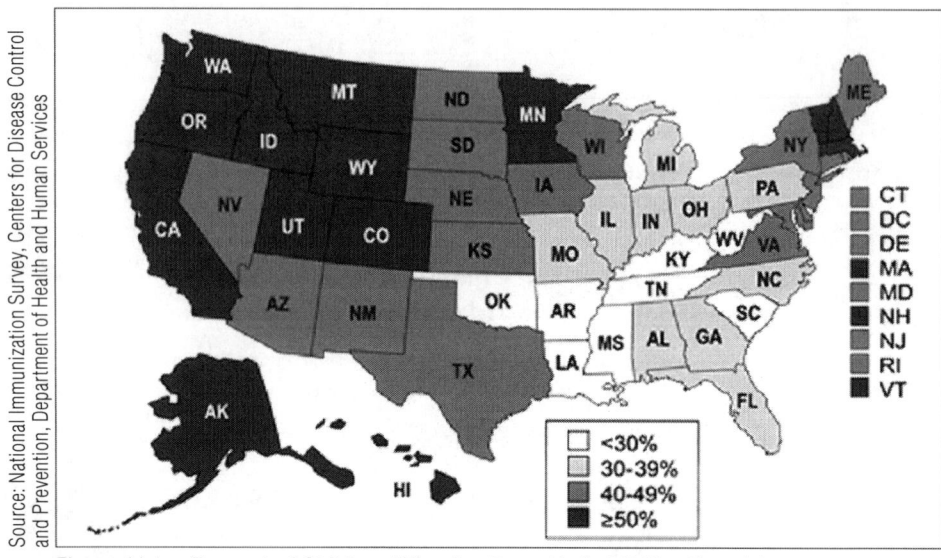

Figure 11.1 Percent of Children Who Are Breastfed at 6 Months of Age among Children Born in 2007

to breastfeed in this country. Even though the rate of breastfeeding in the African American community has improved in the past decade, they remain the least likely to breastfeed.

There are a number of health benefits to the mother if she breastfeeds. These benefits include decreased postpartum bleeding and more rapid uterine *involution* (the uterus shrinks back to size) attributable to the increased concentrations of oxytocin (Chua, Arulkumaran, Lim, Selamat, & Ratnam, 1994). Breastfeeding mothers have been found to return to their pre-pregnancy weight earlier than women who do not breastfeed (Dewey, Heinig, & Nommsen, 1993). That is because producing more milk requires additional energy and that leads to greater postpartum weight loss (Baker et al., 2008). Longer duration of breastfeeding has been associated with lower maternal weight gain 10–15 years later (Gunderson, 2007). Also, breastfeeding has been found to reduce the risk of breast cancer (Collaborative Group on Hormonal Factors in Breast Cancer, 2002) and ovarian cancer (Jernström et al., 2004).

The American Academy of Pediatrics (2005) urges breastfeeding mothers to avoid alcoholic beverages because alcohol is concentrated in breast milk and its use inhibits milk production. An occasional celebratory single, small alcoholic drink is acceptable, but breastfeeding should be avoided for two hours after the drink (Anderson, 1995).

DIFFERENCE BETWEEN BREASTFEEDING AND HAVING A SEXUAL PARTNER SUCK ON A BREAST

Is there a difference? What if you heard that women who breastfed and have had a sexual partner suck on their breast used similar words to describe the sensations—contentment, joy, and pleasure? All of those terms, though, mean different things to different people in different situations. When a woman's genitals

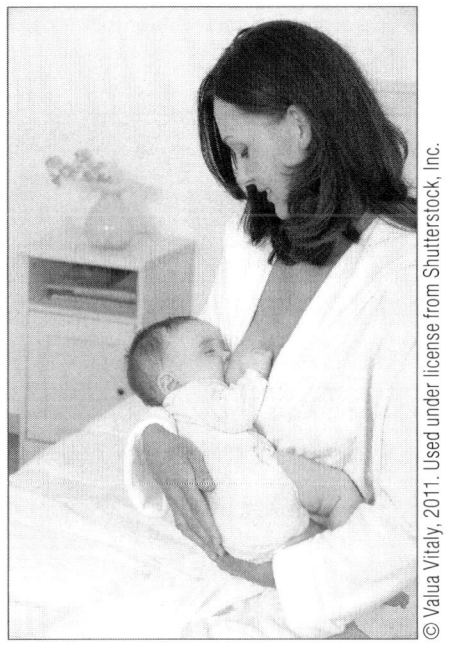 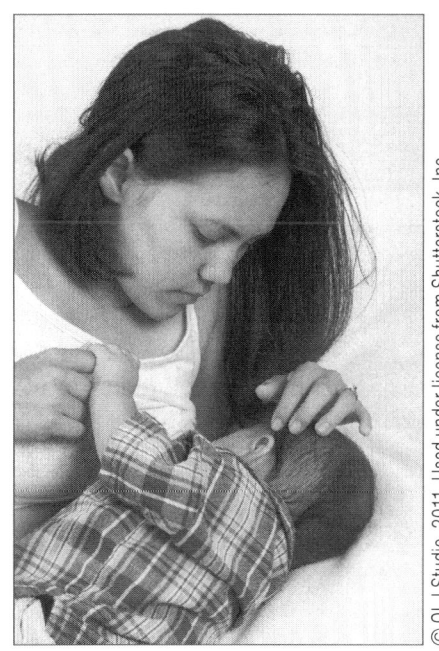

engorge with blood because she is sexually aroused, the sensations can be pleasurable, but when a woman's breasts engorge with milk, the sensations can be uncomfortable, if not painful. The way a baby sucks on the breast and the way a sexual partner sucks on the breast are not the same. The techniques used are usually distinctive because the reason for this behavior has different objectives. Babies suck to get the milk out that they love to drink and a sexual partner sucks to arouse their partner and/or for their own arousal. The way a sexual partner sucks on the breast may not be as forceful, may change in technique throughout the activity and may not necessarily focus only on the nipple but also on other areas of the breast.

Certain hormones play a critical role in breastfeeding. Prolactin is a hormone known to help produce milk. The production of prolactin is suppressed during pregnancy because of the high levels of estrogen and progesterone. When a woman gives birth and these two hormones decrease considerably, prolactin is secreted to produce milk in the mammary glands (Jones & Lopez, 2006). When a woman begins to breastfeed, the hormone oxytocin is released and helps expel the milk from the nipple while the baby is sucking (Jones & Lopez, 2006).

MATERNAL MORTALITY

Maternal mortality can be defined as the death of a woman during pregnancy, childbirth, or the first 42 days after delivery (Hogan et al, 2010). Around the world, the country of Niger has the highest lifetime risk of women dying from pregnancy-related complications (1 in 7). Ireland has the lowest lifetime risk (1 in 48,000).

The lifetime risk in the United States is 1 in 4,800. From 1980 to 2008, the United States and Canada have experienced a 33 percent increase in the maternal mortality rate (Hogan et al, 2010). Forty nations have a lower risk of maternal death than the United States (The World Bank, 2007). The top three causes of

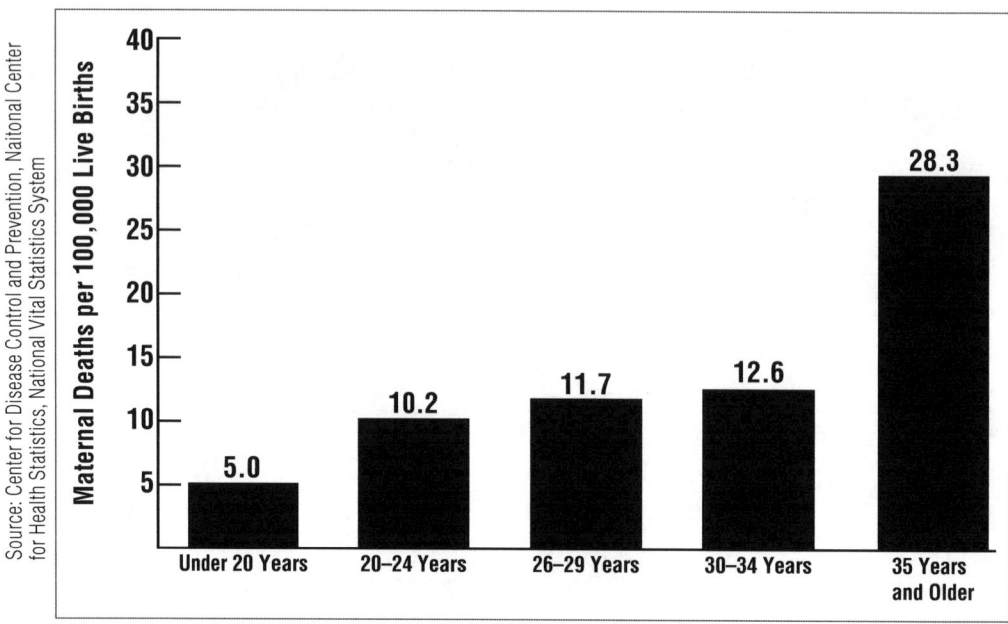

Figure 11.2 Maternal Mortality Rates by Age, 2006

maternal death in the United States are *preeclampsia* (high blood pressure), *eclampsia* (convulsions or seizures), and *postpartum hemorrhage* (severe bleeding). Postpartum hemorrhage is the leading cause of maternal death around the world (McCormick, Sanghvi, Kinzie, & McIntosh, 2002).

Healthy People 2020 has a target of 11.4 maternal deaths per 100,000 live births. In 2007, there were 12.7 maternal deaths per 100,000 live births in the United States. For African American women, though, the ratio was 36.5 deaths per 100,000 births (Kung, Hoyert, Zu, & Murphy, 2008). Also, women older than 35 were more likely to die than any other age group (see Figure 11.2).

INFANT MORTALITY

The rate of infant mortality indicates how healthy a country is. *Infant mortality* is defined as the death of an infant before her or his first birthday. In 2005, the infant mortality rate worldwide was 49.4 per 1,000 live births according to the United Nations and 42.09 per 1,000 live births according to the *CIA World Factbook*. The country with the lowest infant mortality rate was Singapore with 1.92 per 1,000 live births. The country with the highest infant mortality rate was Afghanistan with 135.95 per 1,000 live births. The infant mortality rate in the United States was 6.81 per 1,000 live births and was ranked 30th in the world. Birth defects are the leading cause of infant mortality in the United States (Mathews & MacDorman, 2010). According to the Centers for Health Statistics (Mathews & MacDorman, 2010), infant mortality rates were higher for male infants, African American babies, babies that were part of a multiple pregnancy, and babies born preterm (before 37 weeks gestation) or at low birth weight (below 5½ pounds). One in 8 births in the United States is premature (MacDorman & Mathews, 2008). The lower the gestational age, the more likely that baby will not survive. Babies with a birth defect are also more likely to be born premature and are at risk of dying even if the birth defect is not life-threatening (Callaghan,

MacDorman, Rasmussen, Qin, & Lackritz, 2006). As women age, they are more likely to deliver a baby with chromosomal abnormalities. Birth defects have also been found in babies whose fathers are at an advanced age (Zhu et al., 2005).

Reflections

The United States is considered one of the wealthiest and most powerful countries in the world. Yet we have one of the highest rates of abortion when compared to other developed countries. Why do you think that is the case? Religion strongly influences politics in this country. Why do you think religion affects public policy here in the United States more so than in other developed countries?

We also have low rates of breastfeeding and high rates of c-sections. We have the best medical technology *in the world*, yet our mothers and babies die at an alarming rate. Ironically, more women and infants would die annually if we didn't have the medical facilities we do have. What do you think is needed to improve our country's maternal and infant health?

Critical Thinking Questions

1. A friend has confided in you that she is pregnant and she is asking for your advice. Would your advice differ if your friend were 15 years old rather than 35? How about if she were married versus single? Already had four children? Almost died during her last pregnancy? Why or why not?

2. Do you think if we decreased the rate of unintended pregnancies in the United States, we would indirectly lower the rate of abortions as well? Why or why not?

3. Why is it that a disproportionate number of women of color and in poverty terminate a pregnancy?

4. How do you think public policy has hindered women's ability to prevent unintended pregnancies?

How Much Do You Remember from the Chapter?

(1-4) • Match the stage of development with its correct definition:

1. Blastocyst _____ a. 9 weeks' gestation to birth
2. Embryo _____ b. 3–9 weeks' gestation
3. Fetus _____ c. united sperm and ovum
4. Zygote _____ d. uterine implantation occurs at this stage around 1 week after conception

5. During the first stage of labor, the contractions of the uterus cause the _____.
   a. effacement and dilation of the cervix
   b. baby to come out of the vaginal canal
   c. expulsion of the placenta
   d. woman to have a bowel movement

6. During the second stage of labor, the mother _____ with each contraction, forcing the baby down the vaginal canal.
   a. pants
   b. holds her breath
   c. breathes slowly
   d. pushes

7. The _____ is expelled during the third and final stage of labor.
   a. baby
   b. placenta
   c. uterus
   d. cervix

8. After a birth, a woman will bleed anywhere from _____.
   a. 8–10 weeks
   b. 4–6 days
   c. 1–2 weeks
   d. 4–6 weeks

9. The leading cause of infertility in females is:
   a. blocked fallopian tubes due to PID
   b. incompetent uterus
   c. failure to ovulate
   d. incompetent cervix

10. The leading cause of infertility in males is:
    a. retrograde ejaculation
    b. low seminal fluid
    c. low sperm count
    d. sperm abnormalities

Challenge Yourself!

ACROSS

1. The period of the _____ begins at the 9th week of pregnancy and continues until birth.

4. A baby born _____ is a baby born under 37 weeks' gestation.

5. When implantation occurs, the fertilized egg is called a _____.

6. After the cervix is completely thinned out, it has to dilate _____ centimeters before the mother can begin to push.

9. An at-home pregnancy test detects the hormone _____ to verify that a woman is pregnant.

DOWN

2. The cervix has to become 100% thinned out or fully _____ before dilation can begin.

3. The period of the _____ begins at the 3rd week of pregnancy and extends to the end of the 8th week of pregnancy.

4. The _____ is expelled during the third and final stage of labor.

7. When an egg is fertilized by a sperm, it is called a _____.

8. During the second stage of labor, the mother _____ with each contraction, forcing the baby down the vagina.

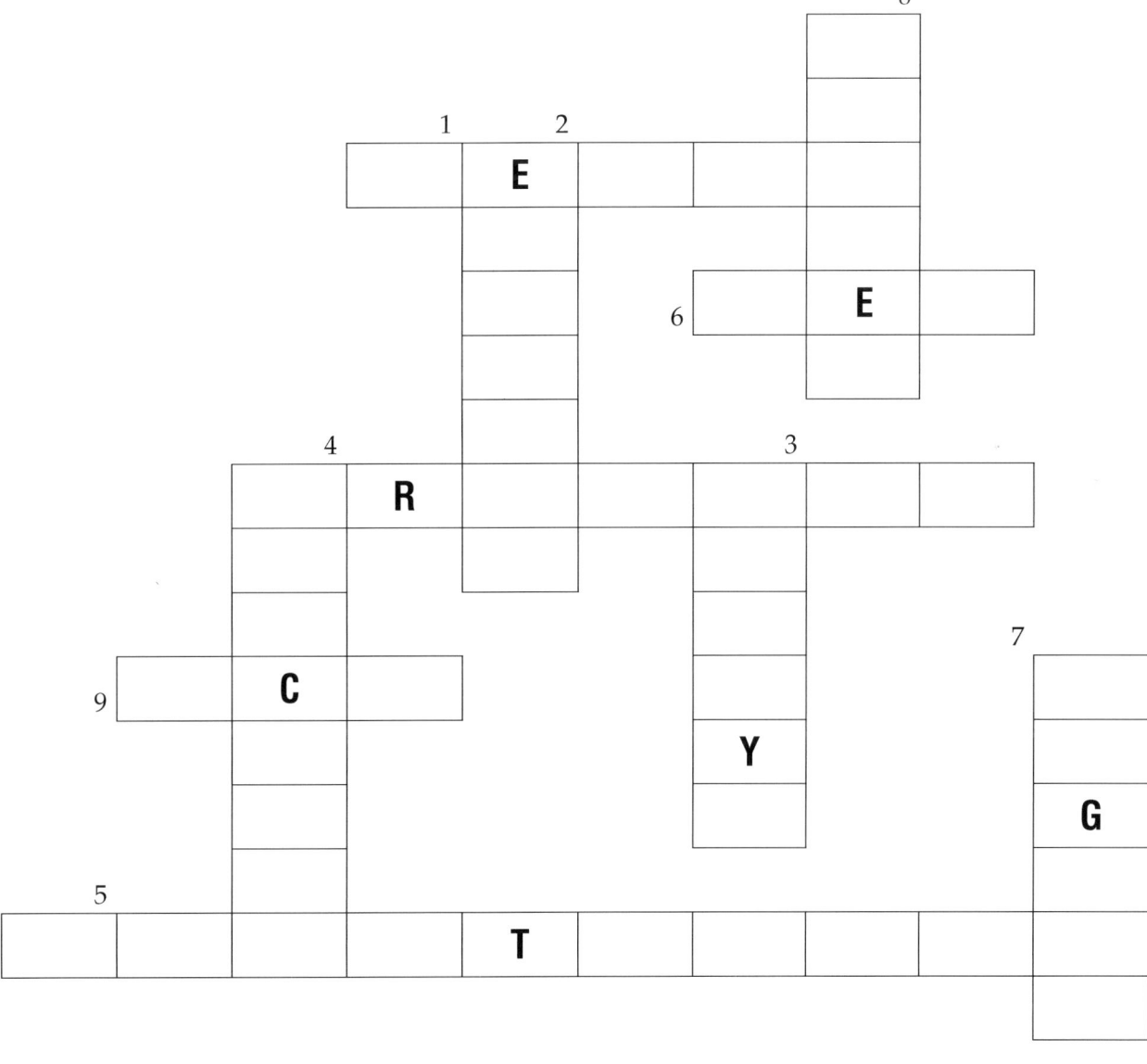

Websites

www.agi-usa.org
The Alan Guttmacher Institute

www.acog.org
The American Congress of Obstetricians and Gynecologists

www.americanpregnancy.org
The American Pregnancy Association

www.asrm.org
The American Society for Reproductive Medicine

www.marchofdimes.com
The March of Dimes

www.cdc.gov/nchs
The National Center for Health Statistics

www.plannedparenthood.org
Planned Parenthood

www.postpartum.net
Postpartum Support International

www.sart.org
Society for Assisted Reproductive Technology

References

The Alan Guttmacher Institute. (2011). *In brief: Facts on induced abortion in the United States.* New York, NY: Author.

American Academy of Pediatrics (AAP). (2005). *Policy statement: Breastfeeding and the use of human milk.* Washington, DC: Author.

American College of Sports Medicine. (2000). *ACSM's guidelines for exercise, testing and prescription* (6th ed.). Philadelphia, PA: Lippincott, Williams, & Wilkins.

American Congress of Obstetricians and Gynecologists (ACOG). (2001). Management of recurrent early pregnancy loss. *ACOG Practice Bulletin, 24.*

American Congress of Obstetricians and Gynecologists (ACOG). (2002). Exercise during pregnancy and the postpartum period. ACOG committee opinion, 267. *Obstetrics & Gynecology, 99,* 171–173.

American Congress of Obstetricians and Gynecologists (ACOG). (2009). *Evaluation of stillbirths and neonatal deaths.* ACOG committee opinion, 383. Washington, DC: Author.

American Congress of Obstetricians and Gynecologists (ACOG). (2010). *How your baby grows during pregnancy.* Washington, DC: Author.

American Diabetes Association. (2004). Gestational diabetes mellitus (position statement). *Diabetes Care, 27,* s88–s90.

Anderson, P. (1995). Alcohol and breastfeeding. *Journal of Human Lactation, 11,* 321–323.

Baker, J., Gamborg, M., Heitmann, B., Lissner, L., Sorensen, T., & Rasmussen, K. (2008). Breastfeeding reduces postpartum weight retention. *American Journal of Clinical Nutrition, 88*(6), 1543–1551.

Baptiste-Roberts, K., Barone, B., Gary, T., Golden, S., Wilson, L., Bass, E. et al. (2009). Risk factors for type 2 diabetes among women with gestational diabetes: A systematic review. *The American Journal of Medicine, 122,* 207–214.

Bloch, M. (2003). Endocrine factors in the etiology of postpartum depression. *Comprehensive Psychiatry, 44*(3), 234–246.

Bonillas, C., & Feehan, R. (2008). Tools for teaching: Normalizing the changes experienced during each trimester of pregnancy. *The Journal of Perinatal Education, 17,* 39–43.

Brown, L. (2007). Elevated risks of pregnancy complications and adverse outcomes with increasing maternal age. *Human Reproduction, 22*(5), 1264–1272.

Brown, S., Burdette, L., & Rodriguez, P. (2008). Looking inward: Provider-based barriers to contraception among teens and young adults. *Contraception, 78,* 355–357.

Callaghan, W., MacDorman, M., Rasmussen, S., Qin C., & Lackritz, E. (2006). The contribution of preterm birth to infant mortality rates in the United States. *Pediatrics, 118,* 1566–1573.

Chang, H., & Suh, C. (2010). Ectopic pregnancy after assisted reproductive technology: What are the risk factors? *Current Opinion in Obstetrics & Gynecology, 22*(3), 202–207.

Chu, S., Bachman, D., Callaghan, W., Whitlock, E., Dietz, P., Berg, C. et al. (2008). Association between obesity during pregnancy and increased use of health care. *The New England Journal of Medicine, 358,* 1444–1453.

Chu, S., Callaghan, W., Kim, S., Schmid, C., Lau, J., England, L. et al. (2007). Maternal obesity and risk of gestational diabetes mellitus. *Diabetes Care, 30,* 2070–2076.

Chua, S., Arulkumaran, S., Lim, I., Selamat, N., & Ratnam, S. (1994). Influence of breastfeeding and nipple stimulation on postpartum uterine activity. *British Journal of Obstetrics & Gynaecology, 101,* 804–805.

Cohen, S. (2006). Toward making abortion 'rare': The shifting battleground over the means to an end. *Guttmacher Policy Review, 9*(1), 1–5.

Collaborative Group on Hormonal Factors in Breast Cancer. (2002). Breast cancer and breastfeeding: Collaborative reanalysis of individual data from 47 epidemiological studies in 30 countries, including 50,302 women with breast cancer and 96,973 women without the disease. *Lancet, 360,* 187–195.

Cottrell, B. (2010). An updated review of evidence to discourage douching. *The American Journal of Maternal Child Nursing, 35*(2), 102–109.

Crooks, R., & Baur, K. (2011). *Our sexuality* (11th ed.). Belmont, CA: Wadsworth/Cengage Learning.

Davis, E. M., Zyzanski, S. J., Olson, C. M., Stange, K. C., & Horwitz, R. I. (2009). Racial, ethnic, and socioeconomic differences in the incidence of obesity related to childbirth. *American Journal of Public Health, 99,* 294–299.

Dewey, K., Heinig, M., & Nommsen, L. (1993). Maternal weight-loss patterns during prolonged lactation. *American Journal of Clinical Nutrition, 58,* 162–166.

Expert Panel on the Identification, Evaluation, and Treatment of Overweight in Adults. (1998). Clinical guidelines on the identification, evaluation and treatment of overweight and obesity in adults: Executive summary. *American Journal of Clinical Nutrition, 68,* 899–917.

Finer, L., & Henshaw, S. (2006). Disparities in rates of unintended pregnancy in the United States, 1994 and 2001. *Perspectives on Sexual & Reproductive Health, 38,* 90–96.

Gartner, L. M., Morton, J., Lawrence, R. A., Naylor, A. J., O'Hare, D., Schanler, R. J. et al. (2005). Breastfeeding and the use of human milk. *Pediatrics, 115,* 496–506.

Gilbert, E., & Harmon, J. (2002). *Manual of high risk pregnancy and delivery* (3rd ed.). St. Louis, MI: Mosby.

Gunderson, E. P. (2007). Breastfeeding after gestational diabetes pregnancy. *Diabetes Care, 30,* 161–168.

Harvard Medical School. (2005). Perimenopause: Rocky road to menopause: Symptoms we call 'menopausal' often precede menopause by years. *Harvard Women's Health Watch, 12*(12), 1–4.

Heffner, L., & Schust, D. (2006). *Reproductive systems at a glance* (2nd ed.). Ames, IA: Blackwell Publishing Professional.

Hogan, M., Foreman, K., Naghavi, M., Ahn, S., Wang, M., Makela, S. et al. (2010). Maternal mortality for 181 countries, 1980–2008: A systematic analysis of progress towards millennium development goal 5. *The Lancet, 375*(9726), 1609–1623.

Honey, E., & Templeton, A. (2002). Prevention of pelvic inflammatory disease by the control of *C. trachomatis* infection. *International Journal of Gynecology & Obstetrics, 78*(3), 257–261.

Institute of Medicine. (1990). *Nutrition during pregnancy: Part I: Nutritional status and weight gain.* Washington, DC: National Academies Press.

Jernström, H., Lubinski, J., Lynch, H., Ghadirian, P., Neuhausen, S., Isaacs, C. et al. (2004). Breast-feeding and the risk of breast cancer in BRCA1 and BRCA2 mutation carriers. *Journal of the National Cancer Institute, 96,* 1094–1098.

Jones, R., Darroch, J., & Henshaw, S. (2002). Patterns in the socioeconomic characteristics of women obtaining abortions in 2000–2001. *Perspectives on Sexual & Reproductive Health, 34*(5), 226–235.

Jones, R., & Henshaw, S.(2002). Mifepristone for early medical abortion: Experiences in France, Great Britain and Sweden. *Perspectives on Sexual & Reproductive Health, 34*(3), 154–161.

Jones, R., & Kooistra, K. (2011). Abortion incidence and access to services in the United States, 2008. *Perspectives on Sexual & Reproductive Health, 43*(1), 41–50.

Jones, R., & Lopez, K. (2006). *Human reproductive biology* (3rd ed.). Burlington, MA: Elsevier.

Kim, S., Dietz, P., England, L., Morrow, B., & Callaghan, W. (2007). Trends in prepregnancy obesity in nine states, 1993–2003. *Obesity, 15,* 986–993.

Kogan, M., Alexander, G., Kotelchuck, M., Macdorman, M., Buckens, P., Martin, J. et al. (2000). Trends in twin birth outcomes and prenatal care utilization in the United States, 1981–1997. *The Journal of American Medical Association, 284*(3), 335–341.

Kung, H., Hoyert, D., Xu, J., & Murphy, S. (2008). Deaths: Final data for 2005. *National Vital Statistics Reports, 56*(10). Hyattsville, MD: National Center for Health Statistics.

Marston, C., & Cleland, J. (2003). Relationships between contraception and abortion: A review of the evidence. *International Family Planning Perspectives, 29*(1), 6–13.

Martin, J., Hamilton, B., Sutton, P., Ventura, S., Menacker, F., Kirmeyer, S. et al. (2009). Births: Final data for 2006. *National Vital Statistics Reports, 57*(7). Hyattsville, MD: National Center for Health Statistics.

MacDorman, M., & Mathews, T. (2008). Recent trends in infant mortality in the United States. *NCHS Data Brief, 9*. Hyattsville, MD: National Center for Health Statistics.

Mathews, T., & MacDorman, M. (2010). Infant mortality statistics from the 2006 period linked birth/infant death data set. *National Vital Statistics Reports, 58*(17). Hyattsville, MD: National Center for Health Statistics.

McClure, E., Nalubamba-Phiri, M., & Goldenberg, R. (2006). Stillbirth in developing countries. *International Journal of Gynecology & Obstetrics, 94*(2), 82–90.

McCormick, M., Sanghvi, H., Kinzie, B., & McIntosh, N. (2002). Averting maternal death and disability: Preventing postpartum hemorrhage in low-resource settings. *International Journal of Gynecology and Obstetrics, 77*, 267–275.

McDowell, M., Wang, C., & Kennedy-Stephenson, J. (2008). Breastfeeding in the United States: Findings from the National Health and Nutrition Examination Survey, 1999–2006. *NCHS Data Brief, 5*. Hyattsville, MD: National Center for Health Statistics.

Menacker, F., & Hamilton, B. (2010). Recent trends in Cesarean delivery in the United States. *NCHS Data Brief, 35*. Hyattsville, MD: National Center for Health Statistics.

Morland, K., Wing, S., & Diez, R. A. (2002). The contextual effect of the local food environment on residents' diets: The atherosclerosis risk in communities study. *American Journal of Public Health, 92*, 1761–1767.

Mosher, W., & Jones. J. (2010). Use of contraception in the United States: 1982–2008. National Center for Health Statistics. *Vital Health Statistics, 23*(29).

Mosley, B., Cleves, M., Siega-Riz, A., Shaw, G., Canfield, M., Waller, D. et al. (2009). Neural tube defects and maternal folate intake among pregnancies conceived after folic acid fortification in the United States. *American Journal of Epidemiology, 169*(1), 9–17.

Murphy, H., Rayman, G., Lewis, K., Kelly, S., Johal, B., Duffield, K. et al. (2008). Effectiveness of continuous glucose monitoring in pregnant women with diabetes: Randomized clinical trial. *British Medical Journal, 337*, 1680–1687.

Myles, T., Gooch, J., & Santolaya, J. (2002). Obesity as an independent risk factor for infectious morbidity in patients who undergo cesarean delivery. *Obstetrics & Gynecology, 100*, 959–964.

Ogden, C., Carroll, M., Curtin, L., McDowell, M., Tabak, C., & Flegal, K. (2006). Prevalence of overweight and obesity in the United States, 1999–2004. *JAMA, 295*, 1549–1555.

Olson, C., Strawderman, M., Hinton, P., & Pearson, T. (2003). Gestational weight gain and postpartum behaviors associated with weight change from early pregnancy to 1 y postpartum. *International Journal of Obesity, 27*, 117–127.

O'Toole, M. L., Sawicki, M. A., & Artal, R. (2003). Structured diet and physical activity prevent postpartum weight retention. *Journal of Women's Health, 2*, 991–998.

Pazol, K., Gamble, S., Parker, W., Cook, D., Zane, S., & Hamdan, S. (2009). Abortion surveillance—United States, 2006. *Morbidity & Mortality Weekly Report, 58*(SS08), 1–35.

Power, M., Cogswell, M., & Schulkin, J. (2006). Obesity prevention and treatment practices of U.S. obstetrician-gynecologists. *Obstetrics & Gynecology, 108*, 961–968.

Rasmussen, K., & Yaktine, A. (2009). *Weight gain during pregnancy: Reexamining the guidelines.* Washington, DC: National Academies Press.

Robinson, H., O'Connell, C., Joseph, K., & McLeod, N. (2005). Maternal outcomes in pregnancies complicated by obesity. *Obstetrics & Gynecology, 106*, 1357–1364.

Roelands, J., Jamison, M., Lyerly, A., & James, A. (2009). Consequences of smoking during pregnancy on maternal health. *Journal of Women's Health, 18*(6), 867–872.

Rosenn, B. (2008). Obesity & diabetes: A recipe for obstetric complications. *Journal of Maternal-Fetal and Neonatal Medicine, 21*, 159–164.

Sedgh, G., Henshaw, S., Singh, S., Bankole, A., & Drescher, J. (2007). Legal abortion worldwide: Incidence and recent trends. *International Family Planning Perspectives, 33*(3), 106–116.

Siega-Riz, A. M., Rodnar, L. M., & Savitz, D. A. (2002). What are pregnant women eating? Nutrient and food group differences by race. *American Journal of Obstetrics & Gynecology, 186*, 480–486.

Siega-Riz, A. M., Siega-Riz, A. M., & Laraia, B. (2006). The Implications of maternal overweight and obesity on the course of pregnancy and birth outcomes. *Maternal & Child Health Journal, 10*, 153–156.

Spandorfer, S., Avrech, O., Colombero, L., Palermo, G., & Rosenwaks, Z. (1998). Effect of parental age on fertilization and pregnancy characteristics in couples treated by intracytoplasmic sperm injection. *Human Reproduction, 13*, 334–338.

Stotland, N., Haas, J., Brawarsky, P., Jackson, R., Fuentes-Afflick, E., & Escobar, G. (2005). Body mass index, provider advice and target gestational weight gain. *Obstetrics & Gynecology, 105*, 633–638.

Ventura, S., Abma, J., Mosher, W., & Henshaw, S. (2009). Estimated pregnancy rates for the United States, 1990–2005: An update. *National Vital Statistics Reports, 58*(4). Hyattsville, MD: National Center for Health Statistics.

Wilcox, A., Baird, D., & Weinberg, C. (1999). Time of implantation of the conceptus and loss of pregnancy. *New England Journal of Medicine, 340*, 1796–1799.

The World Bank. (2007). *Maternal mortality in 2005: Estimates developed by WHO, UNICEF, UNFPA, and the World Bank.* Geneva: Author.

The World Health Organization. (2009). *Training manual for cluster representatives and health volunteers: Module 1: Family Health.* Cairo, Egypt: Author.

Yogev, Y., & Visser, G. (2009). Obesity, gestational diabetes and pregnancy outcome. *Seminars in Fetal & Neonatal Medicine, 14*, 77–84.

Zhang, C., Solomon, C., Manson, J., & Hu, F. (2006). A prospective study of pregravid physical activity and sedentary behaviors in relation to the risk of gestational diabetes mellitus. *Archives of Internal Medicine, 166,* 543–548.

Zhu, J., Madsen, K., Vestergaard, M., Olesen, A., Basso, O., & Olsen, J. (2005). Paternal age and congenital malformations. *Human Reproduction, 20*(11), 3173–3177.

chapter twelve

CONTRACEPTION

CHAPTER OBJECTIVES

On completion of this chapter, students will be able to:

- calculate their reproductive years;
- differentiate among the barrier, hormonal, fertility awareness, spermicide, and sterilization methods of contraception;
- understand how different contraceptive methods prevent pregnancy;
- recognize the effectiveness of each contraceptive method in preventing pregnancy.

ABBREVIATIONS AND ACRONYMS USED IN THIS CHAPTER

ACHES	abdominal, chest, headaches, eye, swelling
FDA	Food and Drug Administration
HPV	human papillomavirus
IUD	intra-uterine device
IUS	intra-uterine system
LARC	long-acting reversible contraceptive
LH	luteinizing hormone
mgs	milligrams
mm	millimeters
STI	sexually transmitted infection(s)

CALCULATING YOUR REPRODUCTIVE YEARS

So … how many kids do you want to have? What age would you like to begin and what age would you like to be done having kids? Many of us do not give it much thought, especially if we are young, have not finished school, are barely starting out on our own, or are not in a committed relationship.

Let's say that a woman wants to start having kids at the age of 25, which just happens to be the average age women in the United States start having kids (Martin et al., 2009). Let's also say that this woman started participating in coitus around the age of 17, which in this country is the average age for women (The Alan Guttmacher Institute, 2002). So, from 17 to 24–25, what contraceptive methods do you think she used *not* to get pregnant? Remember, "hope" is not a reliable contraception method!

According to The Alan Guttmacher Institute (2000), on average, women in this country want to have only two children. Let's say a woman has had both her children by age 30 and does not want to have any more. Now what? She's "done"—does she still have to worry about getting pregnant again? Yes, she does, but for how long? As discussed in chapter 4, most women won't go through menopause until around the age of 50. What will she do for the next *20 years* now that she is done having all the kids she wants to have? Sexual abstinence is an option, but not a very realistic one.

If you think that's crazy, let's figure out how many years men are fertile. Let's say a man was done having kids by the age of 35. Because the majority of men's testicles never stop producing sperm after puberty (Jones & Lopez, 2006), he is

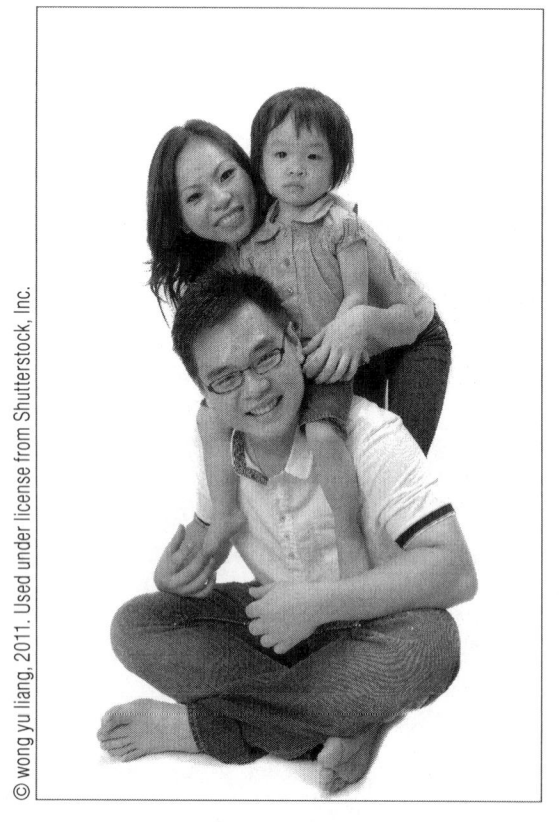
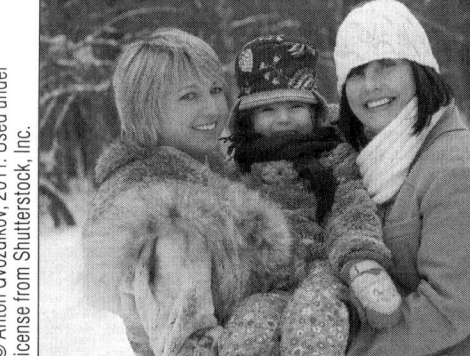

still fertile until he dies, which in this country is around the age of 75 for men (Xu, Kochanek, Murphy, & Tejada-Vera, 2010). That means he still has *40 years* not to get a woman pregnant if he does not want to become a father again! There are really only two reliable contraceptive methods available for men—condoms and male sterilization (these methods are discussed at length later in this chapter). The contraceptive methods available for women, though, are abundant and vary considerably in time spent in using them and cost. Women can choose from hormonal methods that come in a form of an injection, a patch, a vaginal ring, an implant, and an intra-uterine device (IUD), as well as non-hormonal methods. This chapter discusses all of them.

The top two contraceptive methods in the United States since 1982 have been oral contraceptives (known as "the pill") and female sterilization (The Alan Guttmacher Institute, 2010). The pill is a hormonal method that is reversible (i.e., a woman can stop taking it and be able to get pregnant) and is taken by almost 11 million women. Female sterilization, which is permanent (i.e., this method is meant to ensure a woman never gets pregnant again), has been used by over 10 million women (Mosher & Jones, 2010). Women who are childless are more likely to use the pill than sterilization as their form of contraception, whereas women who have three or more children are more likely to be sterilized than be on oral contraceptives (Mosher & Jones, 2010).

As a hormonal method, the pill may contain estrogen and progestin (a synthesized version of progesterone) or only progestin. There is no pill (or other contraceptive method) that contains only estrogen. The estrogen in the pill inhibits ovulation (Nelson, 2007). Ovulation does not occur because the low levels of estrogen in most hormonal contraceptive methods prevent the pituitary gland from releasing luteinizing hormone (LH). As was discussed in chapter 4, LH is needed for ovulation to occur (Hatcher & Brawner Namnoum, 2007). The progestin in the pill thickens a woman's cervical mucus (which creates a barrier to sperm so the sperm can't enter the uterus) and suppresses endometrial growth (that's why women on a hormonal method usually have lighter menstrual bleeding). Unfortunately, there is *no* contraceptive method that is 100 percent effective, completely safe, with no side effects, reversible, separate from sexual activity, inexpensive, easy to obtain, usable by either sex, and not dependent on the user's memory (Crooks & Baur, 2011). Keep in mind that just as no two people tolerate the same medication the same, no two women or two men will necessarily exhibit the same side effects (if any) when using a particular contraceptive method.

LONG-ACTING REVERSIBLE CONTRACEPTIVES (LARCS)

LARC methods are hormonal and non-hormonal options that are highly effective and reversible (a pregnancy is possible when the method is no longer being used). A great advantage to these methods is that women (none exist for men) do not have to rely (or rely at a small degree only) on their memory or correct use (Trussell, 2007b). Currently, the United States has four LARC methods available—three are hormonally-based and one is not. The only non-hormonal, long-acting, reversible contraceptive method is ParaGard®. This contraceptive is an intrauterine device (IUD) that stays in place in the uterus for up to 10 years. It is the longest continuous-use LARC method on the market. One of the hormonal LARCs is also an intrauterine device, called Mirena®. This intrauterine system stays in place in the uterus for up to 5 years. Another hormonal LARC is Implanon®, a subdermal implant (under the skin of a woman's inner arm) that can remain in place for up to 3 years. The last hormonal LARC is an injection given every 12 weeks, called Depo-Provera®. If a pregnancy is planned sooner rather than later, then the first three methods can be removed prior to their expiration. A woman on Depo-Provera® can stop getting the injections to regain her fertility. Each of these methods is described in detail below.

HORMONAL CONTRACEPTIVE METHODS

Hormonal contraceptive methods are very effective. Effectiveness can be defined as calculating how many pregnancies will occur in 100 couples who use that particular method for one year (Trussell, 2007b). The most effective methods have 1–2 pregnancies per 100 couples that consistently use that particular method per year. The least effective methods have 30 pregnancies per 100 couples per year. Most (hormonal) methods have an effectiveness rate of 99.9 percent, but these rates vary when human error is taken into account. Most pregnancies among contraceptive users are caused by inconsistent or incorrect use, not by a failure of the method itself (Trussell, 2007a). The less a person has to think about using a method to prevent a pregnancy, the more effective that method is. Hormonal methods cannot be purchased over-the-counter. All hormonal contraceptives intended to be taken on a long-term basis (i.e., from months to years) are by prescription-only. Emergency contraception does not fall into this category because that hormonal method is not meant to be taken on a regular basis.

Possible Side Effects

Even though the majority of them are not serious, there are side effects a woman should be aware of when on a hormonal contraceptive method (Sulak, Scow, Preece, Riggs, & Kuehl, 2000). They include:

- Nausea
- Weight gain
- Sore or swollen breasts
- Unscheduled withdrawal bleeding
- Lighter menstrual periods
- Mood changes

There are over 100 oral contraceptives available, so a woman can ask her doctor to switch her to a different pill if the symptoms she is experiencing are disconcerting. Other side effects are rare but serious if they occur. Some of these symptoms may indicate a serious health complication like liver disease, stroke, blood clots, high blood pressure, or heart disease (Nelson, 2007). Many of these conditions are not caused by being on a hormonal method, though. Even so, the following side effects can be remembered by the word "ACHES":

A – Abdominal (stomach) pain
C – Chest pain
H – Headaches (severe)
E – Eye problems (blurred vision)
S – Swelling and/or aching in the legs or thighs

If a woman is a smoker or over the age of 35, she needs to speak to her doctor about her contraceptive options because most women who fall in one of these two categories are advised against taking a hormonal method containing estrogen. Hormonal contraceptives should not be considered as an option for women who have experienced blood clots in the arms, legs, or lungs (and it should be discussed with her doctor if a first-degree relative did); serious heart and liver disease; or cancer of the breast or uterus. These women should speak to their doctor about the possibility of carrying a pregnancy to term in the future because a pregnancy can worsen these conditions. The Food and Drug Administration (FDA) encourages women who have experienced negative side effects to prescription drugs (which includes any hormonal and non-hormonal contraceptive available in the United States) to visit www.fda.gov/medwatch or call 1-800-FDA-1088.

The section on hormonal contraceptives begins with a discussion of the least effective method in the most effective category—the pill. This section concludes with a description of the most effective hormonal contraceptive method currently available to women, but *not* the most effective contraceptive on the market!

The Pill

In the 1960s, most oral contraceptives contained anywhere from 2.5–10 milligrams (mgs) of estrogen or progestin (Nelson, 2007). This hormonal contraceptive method has come a long way in the last 50 years. Now, most pills contain less than 1 mg of estrogen or progestin. If a woman is on the pill, she can look at the wrapper or box to identify the exact dosage of estrogen and/or progestin. The names of these hormones differ, though, so instead of reading "estrogen," she may read the word "ethinyl estradiol," and instead of reading "progestin," she may read one of eight words: "desogestrel," "drospirenone," "ethynodiol diacetate," "levonorestrel," "norethindrone," "norethindrone acetate," "norgestimate," or "norgestrel."

Most oral contraceptives come in a pack of 28 pills. There are 28 pills because the pill was developed to mimic an average woman's menstrual cycle to make it easier for women to accept this form of contraception in the 1960s. Twenty-one pills have estrogen and progestin or progestin only (known as "active" days) and the last 7 pills are placebos. The placebo pills do not have hormones in

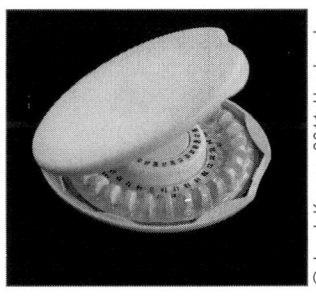
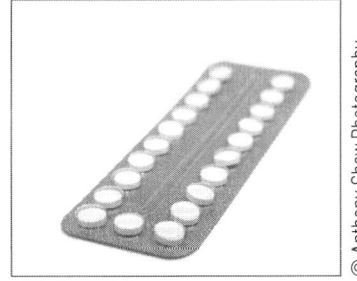
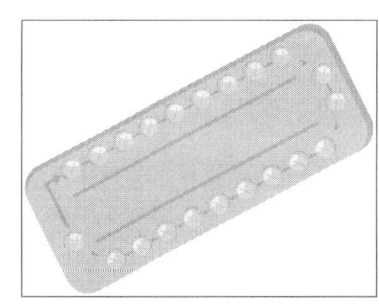

them, but some brands do have iron in their placebo pills. It is while taking the 7 placebo pills that a woman menstruates even though she usually will not menstruate for all seven days. Remember that with any hormonal method, a woman bleeds not because an ovum wasn't fertilized (especially since ovulation should not have occurred), but because the placebo pills do not contain hormones to stop a woman's endometrial lining from growing or shedding (Nelson, 2007).

With oral contraceptives, women are supposed to take a pill every day, usually at the same time every day. For various reasons, women forget to take a pill (or two) during the 21-day "active" period. That is why this method is considered the least effective of the most effective options. Many of us may not understand how difficult it is to take one small pill every day. Yet many women have complex lives with work, school, and family obligations competing for their time. Moreover, women may not appreciate the need for the constant hormonal balance that taking the pill every day at the same time provides. This indifference is more apparent if women never ingest the placebo pills. A woman doesn't have to take the placebo pills because they are mostly there to help her remember that she will be getting her period soon and when she needs to start a new pack. When some women decide not to take the placebo pills, they unfortunately may also forget to start a new pack. With 7 placebo days and a few extra days with no intake of hormones from the pill, a woman's body starts resorting to its old self and she may ovulate, even if she starts a new pack (Baerwald, Olatunbosun, & Pierson, 2006). This event is called "escape ovulation" (Willis, Kuehl, Spiekerman, & Sulak, 2006). That is why you may have heard that some women have gotten pregnant even though they were on the pill.

Also remember that if a woman is on the pill (and probably any hormonal method) and taking antibiotics, she needs to use a backup method for that month because antibiotics interfere with the body's ability to metabolize the pill. Ovulation can occur and increase the risk of an ovum being fertilized by a sperm and implanting itself in the endometrial lining (Nelson, 2007). A woman should not stop taking the pill for that month, though. She may start bleeding when she was not supposed to and then find it difficult to know when she needs to start a new pack. If her male partner is not already doing so, he should wear a condom during that month to protect against an unintended pregnancy, as well as to reduce the couple's risk of any sexually transmitted infection (STI).

To decrease the incidence of "escape ovulation," new oral contraceptives have been developed with more "active" pills and fewer placebo pills. Some pills (such as Loestrin 24Fe® and Yaz®) now have 24 instead of 21 pills with estrogen and progestin and 4 instead of 7 pills with a placebo (Willis et al., 2006). This will hopefully reduce the number of women who get pregnant while on the pill, but women still need to remember to take the pill every day around the same time! According to the FDA, unlike other oral contraceptives, Yasmin® and Yaz® contain the progestin drospirenone, which may increase potassium levels that could cause serious health complications. These oral contraceptives are not recommended for women who have ever had kidney, liver, or adrenal gland diseases.

Some oral contraceptives are considered extended-cycle pills because a woman continues to take active pills past the usual 21 days of most oral contraceptives. For example, women on Seasonale® take a pill for 84 consecutive days with estrogen and progestin and 7 placebo pills (Anderson, Gibbons, & Portman, 2006). Such a pill means that a woman will bleed once every three months (or once a season). Some women reported unscheduled withdrawal bleeding (i.e., spotting between periods), so a similar pill was created to eliminate such events (van Heusden & Fauser, 2002). This pill, called Seasonique® has 84 "active" days and 7 low-dose estrogen pills. There are no placebo pills but because the last 7 days do not contain progestin (which helps thin out the endometrial lining), a woman should experience bleeding only during that timeframe.

Another oral contraceptive relatively new to the market, called Lybrel®, has 28 pills with estrogen and progestin and no placebo pills. With no placebo pills, a woman does not bleed at all because this pill does not allow her endometrial lining to grow. If the endometrium doesn't grow, there's nothing to shed. However, many women see menstrual bleeding as a sign that they are not pregnant. Even though using the pill (or any hormonal method) correctly should be enough to make women feel at ease, that is not always the case. Moreover, some women worry that not bleeding at all on a monthly basis is not healthy or natural. Research studies (Anderson, Gibbons, & Portman, 2006) have reported that concern to be unfounded, but if a woman does not feel comfortable in not bleeding on a monthly basis, then Lybrel® is not the pill for her.

Women who cannot tolerate estrogen in oral contraceptives or are breastfeeding should not be on a hormonal contraceptive method with estrogen (Nelson, 2007). Breastfeeding mothers on a hormonal method with estrogen will have the hormone transferred to the breast milk and ingested by the infant. There is a pill that only has progestin in it, known as the Mini-Pill. The Mini-Pill is believed to be around 95 percent effective, though, so the utmost compliance in taking the Mini-Pill is needed (Raymond, 2007b).

The Patch

The Ortho Evra Patch® is a hormonal contraceptive worn on a woman's skin. The only exception is the breasts because that part of the body usually has too much fatty tissue that does not allow the hormones to be adequately absorbed into

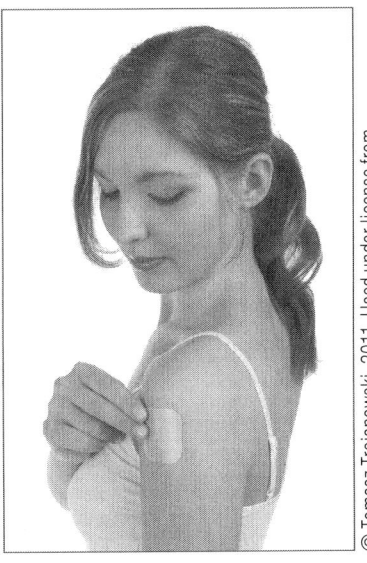
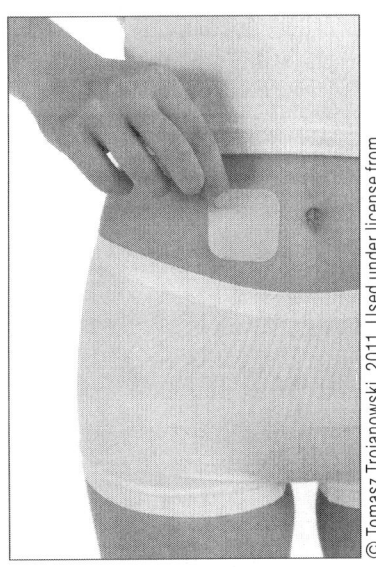

the bloodstream. The hormones (both estrogen and progestin) are in the "sticky part" of the patch. A woman is given three patches in one packet and she changes the patch once a week for three weeks (Nanda, 2007). On the fourth week she does not wear a patch and she will get her period. According to Mosher and Jones (2010), the percentage of women who had ever used the Ortho Evra Patch® rose from 1 percent in 2002 to 10 percent (5.3 million) in 2006–2008. Besides discussing this option with her doctor, a woman can check the manufacture's website at www.orthoevra.com for more information.

The Vaginal Ring

The NuvaRing® is a hormonal contraceptive ring (about the size of a silver dollar) that a woman inserts into her vagina and places it by her cervix (Nanda, 2007). Before you think this is a daunting task, remember that a woman's vagina is not an endless tunnel—she will get to the end sooner than she thinks! She leaves the ring in place for three weeks. Even though for most women it will not fall out, if she feels it in her vagina then she hasn't put it in as far as it can go. On the fourth week she does not wear a vaginal ring and she gets her period. To help a woman remember how long she's had the vaginal ring inside her and when to put in a new one, her doctor provides her with a digital hourglass that helps her keep track. Each NuvaRing® packet comes with stickers that she can place on her calendar to remember when she put the vaginal ring in and when she needs to take it out. Besides discussing this option with her doctor, a woman can check the manufacture's website at www.nuvaring.com for more information.

The Shot

Depo-Provera® is a hormonal contraceptive injection that a woman gets every 12 weeks. This contraception does not contain estrogen, it is progestin only. Because of this, most women will cease menstruating completely after 6–12 months of being on this method (Goldberg & Grimes, 2007). Menstrual bleeding will return anywhere from 3–6 months after stopping this hormonal method. This method may also decrease the calcium in a woman's bones (Goldberg & Grimes, 2007). A woman on Depo-Provera® should take a calcium supplement and exercise to defray calcium loss. These side effects are completely reversed when a woman stops using this method (Trussell, 2007b). Besides discussing this option with her doctor, a woman can check the manufacture's website at www.pfizer.com/products/rx/rx_product_depo_provera.jsp for more information.

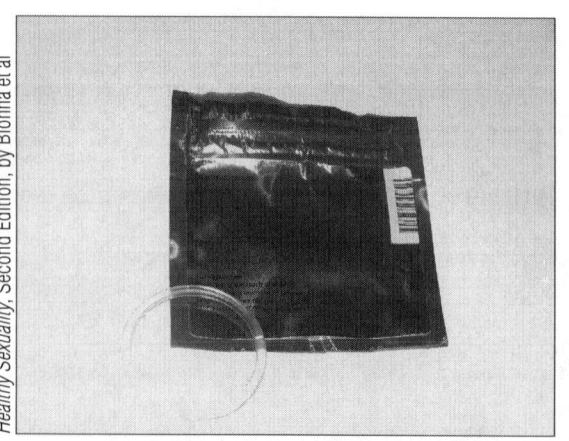

Implants

Implanon® is a hormonal contraceptive that is a small rod (2 mm in diameter and 40 mm in length) implanted under the skin of a woman's inner arm by a doctor (Raymond, 2007a). The implant provides three years of contraceptive protection. Even though it lasts for three years, a woman can have the implant removed at any time before then if she decides to plan a pregnancy earlier than anticipated. This contraception does not contain estrogen, it is progestin only. Because this method has to be implanted under the skin (a procedure that takes less than five minutes), the doctor needs to be trained. A woman can ask her doctor if she/he is trained and offers this method in the practice. She can learn more about this contraception by visiting the manufacture's website at www.implanon-usa.com for more information. England has recently taken Implanon® off the market because of a higher-than-expected incidence of pregnancies with this method.

Nexplanon® is similar to Implanon®, but not available in the United States. The difference between the two is that the Nexplanon applicator is designed for ease of insertion and the rod is *radiopaque* (does not let X-rays or other types of radiation penetrate) so it is easily identifiable. To learn more about this contraception, visit the manufacture's website at www.nexplanontraining.co.uk/FAQ.aspx for more information.

Jadelle® is a hormonal contraceptive that is two small rods (approximately 2.5 mm in diameter and 43 mm in length) implanted under the skin of a woman's inner arm by a doctor. The implants provide five years of contraceptive protection (Raymond, 2007a). Unfortunately, this method is currently unavailable in the United States. To learn more about this contraception, visit the Population Council's website at www.popcouncil.org/what/jadelle.asp for more information.

Intra-Uterine System (IUS)

Mirena® is a hormonal contraceptive this is inserted in a woman's uterus by a doctor. This is done by inserting the T-shaped device (around the size of a quarter) in the vagina, then the cervix to the uterus (Grimes, 2007). A woman is usually not given general anesthesia for this procedure. Local anesthesia (to the cervix) is possible. Most women are asked to take an over-the-counter pain-reliever before the procedure. Insertion takes place when a woman is menstruating because the cervical os is slightly open to allow menstrual flow (Grimes, 2007). This contraception does not contain estrogen; it is progestin only. The IUS can remain in the uterus for up to five years. To aid in detection and removal of the device, two white threads are tied through the tip. A doctor cuts the thread enough to have only a small amount protrude through the os. Similar to Implanon®, a woman can have the IUS removed before the five years is up if she decides to plan a pregnancy earlier than anticipated. The majority of gynecologists have been trained to insert Mirena®, so it should not be a problem finding a trained physician. Besides discussing this option with her doctor, a woman can check the manufacture's website at www.mirena-us.com for more information.

CHOOSING A HORMONAL METHOD

As you can see, women have a variety of hormonal methods to choose from. Men, though, currently do not have any hormonal contraceptive methods available for them. Why do you think that is the case? Given the choices available to women, and if a woman decides to use one of these options, she needs to ask herself which method seems right for her. Can she take a pill every day at the same time without forgetting? Would she prefer to get a shot every 12 weeks? Can she put her fingers in her vagina to insert the NuvaRing®? Does she mind having a patch on some part of her body and changing it once a week? Is she comfortable having a device somewhere inside her body for years at a time? A woman needs to pick the method she can realistically and consistently use. If not, then it is not going to help prevent a pregnancy.

If a woman is a smoker, she should not be on any hormonal method with estrogen. Why? The pill adds stress to the blood vessels as it produces extra estrogen in the woman's body (Nelson, 2007). For a healthy woman, this should not be a concern. For a woman who smokes, however, this increased stress is combined with what smoking does to the body. Nicotine causes high blood pressure and increases the heart rate (Nelson, 2007). This also stresses the blood vessels. Therefore, a woman who smokes while on a hormonal method with estrogen is overexerting her blood vessels in two ways. This combination can cause heart attacks, blood clots, and strokes. This becomes even more likely for women who are heavy smokers (smoking more than 15 cigarettes a day), as well as women over age 35.

Some women change contraception methods depending on their lifestyle. Maybe taking a pill every day is possible right now, but what if her work and home life become more demanding? Maybe she needs to switch to a method that she doesn't have to think about often but is just as effective. Never forget that there is someone else who can help prevent a pregnancy and that's the man she is sexually active with! Part of a healthy (heterosexual) sexual relationship is communicating about how to prevent unintended pregnancies together. Given the few contraceptive options available to men who are in sexual relationships with women, they need to realize that they are or will be surrendering their reproductive health to their female sexual partner. If men want to decide when they want to become fathers or not, they have to take a more active role in preventing unintended pregnancies by using condoms consistently or getting sterilized (the latter is usually not available to men younger than 25 and childless).

Preventing a Pregnancy and STI Exposure

There is no hormonal contraceptive method that reduces a person's risk of being infected by an STI (Marrazzo, Guest, & Cates, 2007). Besides trying to keep yourself from getting pregnant (or getting someone pregnant), you also need to reduce your risk of exposing yourself to an STI (discussed in chapter 7). Along with being in a monogamous relationship with an uninfected partner, only barriers like the female and male condom can help reduce your risk. Using a hormonal and barrier method simultaneously can improve the chances of preventing an unintended pregnancy and reducing one's risk to an STI. Keep in mind that some STIs can be passed on by skin-to-skin contact (meaning no seminal and/or vaginal fluid transmission is needed to become infected), like genital herpes and HPV (Marrazzo, Guest, & Cates, 2007).

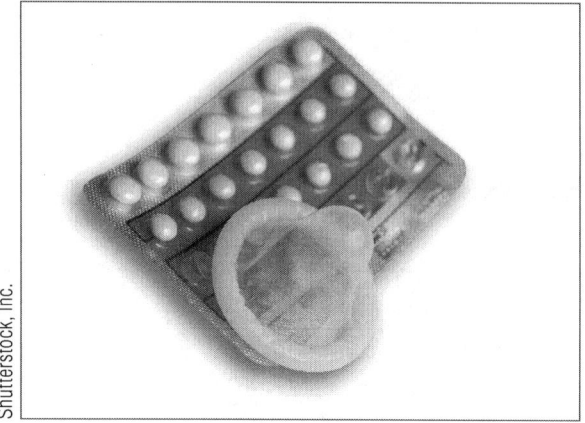

NON-HORMONAL CONTRACEPTIVE METHODS

Non-hormonal contraceptive agents or devices work by preventing sperm from reaching an ovum or by preventing implantation if fertilization does occur. Even though the majority of these methods are not as effective as hormonal options to prevent a pregnancy, the most effective method falls in this category, as do the permanent, non-reversible contraceptive choices currently available (Pollack, Thomas, & Barone, 2007). This section begins with the least effective method of contraception and concludes with the most effective contraceptive on the market.

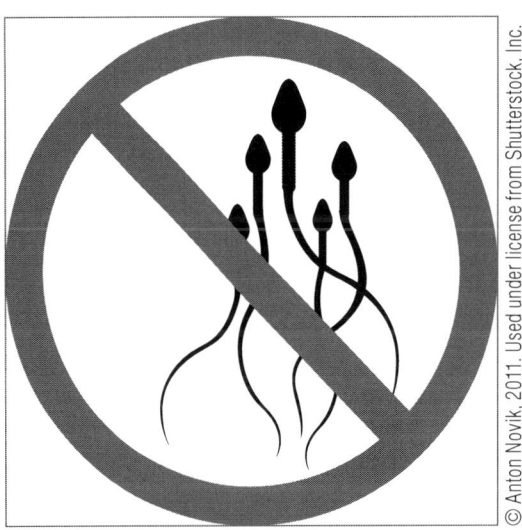

Fertility Awareness Methods

Fertility awareness methods are considered the least effective method in preventing unintended pregnancies because daily adherence is needed for continued protection and some days out of the month are considered "non-coital" days. Thus, spontaneous sexual activity is not always realistic and a woman's menstrual cycle can deviate from its normal schedule due to illness, medication, and stress (Jennings & Arevalo, 2007). Using more than one fertility awareness method concurrently can improve the chances of preventing an unintended pregnancy, though.

In using the Standard Days Method®, women follow their "safe" and "unsafe" days to participate in coitus by using CycleBeads®. CycleBeads® is a color-coded string of beads that represents the days of a woman's cycle. A woman moves a ring over the beads to track *each day* of her cycle. The color of the beads indicates whether a particular day may result in a pregnancy if coitus is initiated. Women do not have to buy the beads to use this method because the makers of CycleBeads® have created an app to help women follow their menstrual cycle and calculate their most fertile days.

In using the Cervical Mucus Ovulation Detection method, women check the quantity and quality of cervical mucus expelled from the vaginal opening with their fingers or tissue paper *every morning*. Cervical mucus changes in color and consistency throughout the menstrual cycle. Before ovulation, the mucus is cloudy, white or yellow, and sticky. During ovulation, the mucus is clear, wet, stretchy, sticky, and slippery (Jennings & Arevalo, 2007).

In using the Basal Body Temperature Method, women check their temperature *every day* before they get out of bed. A woman's body temperature rises as she nears ovulation. With this method, a woman is expected to refrain from coitus starting on the first day of her menstrual bleeding until she has documented three consecutive days of sustained body temperature (Jennings & Arevalo, 2007).

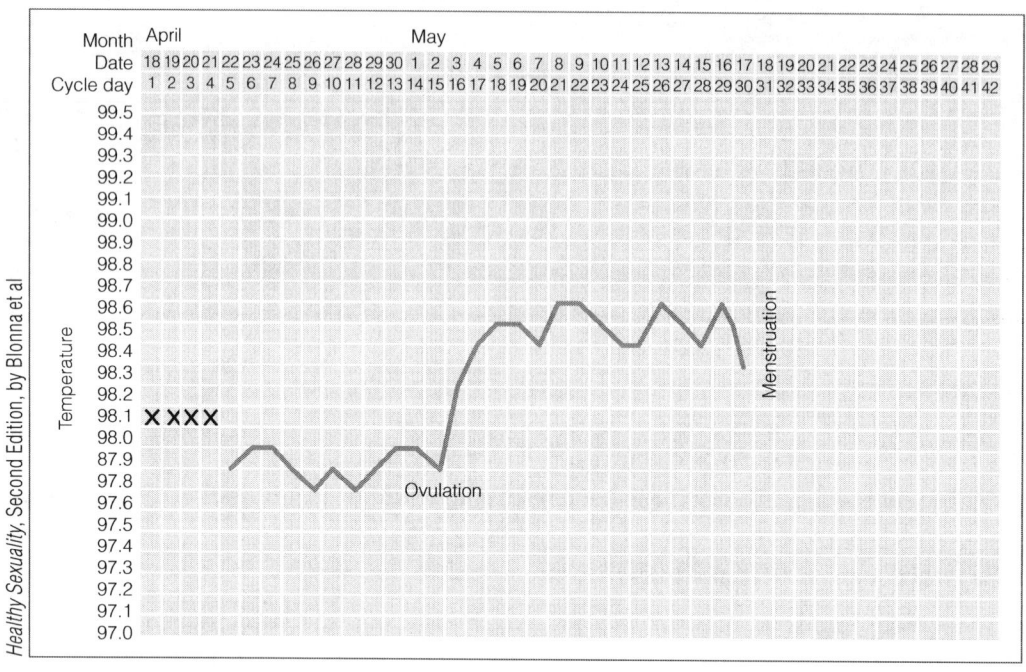

Spermicides

Spermicide contains a chemical that kills sperm. This substance may be purchased in the form of foam, jelly, cream, suppository, film, or sponge that is placed inside the vagina near the cervix before coitus. Some types must be put in place 30 minutes ahead of time (read the package for instructions). Spermicides have a higher unintended pregnancy rate than other barrier methods (Cates & Raymond, 2007). Spermicides should always be used with another form of contraception, such as a condom to increase protection. Keep in mind that frequent use may cause tissue (vaginal, cervical, or penile) irritation, which can increase the risk of vaginal infections and the transmission of STIs.

Barrier Methods

Barriers have been developed to prevent sperm from fertilizing an egg by either blocking the entrance to the cervix through a removable device surrounding the cervix or a sheath that covers the penis or vagina. Cervical devices currently available in the United States are the diaphragm, the cervical cap, Lea's shield, FemCap, and the contraceptive sponge. These cervical barriers allow seminal

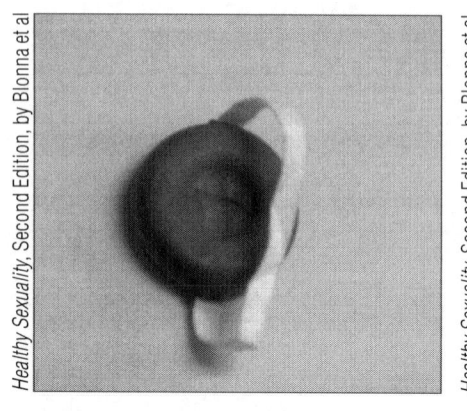
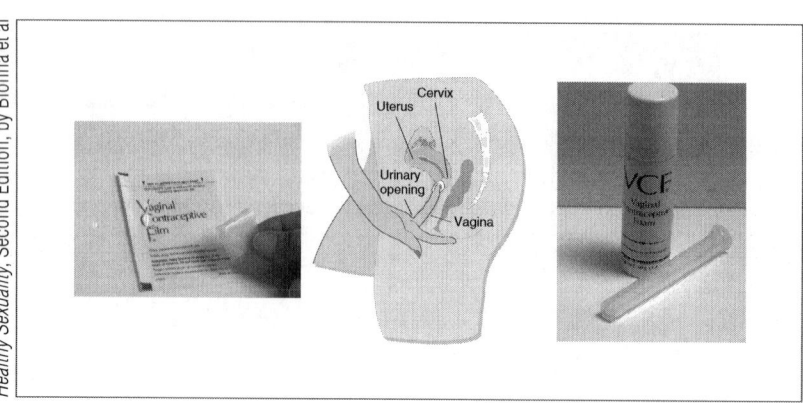

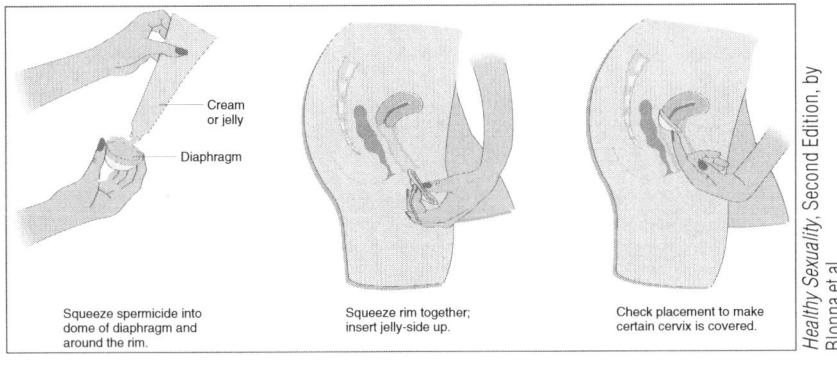
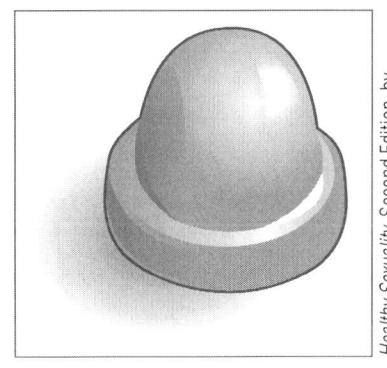

fluid to enter the vagina but the device covering the cervix does not allow the sperm to enter the upper reproductive tract (Cates & Raymond, 2007).

Cervical Barriers

Diaphragms, Lea's shield, FemCap, and cervical caps come in different sizes, thus they must be fitted by an experienced health care provider. The woman is taught how to insert the device herself for future use. The device is not left in the cervix permanently. Some of these cervical barriers have to be inserted hours before coitus is anticipated. After insertion, the device is left in place by the cervix for 6–8 hours after coitus. Spermicide is also used with these cervical devices. Thus, spontaneous sexual activity may be difficult with some of these methods. Condoms and the contraceptive sponge do not require a prescription. Barrier methods do not have many side effects, unless you or your sexual partner is allergic to the material (latex) some of these methods are made from (Cates & Raymond, 2007).

Coitus Interruptus (Withdrawal Method)

With the withdrawal method, the man does not ejaculate inside a woman's vagina during coitus (Kowal, 2007). Recent research suggests that more couples use this method than previously documented (Jones, Fennell, Higgins, & Blanchard, 2009). Even so, this method is not for the faint of heart, given a typical use failure rate of 18 percent, but ranging from 14–24 percent (Kost et al., 2008). Many couples report "pulling out" along with using another contraceptive method, like the pill or the condom (Jones et al., 2009).

Female & Male Condoms

During coitus, physical barrier contraceptives, such as the female and male condoms prevent sperm from fertilizing an egg by blocking the presence of semen in the female lower reproductive tract (Warner & Steiner, 2007). The male condom is the third most popular contraception method in the United States (The Alan Guttmacher Institute, 2010). A male condom is worn on an erect penis to physically block his semen from entering another person's body during coitus, fellatio, or anal sex (Warner & Steiner, 2007). After ejaculation, the semen remains within the sheath of the male condom.

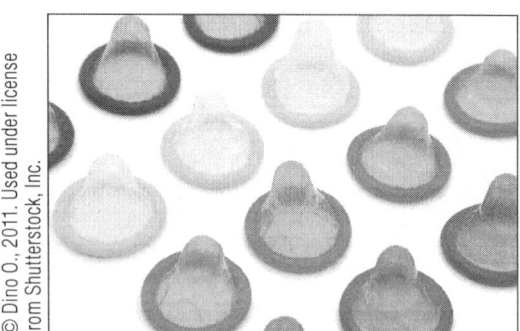

| Pinch or twist the tip of the condom, leaving one-half inch at the tip to catch the semen. | Holding the tip, unroll the condom. | Unroll the condom until it reaches the pubic hairs. |

A female condom is worn internally by the receptive partner to physically block semen from entering that person's body and can be worn up to eight hours before coitus. After ejaculation, the semen remains within the sheath of the female condom. Unlike all hormonal methods, condoms do not require a prescription and side effects are minimal. It is possible, though, for either sexual partner to have an allergic reaction to latex, the material that the majority of male condoms are made. Female and some male condoms are made of polyurethane. A new female condom has been developed from synthetic nitrile. If a condom is the method of contraceptive choice for a couple, a penis should never be near or enter the vaginal opening unless a condom is worn by either partner. It is not recommended for both partners to have a condom on at the same time or for a male partner to wear more than one condom simultaneously—the thrusting is believed to weaken the integrity of the condoms, thus increasing the risk of breakage.

Intra-Uterine Device (IUD)

ParaGard® is an IUD that can be inserted into the uterus by a doctor. Insertion of ParaGard® follows the same procedure as Mirena®. Unlike Mirena®, though, this method does not contain hormones and

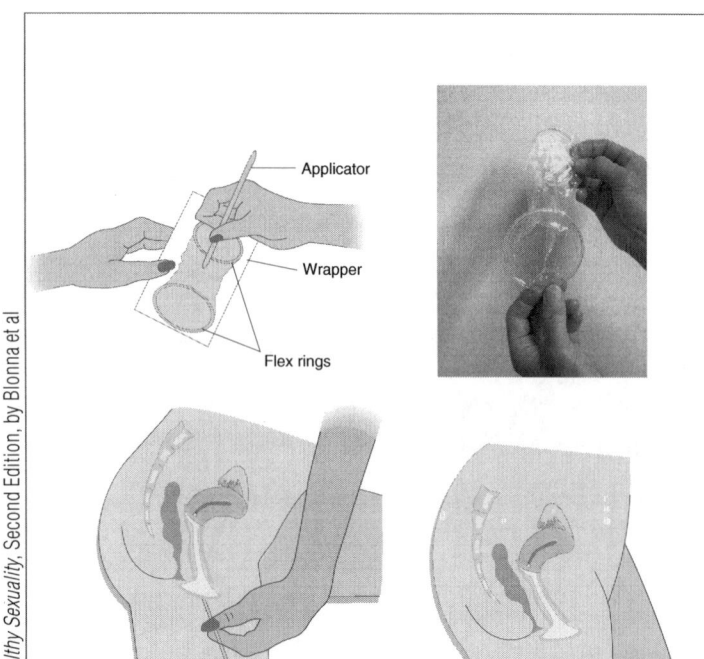

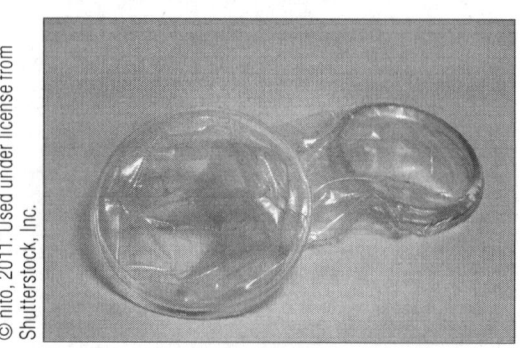

it can stay in place for up to 10 years. ParaGard® has copper throughout and works by creating a hostile uterine environment to sperm (Grimes, 2007). Besides discussing this option with her doctor, a woman can check the manufacture's website at www.paragard.com/ for more information.

GyneFix® is another IUD that can be inserted into the uterus by a doctor. It differs in shape and size when compared to ParaGard® or Mirena®. It has no "arms" (which give ParaGard® and Mirena® the T shape) and it is smaller. It contains no hormones and can stay in place for up to five years. It is currently unavailable in the United States.

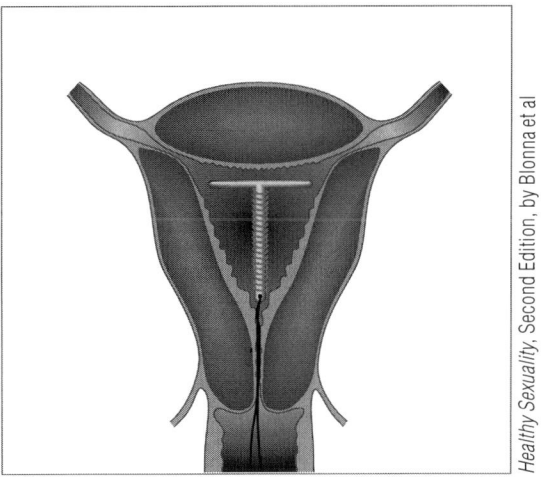

Female Sterilization

As previously mentioned, female sterilization has been in the top two spots as one of the most widely used contraceptive methods in the United States since 1982. The percentage of women who rely on female sterilization as their form of contraception increases as a woman gets older (Mosher & Jones, 2010). There are two procedures to permanently end a woman's ability to become pregnant: a hysteroscopic tubal sterilization (known as Essure®) and tubal ligation (Jones & Lopez, 2006).

With tubal ligation, the fallopian tubes are cut, burned, or blocked with rings, bands, or clips. Carbon dioxide is pumped into the abdominal cavity to render the fallopian tubes more visible to the doctor performing the surgery (Jones & Lopez, 2006). A woman is usually given general anesthesia, but local anesthesia is on the rise, with many of these procedures taking place in an outpatient setting. During the procedure, an incision is made in the navel and either two punctures are done on either side of the abdomen where the fallopian tubes are or another incision is made above the mons pubis. A woman will experience pain, tenderness, and bloating for about a week after the surgery. The surgery is effective immediately.

For Essure®, a doctor inserts a coil through the vagina, cervix, and uterus and into the fallopian tubes. A camera is also inserted to help the doctor navigate through the vagina, cervix, and uterus into the fallopian tubes, as well as to provide immediate visual confirmation of placement. A woman is not given general anesthesia, but

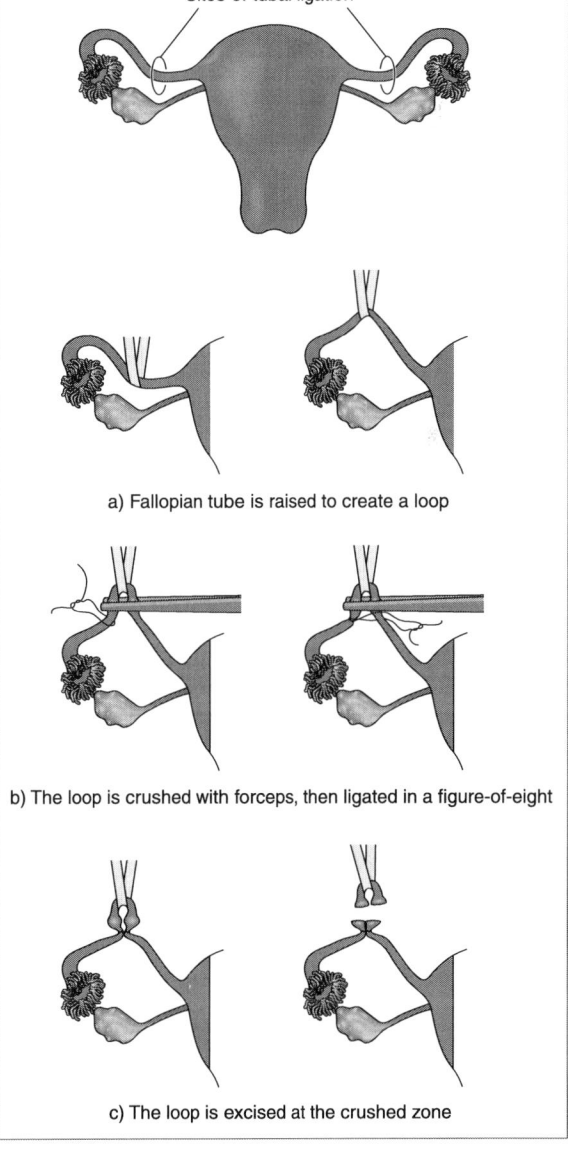

she does receive local anesthesia in the cervix. Most women are asked to take an over-the-counter pain reliever before the procedure. She will probably feel cramping throughout the procedure and for a few hours after. During the three months following the procedure, the fallopian tubes form scar tissue around the inserted coil that prevents sperm from reaching the ovum (Pollack, Thomas, & Barone, 2007). During this time, a woman must continue using another method of contraception to prevent a pregnancy. After three months of undergoing this procedure, a woman gets an Essure Confirmation Test. This test is usually done in a hospital because a dye is placed in the uterus and a special type of X-ray is used to ensure that the coils are in place and the fallopian tubes are completely blocked (Jones & Lopez, 2006). Besides discussing this option with her doctor, a woman can check the manufacture's website at www.essure.com/ for more information.

Male Sterilization

A vasectomy is considered the most effective contraception available. It is the fourth most popular contraception method in the United States (The Alan Guttmacher Institute, 2010). A vasectomy is a permanent form of contraception that prevents the release of sperm when a man ejaculates (Pollack, Thomas, & Barone, 2007). During a vasectomy, the scrotal skin is cut, the vas deferens is located in each testicle and severed. The two ends of the vas deferens are tied, stitched, or sealed. Electrocautery (cutting with heat) may be used to seal the ends. Scar tissue from the surgery also helps block the tubes.

During this procedure, a man is given local anesthesia in each testicle. He is rarely, if ever, given general anesthesia. The procedure takes around 20–30 minutes. The man is asked to relax at home for the next 2–3 days and refrain from lifting anything heavy for one week. His testicles will ache and be tender, and he might experience scrotal swelling (Pollack, Thomas, & Barone, 2007).

After a vasectomy, it usually takes around 15–20 ejaculations to completely clear sperm from the semen (Jones & Lopez, 2006). Thus, a man will have to use another form of reliable contraception for the first three months after the procedure. After three months (or 20 ejaculations—whichever comes first), the man returns to the doctor who performed the vasectomy to confirm that the reproductive tract has been cleared of sperm (Pollack, Thomas, & Barone, 2007). This is done by having the man ejaculate in a cup and the seminal fluid is analyzed for the existence of sperm.

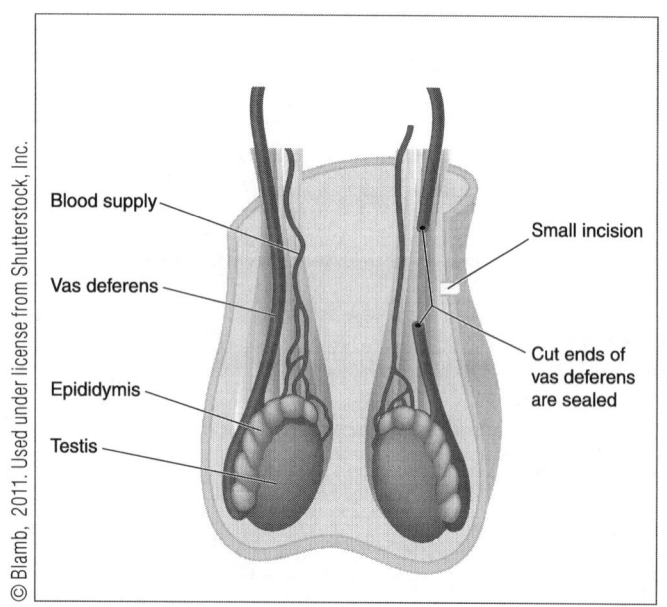

The testicles continue to produce sperm after a vasectomy, but the sperm are reabsorbed by the body. Sperm is also reabsorbed if ejaculation does not occur after a while, regardless of whether a male has had a vasectomy or not (Jones & Lopez, 2006). Because only 1 percent of ejaculation is sperm and the tubes are blocked before the seminal vesicles and prostate gland (where the majority of seminal fluid is produced), a man will still ejaculate about the same amount of fluid (Pollack, Thomas, & Barone, 2007).

MEN AND CONTRACEPTION

Because there are so many more contraceptive options for women and because society assumes women should take primary responsibility in preventing unintended pregnancies, many men may be ambivalent about their role in their own reproductive health. There are only three contraceptive options (and one of them is not considered as reliable) for men and all are non-hormonal methods. Why do you think we have not developed reliable hormonal contraceptives for men?

Men will have to ask themselves which method is right for them given their current circumstances. Are they currently in a casual relationship that deems condom use necessary? Is it possible to seriously consider condom use as the main form of contraception if the relationship is considered monogamous and long term? Why or why not? What if a female sexual partner admits to be using a reliable form of contraception, like the pill, will the man surrender full responsibility of preventing an unintended pregnancy to her? What if he's 30 years old and has had all the children he wants to have, would he seriously consider having a vasectomy?

Emergency Contraception

Emergency contraception works after coitus has occurred to help avoid an unintended pregnancy. This is an option if no contraceptive method was used or if a couple suspects their usual method failed. Plan B, Plan B One-Step, and a generic version of Plan B called Next Choice all contain a high dose of progestin. Emergency contraception inhibits ovulation, thus decreasing the chance of fertilization from a specific coital act. Emergency contraception is *not* a form of abortion. On the contrary, it helps prevent abortion by preventing unintended pregnancies (Stewart, Trussell, & Van Look, 2007). No prescription is needed for women who are 17 years and older. Emergency contraception must be used within 120 hours of coitus. According to Mosher and Jones (2010), between 2002 and 2006–2008, the percentage of women who had used emergency contraception rose from 4 to 10 percent (5.2 million).

Reflections

The purpose of this chapter is to provide information about the variety of options available for preventing an unintended pregnancy. With an unplanned pregnancy rate of almost 50 percent in the United States (Ventura, Abma, Mosher, & Henshaw, 2009), a number of issues need to be addressed to increase the percentage of planned pregnancies while decreasing the incidence of unintended pregnancies. Obtaining reliable, medically accurate information on the contraceptive methods available in the United States is a good start to help prevent unintended pregnancies and plan future pregnancies. Access to affordable and reliable contraceptive options to all women and men also needs to become a reality.

Critical Thinking Questions

1. Other countries, such as Sweden, Denmark, the Netherlands, England, and France, have lower rates of unintended pregnancies than the United States. Why do you think that is?

2. How do you think access to reliable methods and comprehensive sexuality education, along with an awareness of adolescent sexuality, helps to prevent unintended pregnancies?

3. What role, if any, do you think religion played in your parents' contraceptive use? How about your own?

4. If there were a hormonal method like the Pill for men, do you think they would take it? Why or why not? If such an option were available, do you think women would surrender control of their reproductive health to men? Why or why not?

How Much Do You Remember from the Chapter?

(1–20) • Match the contraceptive with the type of method it is:

1. Essure _____
2. NuvaRing _____
3. Cycle Beads _____
4. Male condom _____
5. ParaGard _____
6. Cervical cap _____
7. Tubal ligation _____

a. barrier
b. hormonal
c. intra-uterine
d. sterilization
e. fertility awareness
f. cervical barrier
g. spermicide

8. Today Sponge _____
9. Female condom _____
10. Mirena _____
11. Cervical mucus _____
12. Implanon _____
13. Diaphragm _____
14. Vaginal film _____
15. Vasectomy _____
16. Depo-Provera _____
17. Vaginal foam _____
18. Ortho Evra Patch _____
19. Body temperature _____
20. Jadelle _____

Challenge Yourself!

(1–15) • Match the contraceptive with its level of effectiveness:

MOST EFFECTIVE

1. _____
2. _____
3. _____
4. _____
5. _____
6. _____
7. _____
8. _____
9. _____
10. _____
11. _____
12. _____
13. _____
14. _____
15. _____

LEAST EFFECTIVE

a. Oral contraceptives
b. Fertility awareness method
c. Implanon
d. Female condom
e. Mirena
f. Spermicides
g. Male sterilization
h. The patch
i. NuvaRing
j. Cervical barriers
k. Jadelle
l. Male condom
m. ParaGard
n. Depo-Provera
o. Female sterilization

Websites

www.acha.org
American College Health Association

www.acog.org
American College of Obstetrics and Gynecology

www.asrm.org
American Society for Reproductive Medicine

www.cdc.gov
Centers for Disease Control and Prevention

www.cdc.gov/nchs/
National Center for Health Statistics

www.nfprha.org/facts/contraception
National Family Planning and Reproductive Health Association

www.ppfa.org
Planned Parenthood Federation of America

www.siecus.org
Sexuality Information and Education Council of the United States (SICEUS)

References

The Alan Guttmacher Institute. (2000). *Fulfilling the promise: Public policy and U.S. family planning clinics.* New York, NY: Author.

The Alan Guttmacher Institute. (2002). *In their own right: Addressing the sexual and reproductive health needs of American men.* New York, NY: Author.

The Alan Guttmacher Institute. (2010). *Facts on contraceptive use in the United States.* New York, NY: Author.

Anderson, F., Gibbons, W., & Portman, D. (2006). Safety and efficacy of an extended-regimen oral contraceptive utilizing continuous low-dose ethinyl estradiol. *Contraception, 73,* 229–234.

Baerwald, A., Olatunbosun, O., & Pierson, R. (2006). Effects of oral contraceptives administered at defined stages of ovarian follicular development. *Fertility & Sterility, 86,* 27–35.

Cates, W., & Raymond, E. (2007). Vaginal barriers and spermicides. In R. Hatcher, J. Trussell, A. Nelson, W. Cates, F. Stewart, & D. Kowal (Eds.), *Contraceptive technology* (19th ed., pp. 317–336). New York, NY: Ardent Media.

Crooks, R., & Baur, K. (2011). *Our sexuality* (11th ed.). Belmont, CA: Wadsworth/Cengage Learning.

Goldberg, A., & Grimes, D. (2007). Injectable contraceptives. In R. Hatcher, J. Trussell, A. Nelson, W. Cates, F. Stewart, & D. Kowal (eds.), *Contraceptive technology* (19th Ed., pp. 157–170). New York, NY: Ardent Media.

Grimes, D. (2007). Intrauterine devices (IUDs). In R. Hatcher, J. Trussell, A. Nelson, W. Cates, F. Stewart, & D. Kowal (Eds.), *Contraceptive technology* (19th ed., pp. 117–139). New York, NY: Ardent Media.

Hatcher R., & Brawner Namnoum, A. (2007). The menstrual cycle. In R. Hatcher, J. Trussell, A. Nelson, W. Cates, F. Stewart, & D. Kowal (Eds.), *Contraceptive technology* (19th ed., pp. 7–18). New York, NY: Ardent Media.

Jennings, V., & Arevalo, M. (2007). Family awareness-based methods. In R. Hatcher, J. Trussell, A. Nelson, W. Cates, F. Stewart, & D. Kowal (Eds.), *Contraceptive technology* (19th ed., pp. 343–336). New York, NY: Ardent Media.

Jones, R., Fennell, J., Higgins, J., & Blanchard, K. (2009). Better than nothing or savvy risk-reduction practice? The importance of withdrawal. *Contraception, 79*, 407–410.

Jones, R., & Lopez, K. (2006). *Human reproductive biology* (3rd ed.). Burlington, MA: Elsevier.

Kost, K., Singh, S., Vaughan, B., Trussell, J., & Bankole, A. (2008). Estimates of contraceptive failure from the 2002 National Survey of Family Growth. *Contraception, 77*(1), 10–21.

Kowal, D. (2007). Coitus interruptus (withdrawal). In R. Hatcher, J. Trussell, A. Nelson, W. Cates, F. Stewart, & D. Kowal (Eds.), *Contraceptive technology* (19th ed., pp. 337–342). New York, NY: Ardent Media.

Marrazzo, J., Guest, F., & Cates, W. (2007). Reproductive tract infections, including HIV and other sexually transmitted infections. In R. Hatcher, J. Trussell, A. Nelson, W. Cates, F. Stewart, & D. Kowal (Eds.), *Contraceptive technology* (19th ed., pp. 499–558). New York, NY: Ardent Media.

Martin, J., Hamilton, B., Sutton, P., Ventura, S., Menacker, F., Kirmeyer, S. et al. (2009). Births: Final data for 2006. *National Vital Statistics Reports, 57*(7). Hyattsville, MD: National Center for Health Statistics.

Mosher, W., & Jones, J. (2010). Use of contraception in the United States: 1982–2008. *Vital Health Statistics, 23*(29). Hyattsville, MD: National Center for Health Statistics.

Nanda, K. (2007). Contraceptive patch and vaginal contraceptive ring. In R. Hatcher, J. Trussell, A. Nelson, W. Cates, F. Stewart, & D. Kowal (Eds.), *Contraceptive technology* (19th ed., pp. 271–296). New York, NY: Ardent Media.

Nelson, A. (2007). Combined oral contraceptives. In R. Hatcher, J. Trussell, A. Nelson, W. Cates, F. Stewart, & D. Kowal (Eds.), *Contraceptive technology* (19th ed., pp. 193–270). New York, NY: Ardent Media.

Pollack, A., Thomas, L., & Barone, M. (2007). Female and male sterilization. In R. Hatcher, J. Trussell, A. Nelson, W. Cates, F. Stewart, & D. Kowal (Eds.), *Contraceptive technology* (19th ed., pp. 361–402). New York, NY: Ardent Media.

Raymond, E. (2007a). Contraceptive implants. In R. Hatcher, J. Trussell, A. Nelson, W. Cates, F. Stewart, & D. Kowal (Eds.), *Contraceptive technology* (19th ed., pp. 145–156). New York, NY: Ardent Media.

Raymond, E. (2007b). Progestin-only pills. In R. Hatcher, J. Trussell, A. Nelson, W. Cates, F. Stewart, & D. Kowal (Eds.), *Contraceptive technology* (19th ed., pp. 181–192). New York, NY: Ardent Media.

Stewart, F., Trussell, J., & Van Look, P. (2007). Emergency contraception. In R. Hatcher, J. Trussell, A. Nelson, W. Cates, F. Stewart, & D. Kowal (Eds.), *Contraceptive technology* (19th ed., pp. 87–116). New York, NY: Ardent Media.

Sulak, P., Scow, R., Preece, C., Riggs, M., & Kuehl, T. (2000). Hormone withdrawal symptoms in oral contraceptive users. *Obstetrics & Gynecology, 95*, 261–266.

Trussell, J. (2007a). Choosing a contraceptive: Efficacy, safety and personal considerations. In R. Hatcher, J. Trussell, A. Nelson, W. Cates, F. Stewart, & D. Kowal (Eds.), *Contraceptive technology* (19th ed., pp. 19–48). New York, NY: Ardent Media.

Trussell, J. (2007b). Contraceptive efficacy. In R. Hatcher, J. Trussell, A. Nelson, W. Cates, F. Stewart, & D. Kowal (Eds.), *Contraceptive technology* (19th ed., pp. 747–756). New York, NY: Ardent Media.

van Heusden, A., & Fauser, B. (2002). Residual ovarian activity during oral steroid contraception. *Human Reproduction Update, 8,* 345–358.

Ventura, S., Abma, J., Mosher, W., & Henshaw, S. (2009). Estimated pregnancy rates for the United States, 1990–2005: An update. *National Vital Statistics Reports, 58*(4). Hyattsville, MD: National Center for Health Statistics.

Warner, L., & Steiner, M. (2007). Male condoms. In R. Hatcher, J. Trussell, A. Nelson, W. Cates, F. Stewart, & D. Kowal (Eds.), *Contraceptive technology* (19th ed., pp. 297–316). New York, NY: Ardent Media.

Willis, S., Kuehl, T., Spiekerman, A., & Sulak, P. (2006). Greater inhibition of the pituitary-ovarian axis in oral contraceptive regimens with a shortened hormone-free interval. *Contraception, 74,* 100–103.

Xu, J., Kochanek, K., Murphy, S., & Tejada-Vera, B. (2010). Deaths: Final data for 2007. *National Vital Statistics Reports, 58*(19). Hyattsville, MD: National Center for Health Statistics.

chapter thirteen

SEX AS A BUSINESS

CHAPTER OBJECTIVES
On completion of this chapter, students will be able to:
- discuss what encompasses the sex industry;
- list reasons why a customer goes to a prostitute;
- comprehend the ways pornography has changed throughout the years;
- describe the different types of female and male prostitutes.

ABBREVIATIONS AND ACRONYMS USED IN THIS CHAPTER
CE   common era (formerly AD)

SELLING SEX

Selling sex is a billion-dollar business. In 2006, American spent over $13 billion on X-rated printed material, videos and DVDs, live sex shows, strip clubs, adult cable shows, online pornography, and commercial telephone sex (Weitzer, 2010). Less conservative views on sexuality, less stringent laws on what is considered obscene, and the Internet have all helped to fuel this thriving enterprise. Selling sex is not only about watching a pornographic video online or purchasing the services of a prostitute, though. Buying a romance novel at a local bookstore, or lingerie at the mall, or purchasing a back massager online that will be used as a vibrator all can count as taking part in the sex industry, and thus $13 billion understates how much we are willing to pay to get it on!

Sex work refers to the exchange of sexual services, performances, or products for material compensation (Weitzer, 2010). Sex work can include direct and indirect sexual gratification. For example, prostitution and lap dancing are considered direct physical contact between buyers and sellers. Pornography, stripping, telephone sex, live sex shows, and erotic webcam performances are considered indirect sexual stimulation (Weitzer, 2010). This chapter focuses on prostitution and pornography.

HISTORICAL PERSPECTIVE ON PROSTITUTION

In many societies throughout history, women have often been confined to the home and limited in the type of occupations they could pursue (Bullough & Bullough, 1987). Women who were rejected for marriage because they were considered to have already participated in sexual activity, or for whatever reason had no home, husband, or supporting male relative had limited opportunities for financial stability. Many women were then forced to turn to prostitution to

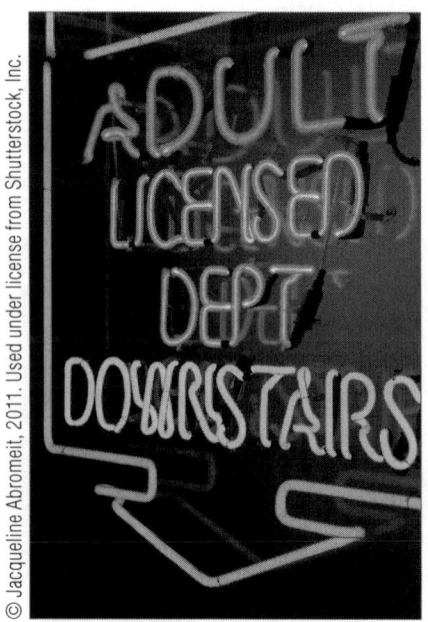
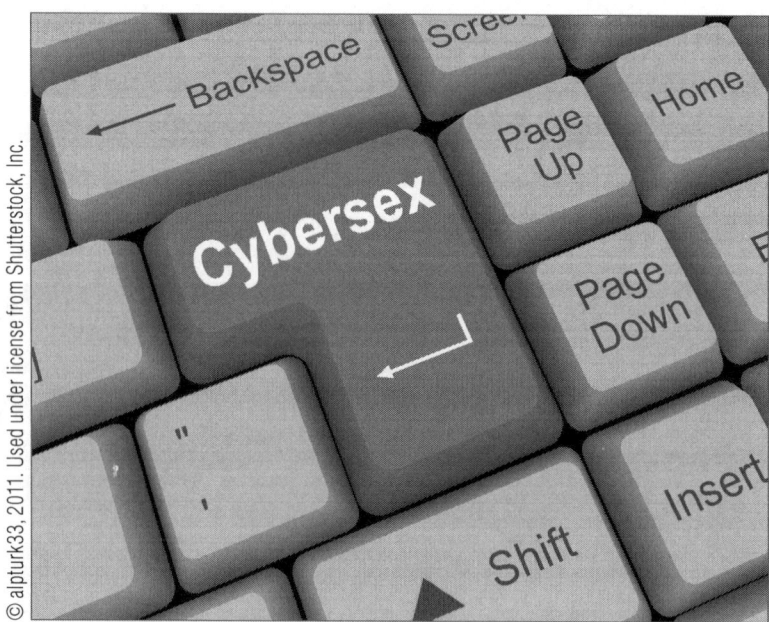

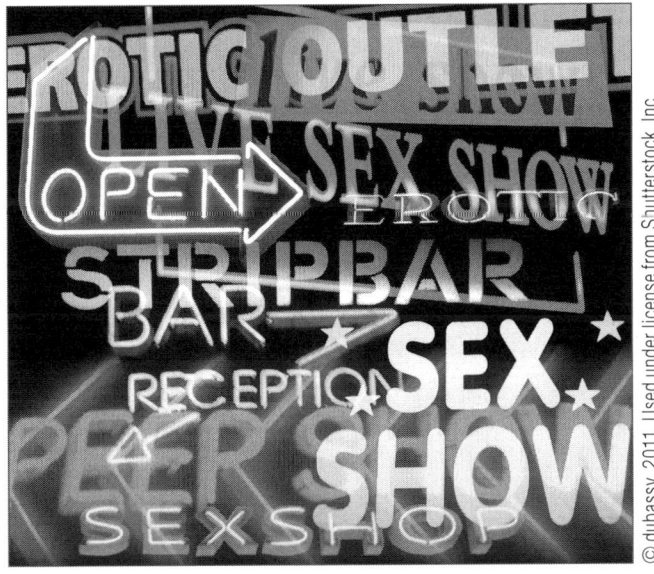 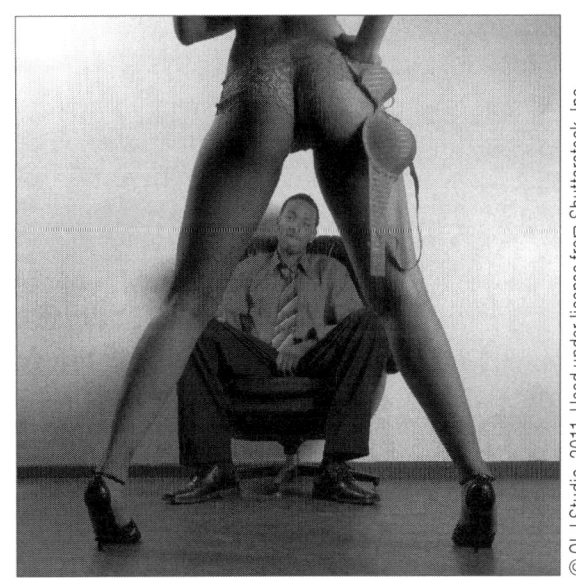

support themselves (Bullough & Bullough, 1987). Prostitution, though, is neither universal nor found in all societies (Ringdal, 2004). Yet, depending on the time and culture, commercial sex workers have either been severely stigmatized for "choosing" this profession or tolerated for providing a "necessary" sexual outlet to men (given the perception that men were "highly" sexual, but wives were not). For example, in Ancient Greece and Italy, prostitutes were valued not only for the sexual gratification they provided for men, but for their social companionship. In Medieval Europe, women who provided sexual services to men were welcomed in bathhouses. During the Victorian Era of the 1800s, prostitution was viewed as a scandalous, but necessary outlet for men (Crooks & Baur, 2011).

PROSTITUTION

How would you define prostitution? What constitutes sex for money? Does paying for dinner and then participating in sexual activity afterward refer to prostitution? Does rising up the corporate ladder by "sleeping" with one's boss smack of prostitution? How would you feel if you were sexually intimate with another person and that individual left money on the nightstand with a note that said "thank you"? Would you take that as a compliment or be ashamed and offended by it? Do you think women and men would differ in their reactions to these scenarios?

Prostitution is difficult to define (Bullough & Bullough, 1987). Is it simply sexual services for money? What if money was not negotiated, but illicit drugs were the currency? What if only mutual services were rendered in the form of bartering? What if an individual participates in sexual activity with another person because that person pays for needed expenses, like the rent, groceries, or clothing? Is that prostitution? Would your opinion differ if you thought the couple was married to each other?

Even though much of what has been discussed thus far in regard to prostitution has implied that a woman is a prostitute and the man is the customer, male prostitutes are just as prevalent as female prostitutes across the globe (Ringdal,

2004). However, the *customer* of a commercial sex worker is more likely to be a man. In the United States, these men are more likely to be white, middle-aged, middle-class, and married. Women are not very likely to purchase the sexual services of another individual. This could be because there is a societal stigma for women to do so, or because sexual partners would easily and willingly provide their sexual services to women for free. Even so, sexual tourism in which women travel for the sexual services of another is increasing around the world (Crooks & Baur, 2001).

Why do women and men become prostitutes? Most commercial sex workers feel they have no choice in life but to sell their body for the sexual gratification of others. It is not as if they fantasized about becoming a commercial sex worker when they were 10 years old. Some have been enslaved to do so, and others participate on a part-time basis (Bullough & Bullough, 1987). The main reason for their involvement in this profession is for the financial incentives. Prostitution can be broadened to include other types of commercial sex work, such as phone sex, nude dancing, erotic massage, Internet sex, and being in pornographic films (Crooks & Baur, 2011).

Why do customers of commercial sex workers look for the purchase of the sexual services of others? Is it surprising to realize that many men who seek such services are married? In 2006, ten to fifteen percent of men in Australia, England, and the United States reported purchasing sexual services from a prostitute (Weitzer, 2010). What does prostitution offer their customers? For example, purchased sexual transactions can offer the customer sexual contact. What if the individual is not currently in a sexual relationship or cannot participate in sexual activity with their current partner (due to illness, for example)? Prostitution also allows no intimacy or commitment. Most individuals seeking to purchase sexual services are only looking for the immediate sexual gratification of such a transaction and nothing else. Sexual variety can be another reason that individuals seek out commercial sex workers. Many prostitutes are more willing to participate in exotic sexual behaviors than a customer's spouse or sexual partner. Lastly, it may be more convenient for the customer, as commercial sex workers are less likely to reject an individual's proposition for sexual services for the right price.

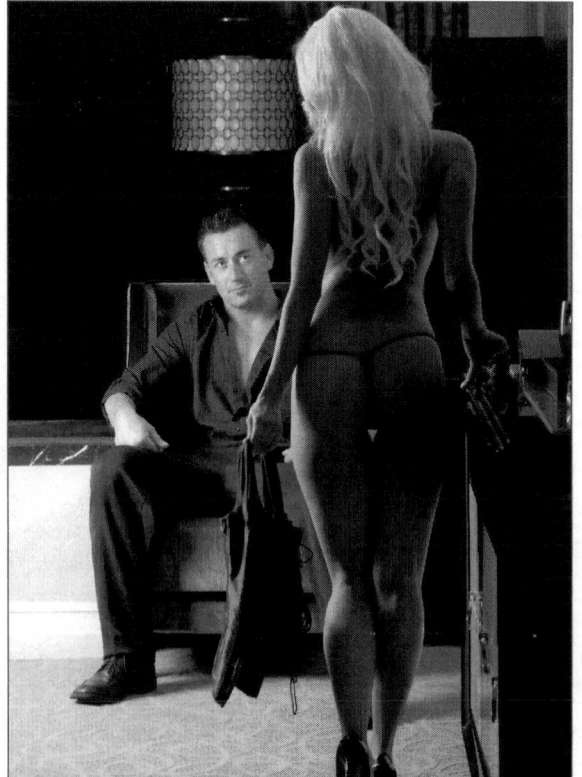

Types of Female Prostitutes

Call girls are women who offer companionship and sexual services to wealthy men (Crooks & Baur, 2011). Their services to a select few make their worth highly sought after and profitable. It is not unheard of for a call girl to make $10,000 over a weekend. Some may have a *madam*, which is usually a woman who procures young, attractive, intelligent women for men seeking discretion and particular needs

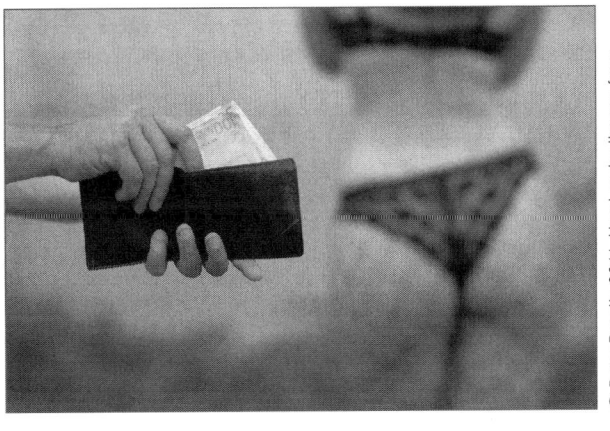 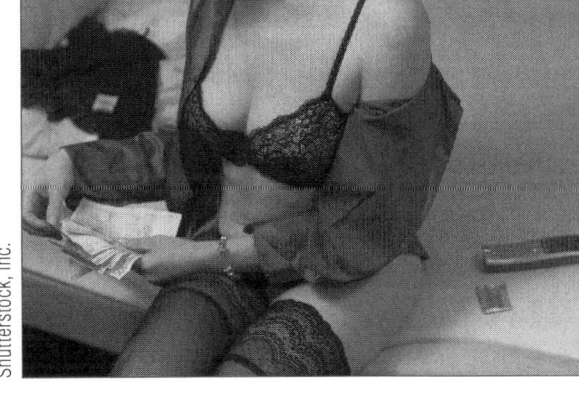

(i.e., a woman who is 5'10", who is a brunette, and can speak several languages). Call girls are often taken on business trips around the world and can be seen as trophies on the arms of older men. Of course, public discovery of a call girl can destroy a customer's family life and career, especially for those in politics.

A *brothel* is a place where commercial sex workers work in an establishment and customers come to them for their services (Crooks & Baur, 2011). Brothels are only legal in certain parts of Nevada (Las Vegas and Reno are not located in these areas). Women who work in brothels are provided 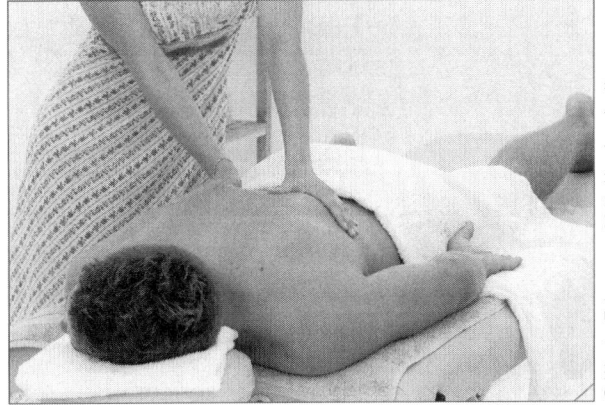 with medical services and their customers are required to wear condoms. Even though the female prostitutes in brothels are required to be tested for sexually transmitted infections frequently, their male customers are not (Bullough & Bullough, 1987).

Some *massage parlors* provide more than just back massages (Crooks & Baur, 2011). Women may be asked to perform specific sexual acts for a fee. Advertisements for such services are usually through word-of-mouth to maintain a certain level of clientele, as well as keep a low profile from law enforcement.

Streetwalker is a term for a woman who solicits customers on the street (Crooks & Baur, 2011). The sexual transaction can happen in a car, in an alley,

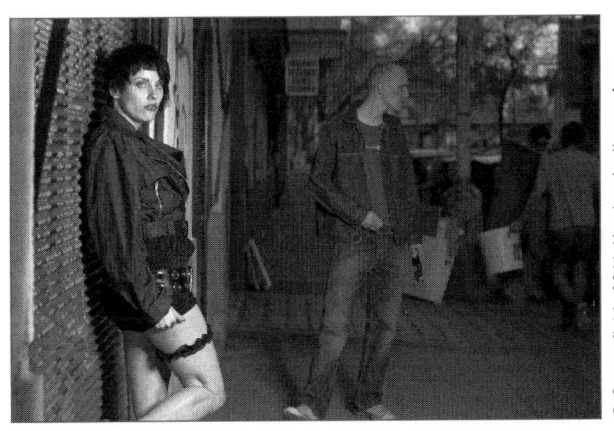 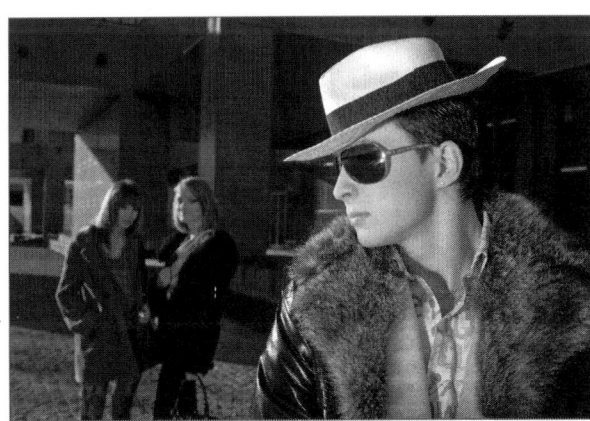

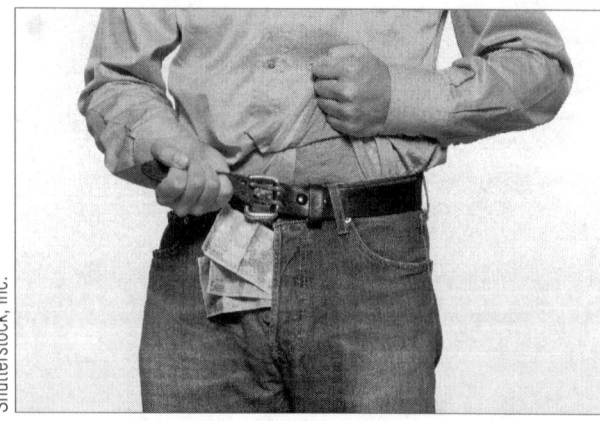

or at a "pay-by-the-hour," "no-tell" motel. Given their public visibility, it is not surprising that streetwalkers are more likely to be arrested than any other type of female prostitute. Some streetwalkers may have a *pimp*, an individual who finds customers, provides protection, or enslaves them into this profession.

Types of Male Prostitutes

Gigolos are the only known form of commercial male sex worker that caters to women (Crooks & Baur, 2011). The women may be single, married, divorced, or widowed and many are wealthy. Many women who procure the services of gigolos do so for the companionship as well as for the sexual services the men provide. It can be a profitable profession for these men.

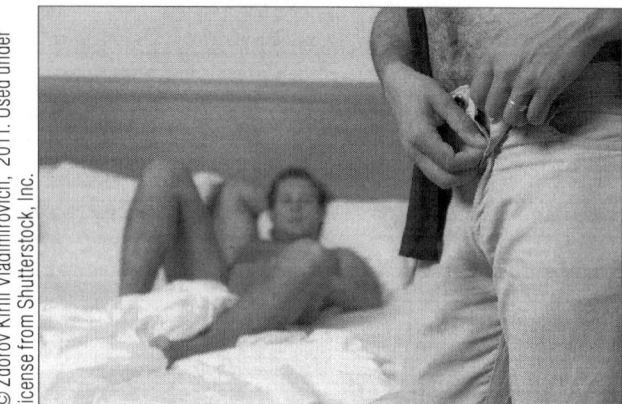

Call boys are similar to call girls. They offer companionship and sexual services to wealthy men (Crooks & Baur, 2011). Many times their discreet services are rendered only for a select few men, usually wealthy businessmen, politicians, or actors (to name a few). Even though same-sex relationships are not as stigmatized as they once were in this country, many customers do not "show off" their call boy on business trips.

Kept boys are usually young men in their early to late teens who are financially supported by an older man (Bullough & Bullough, 1987). Kept boys provide sexual services in return for lodging, food, and clothing. Many times, these young men ran away from a physically or sexually abusive household or relationship.

Hustlers are similar to streetwalkers (Crooks & Baur, 2011). These men solicit customers not only on the streets, but also in bars or in parks. The sexual transactions can occur in a bathroom, an alley, a car, or by a tree. They are more likely to be arrested than other types of male prostitutes because of their

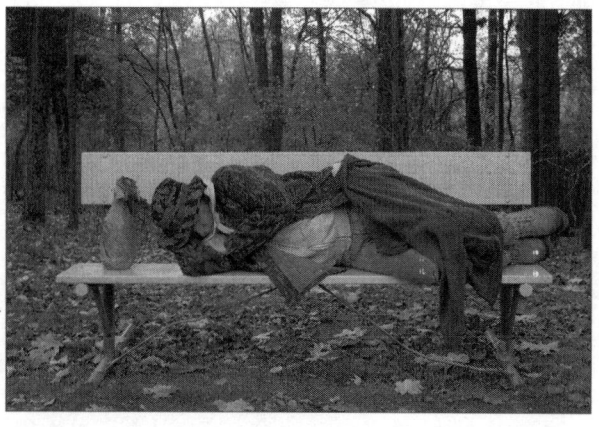
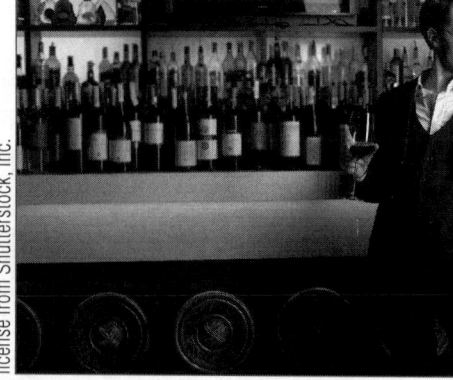

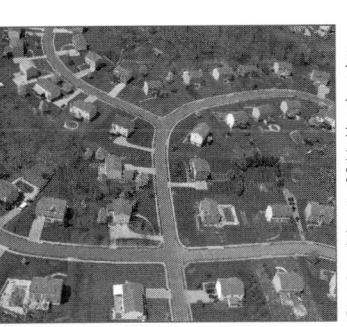
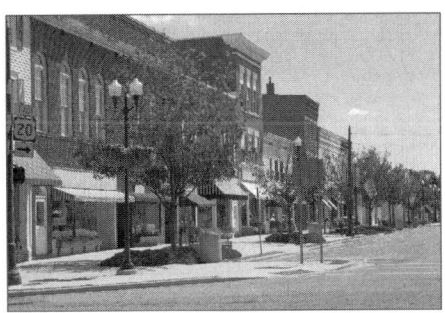

visibility. Hustler can also refer to those who make their living by selling drugs, rolling dice, etc.

Prostitution exists in the suburbs, urban cities, and rural towns. Some types of prostitutes are more visible than others, depending on the location. For example, streetwalkers are seen more often on street corners of big cities, but that doesn't mean they are not found in small towns. Do you think the majority of commercial sex workers have willingly chosen this profession or were they coerced into it? Do you think prostitution should be legalized? Do you think legalization would reduce the numbers of prostitutes or individuals who seek their sexual services, or increase the numbers?

PORNOGRAPHY

Pornography can be defined as any material that can be seen, read, or heard depicting sexual activity or genital exposure for the purpose of sexual arousal (Crooks & Baur, 2011). Such a definition can be perceived as broad and confusing at the same time. Would most women who purchase romance novels believe they are reading pornographic material? Are artwork and statues depicting naked individuals considered pornographic? Does pornography only encompass materials that society deems *unacceptable*?

Sexually explicit material has been in existence for centuries. Take for example Ancient Greek and Roman societies that decorated housewares (e.g., plates and bowls) and constructed architecture that depicted sexual themes. Also, the

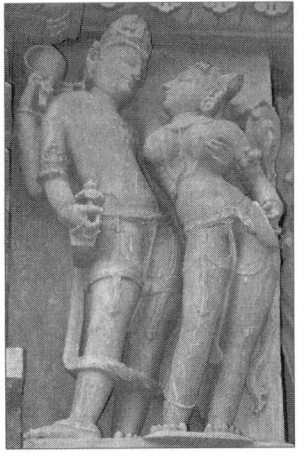
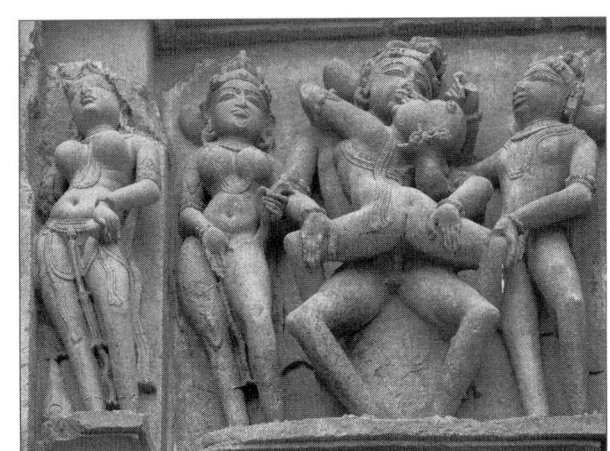

Indian love manual *Kama Sutra*, dating back to 400 CE, described specific sexual techniques that would enhance sexual pleasure and a couple's spirituality (Crooks & Baur, 2011).

In the U.S., the first published magazine to include sexually explicit imagery was *Playboy* in the 1950s. The first pornographic film that attracted mainstream audiences was *Deep Throat* in the 1970s (Crooks & Baur, 2011). Nowadays, numerous countries produce and distribute thousands of X-rated films online, as DVDs, and through pay-per-view television stations. The pornographic industry is estimated to make $10 to $20 billion a year—more than professional baseball, basketball, and football *combined* (Byassee, 2008).

Each country has its own laws that restrict the production or dissemination of sexually explicit material. Throughout U.S. history, the federal government has attempted, with little success, to undermine the production, distribution, and tolerance of pornographic material. What is considered obscene to one person may be considered erotic to another. Local governments, though, are able to restrict access to printed material that elected officials find offensive. However, it is almost impossible to restrict access to sexually material on the Internet, although some countries like China have had better success in imposing Internet restrictions than others. Pornographic material that includes children, though, is restricted around the country and in many other nations. Child pornography is not protected under the U.S. Constitution's First Amendment that guarantees freedom of speech and freedom of the press (Crooks & Baur, 2011).

The genre of sexually explicit films developed to arouse men who are attracted to women is comparable in size to production and consumption of pornographic films geared toward men attracted to men (Crooks & Baur, 2011). The sex industry produces both low-budget and well-made films for their viewers. Many films focused on arousing men (who are attracted to women) portray women in subservient positions. For instance, such films tend to show a man ejaculating on a woman's face, having numerous men penetrating any opening they can find on one woman, as well as scenes in which the woman is choked, slapped (usually on her buttocks), her hair pulled, and called demeaning names (Dines, Jensen, & Russo, 1998). There are some production companies that focus

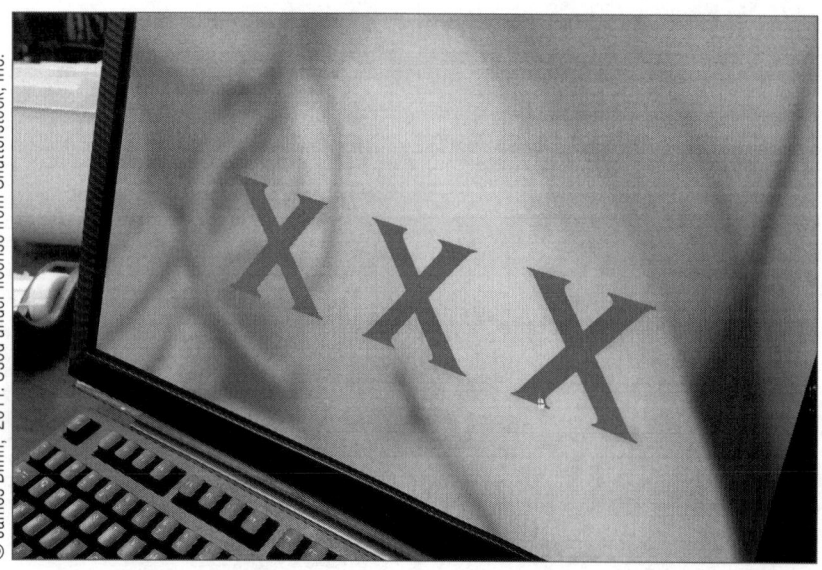
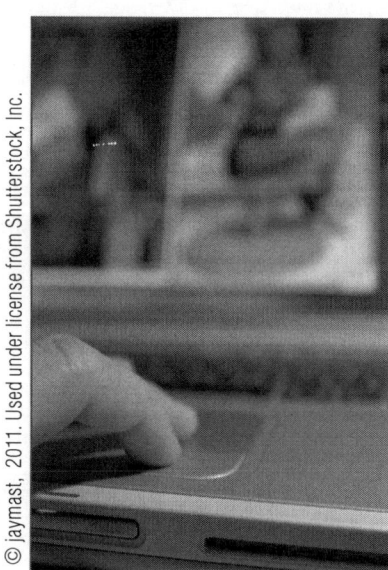

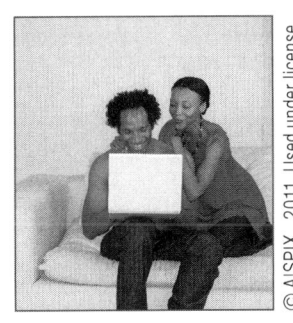 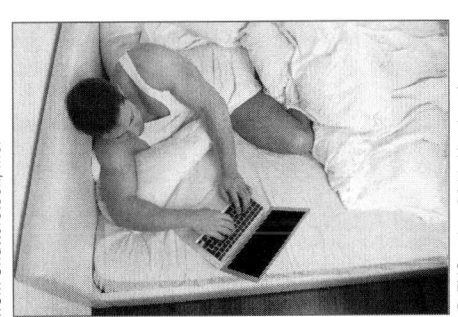 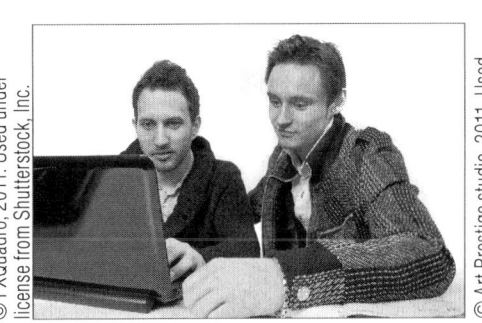

on producing films that focus on highlighting women's pleasure and assertiveness, but most films with female and male adult film stars are developed to portray men's sexual pleasure and assertiveness instead of equal sexual gratification. For example, how many films do you think exist that show men asking women to "fuck them in the ass," or enjoying a woman's ejaculation all over his face? Not too many. There are very few movies directed toward women attracted to women.

In the U.S., around 40 million people visit pornographic sites online at least once a month. Twenty-five percent of daily Internet search requests and 35 percent of all downloads are for sexually explicit material (Maltz & Maltz, 2008). Interestingly, residents from conservative U.S. states have been found to have higher rates of accessing pornography online than people who live in less conservative U.S. states (Callaway, 2009).

Reflections

Sexually explicit material can be used to enhance a couple's sex life, learn new sexual techniques, be exposed to a variety of sex acts, increase sexual arousal, or for entertainment (to name a few reasons). Yet some worry that "pornography has moved from helping couples become more sexually intimate with each other to arousing the user to have a sexual relationship *with it*" (Maltz & Matlz, 2008, p. 1).

After centuries of debate, prostitution and pornography remain contentious issues in the U.S. Society has the responsibility to protect individuals from coercion into the sex industry. But society also has the responsibility to protect and respect individuals who freely choose to participate in prostitution and pornography. Like so many other social issues discussed in previous chapters, strategies are needed to establish common ground to progress to constructive dialogue.

Critical Thinking Questions

1. Do you find prostitution demeaning or empowering? Does your answer differ for the seller or the buyer?
2. Can strippers be considered a type of prostitute?
3. Should a high-ranking individual such as a politician be forgiven by the public after being found guilty of consorting with a prostitute? Should it matter, especially if the politician was doing a fine job representing their constituents? Would it matter if they were in a committed relationship or not? Would it matter if they were hypocritically fighting to restrict prostitution?
4. What if the politician was caught purchasing sexually explicit material? Would it matter if it contained pornographic images of individuals that did not reflect the politician's sexual orientation? Would it matter if the politician was in a committed relationship or not? Would it matter if she/he was fighting to restrict pornography?
5. What cultural stereotypes about gender does pornography perpetuate?
6. To what extent should the U.S. censor pornography, if at all?
7. What would you do if your loved one was addicted to Internet porn?

How Much Do You Remember from the Chapter?

1. Which of the following *best* characterizes the type of man who would patronize a female prostitute?
    a. white, middle-aged, upper-class, married
    b. Hispanic, young, lower-class, unmarried
    c. African American, young, middle-class, married
    d. white, middle-aged, middle-class, married

2. Which of the following would *most likely* explain why women become prostitutes?
    a. financial necessity
    b. high sexual drive
    c. strong desire to please men
    d. strong desire to please themselves

(3–6) Match the type of *female* prostitute with the correct definition:

3. Call girls _____
4. Streetwalkers _____
5. Brothels _____
6. Massage parlors _____

a. require customers to use condoms
b. more likely to be arrested
c. very profitable
d. "quick service" version of a brothel

(7–10) Match the type of *male* prostitute with the correct definition:

7. Hustlers _____   a. cater only to women
8. Gigolos _____   b. very profitable
9. Kept boys _____   c. solicit customers on the street
10. Call boys _____ d. supported by an older man

Challenge Yourself!

Search online for your state's laws on prostitution or pornography. Does the severity of the punishment differ for the seller and the buyer? Does your state ban specific material considered pornographic (for example, there are some states that have banned certain magazines, like *Playboy*, or reproductive health manuals, like *Our Bodies, Ourselves*). Compare these laws with a neighboring state. How do they differ?

Websites

www.bayswan.org/index.html
Prostitutions Education Network

References

Bullough, V., & Bullough, B. (1987). *Women and prostitution: A social history*. Buffalo, NY: Prometheus Books.

Byassee, J. (2008). Not your father's pornography. *First Things: A Monthly Journal of Religion & Public Life, 179*, 15–19.

Callaway, E. (2009, February 28). *Porn in the USA: Conservatives are biggest consumers*. Retrieved from abcnews.go.com/print?id=6977202

Crooks, R., & Baur, K. (2011). *Our sexuality* (11th ed.). Belmont, CA: Wadsworth/Cengage.

Dines, G., Jensen, R., & Russo, A. (1998). *Pornography: The production and consumption of inequality*. New York, NY: Routlege.

Maltz, W., & Maltz, L. (2008). *The porn trap: The essential guide to overcoming problems caused by pornography*. New York, NY: HarperCollins Publishers.

Ringdal, N. (2004). *Love for sale: A history of prostitution*. New York, NY: Grove/Atlantic, Inc.

Weitzer, R. (2010). Sex work: Paradigms and policies. In R. Weitzer, *Sex for sale: Prostitution, pornography and the sex industry* (2nd ed., pp. 1–46). New York, NY: Routledge.

chapter fourteen

PARAPHILIAS

CHAPTER OBJECTIVES
On completion of this chapter, students will be able to:
- understand the difference between coercive and noncoercive paraphilias;
- list the treatment options available for coercive paraphilias;
- ascertain the reasons why successful treatment is low.

ABBREVIATIONS AND ACRONYMS USED IN THIS CHAPTER

APA	American Psychiatric Association
BDSM	**b**ondage, **d**iscipline, **s**ado**m**asochism
DSM-IV-TR	**D**iagnostic and **S**tatistical **M**anual of Mental Disorders (**4**th edition, **t**ext **r**evised)
S&M	**s**ado**m**asochism

THE SOCIAL CONSTRUCT OF SEXUAL INTERACTIONS

What is deemed acceptable and unacceptable sexual behavior has varied considerably throughout history and has been influenced by such socially constructed factors as gender, culture, politics, and religion (Philaretou, Phellas, & Karayianni, 2006). Before Kinsey's publications on the sexual activity of men and women (Kinsey, Pomeroy, & Martin, 1948; Kinsey, Pomeroy, Martin, & Gebhard, 1953), the general viewpoints on individual sexual interactions were conservative. For example, it was commonly believed that most women and men waited for coitus until marriage and usually only for reproduction, women did not crave sexual activity, same-sex sexual intimacy occurred between a small minority of people, and most people (regardless of age, sex, and marital status) did not masturbate. Thus, at one time, participating in coitus outside of marriage would have been considered immoral, masturbation would have been deemed a deviant act, and individuals attracted to the same sex would have been considered mentally unstable. The *Kinsey Reports*, along with the work by Masters and Johnson (1966) and others, refuted each of these viewpoints and influenced more progressive social and cultural values related to sexuality in the U.S. and Europe (Roach, 2008). That is not to say that certain other sexual behaviors are no longer viewed as immoral, deviant, or unhealthy by some individuals and in a few countries (especially in Africa, Asia, and the Middle East), because they continue to be perceived as such. Do you think there are behaviors that, regardless of where you are in the world, would probably be considered strange, weird, or unacceptable forms of sexual interaction by the general population? What would you deem strange, weird, or unacceptable and why?

PARAPHILIA

Paraphilia (pair-uh-FILL-ee-uh), or atypical sexual behavior, can be defined as uncommon, extreme types of sexual expression. The *Merriam-Webster Collegiate Dictionary* (2008) defines paraphilia as a pattern of recurring mental imagery or behavior that is sexually arousing and involves unusual and socially unacceptable sexual practices. Many of these behaviors are outside what our society identifies as normative (i.e., they are not considered very common in the general population). The term was coined by Wilhelm Stekel in the 1920s (Stekel, 1930).

According to the American Psychiatric Association (APA, 2000), paraphilias can be expressed as sexual urges, fantasies, or behaviors. For example, someone might have an urge to peek into someone's window to see if anyone is naked. Or someone might fantasize about participating in sexual activity with a corpse. Or someone might urinate in a sexual partner's mouth for sexual pleasure. Paraphilias fall on a continuum, ranging from those who exhibit a fleeting thought or fantasy of an atypical behavior, to others for whom the paraphilic acts have consumed their lives (Hanson, 2010). It is common for those who engage in one type of paraphilic behavior to report participating in other atypical sexual behaviors as well (Heil & English, 2009).

The latest edition of the *Diagnostic and Statistical Manual of Mental Disorders* (DSM-IV-TR) includes eight paraphilias, each with its own category for diagnosis (APA, 2000):

Table 14.1 PARAPHILIAS INCLUDED IN THE DSM-IV-TR

Name	Definition
exhibitionism	aroused by exposure of one's genitals to an unsuspecting person
fetishism	aroused by an inanimate object
frotteurism	aroused by touching or rubbing one's genitals against strangers
pedophilia*	aroused by sexual contact with children
sexual masochism	consenting to receiving pain for sexual arousal
sexual sadism	aroused by inflicting pain on a consenting or nonconsenting individual
transvestic fetishism*	aroused by dressing as the other gender
voyeurism	aroused by secretly watching others in the nude or participating in sexual activity

* Not discussed in this chapter

The DSM-IV-TR also includes eight other paraphilias, listed in Table 14.2, that do not meet the criteria for any of the above-mentioned atypical sexual behaviors:

Table 14.2 PARAPHILIAS THAT DO NOT MEET THE CRITERIA IN TABLE 14.1, BUT ARE INCLUDED IN THE DSM-IV-TR

Name	Definition
coprophilia	aroused by feces
klismaphilia*	aroused by enemas
necrophilia	aroused by corpses
telephone scatologia*	aroused by obscene phone calls
partialism	aroused by exclusive focus on one part of the body
urophilia	aroused by urine
vomerophilia	aroused by vomit
zoophilia	aroused by animals

* Not discussed in this chapter

In an effort to decrease the social stigma attached to certain atypical sexual behaviors, Sweden removed transvestic fetishism, fetishism, and sadomasochism from its official list of mental disorders in 2008 (Kruger, 2010).

The majority of the paraphilias are found mostly in men (Lowenstein, 2002). It is not entirely known why that is the case. It could be because men are more often apprehended or caught during the behavior by police, family, friends, or strangers than women. It could also be that women are able to conceal their paraphilias more successfully than men.

NONCOERCIVE PARAPHILIAS VS. COERCIVE PARAPHILIAS

People who participate in noncoercive paraphilias with someone else need that other person to provide consent to participate (APA, 2000). Research has found that many individuals who consent to participate in an atypical sexual behavior do not experience distress or endure significant psychosocial harm (Richters, de Visser, Rissel, Grulich, & Smith, 2008). People who participate in coercive paraphilias purposely do not seek consent. Part of the arousal is to deceive or cause (physical, mental, emotional) harm to others (APA, 2000). There are numerous noncoercive and coercive paraphilias, but only eight noncoercive paraphilias and five coercive paraphilias are discussed in this chapter (review *Art and Popular Culture Encyclopedia*, 2009 for a full list).

NONCOERCIVE PARAPHILIAS

Fetish

An individual with a *fetish* (FET-ish) is aroused by an inanimate object (APA, 2000). Objects that seem to be popular are women's underwear, silk sheets, shoes (like stiletto shoes), and/or rubber boots. Do not be alarmed if you are sexually aroused by any of the items listed above. To some degree, many individuals have a fetish. The difference is that someone with a *true* fetish *prefers* the object over human contact (Lowenstein, 2002).

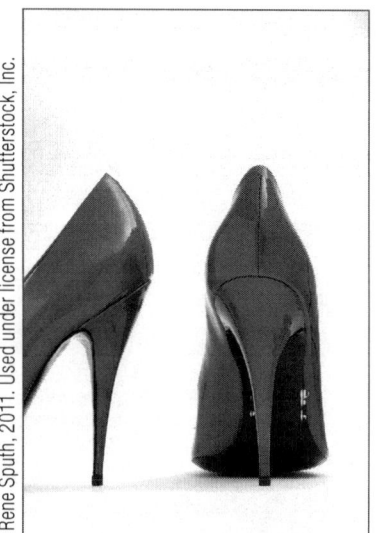

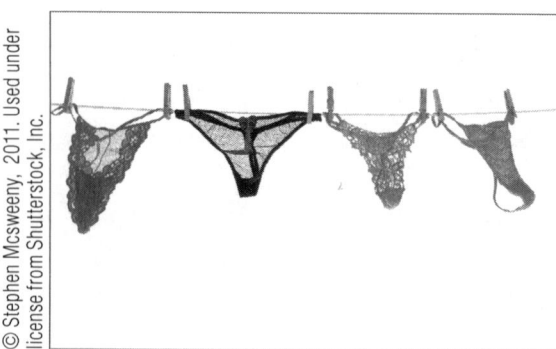

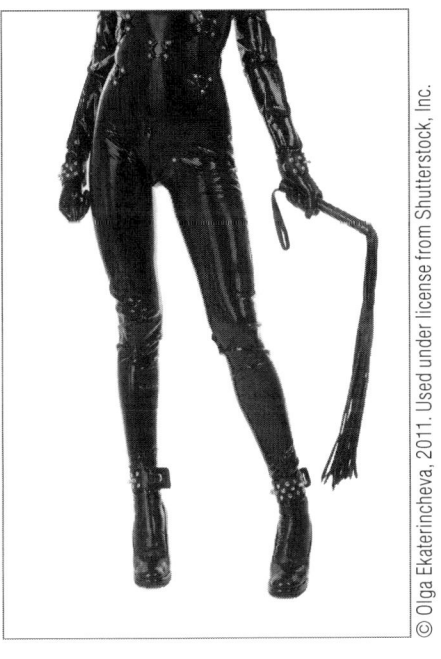
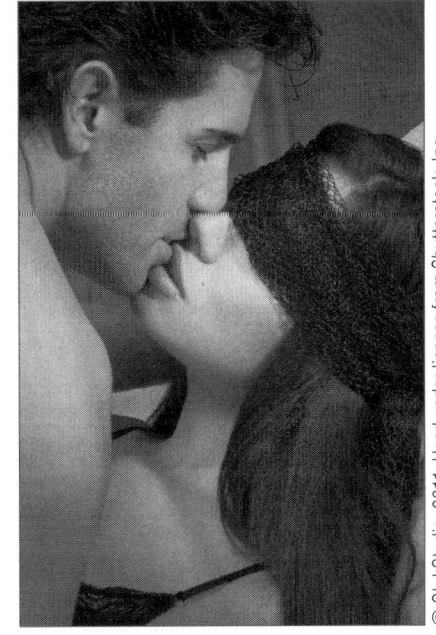

Sadomasochism

Sadomasochism (SAY-doh-ma-suh-kis-um), also known as *S&M* and *bondage, discipline, sadomasochism* (BDSM), can be defined as including "all sexual identities and practices involving pain play, bondage, dominance and submission and erotic power exchange" (Langdridge & Barker, 2007, p. 6). The term *pain* does not have to be taken literally, even though some individuals who participate in S&M want to experience physical or emotional pain. There are individuals who would prefer to be "hit" with a feather than with a whip, for example.

Sadomasochism is considered two distinct paraphilias that are similar and overlap one another. A *sexual sadist* is someone who consents to inflict pain for sexual arousal on a consenting individual or individuals. Sexual sadism can also be categorized as a coercive paraphilia if an individual intentionally inflicts psychological or physical suffering on a nonconsenting partner to produce sexual excitement (APA, 2000). A *sexual masochist* is someone who consents to receive pain for sexual arousal from someone who consents to inflict it (APA, 2000). Table 14.3 includes a list of possible BDSM behaviors (Williams, 2006).

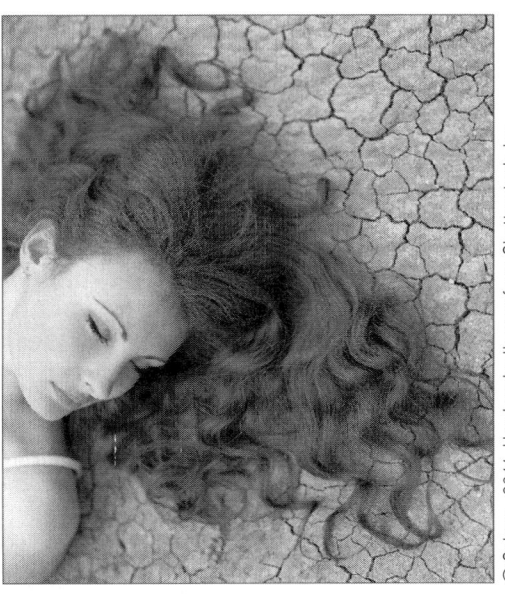

Partialism

Many individuals prefer a certain nongenital body part to look a certain way on a potential sexual partner. But in *partialism*, an individual *needs* a particular nongenital body part to look a specific way to become sexually aroused (Lowenstein, 2002). Common body parts are hair (length, color, or style), female breasts (cup size and/or size of the areola), or feet (shoe size and/or cleanliness of toes).

Chapter Fourteen **263**

Table 14.3 A SAMPLING OF BEHAVIORS OFTEN ASSOCIATED WITH BDSM

Anal sex

Bondage/restraints

Body suspension

Breath play (erotic asphyxia or hypoxyphilia)

Caning (hitting with a thin stick)

Catheters

Clothespins and clamps (attached to various parts of the body)

Cockbinding

Conventional sex toys (vibrators)

Cuttings (superficial)

Dildos

Electrical play (with medical TENS unit or violet wand)

Face slapping/humiliation

Fire play (fire quickly applied via alcohol solution and extinguished on bare skin)

Fisting (careful insertion of a hand into the vagina or anus)

Flogging/whipping

Gags

Hoods

Hot wax (dripped on skin)

Ice

Knife play (used for surface play to evoke fear, excitement)

Mummification or immobilization

Needle play (carefully inserted under the outer layers of skin)/piercings

Role play (teacher–student, doctor–patient, police–criminal, etc.)

Spanking

Skin branding

Vaginal sex

Weights (attached to piercings, nipples, or genitalia

Source: Williams, D. (2006). Different (painful!) strokes for different folks: A general overview of sexual sadomasochism (SM) and its diversity, *Sexual Addiction & Compulsivity*, 13, 333–346.

Coprophilia

There are certain bodily fluids that individuals may find arousing during sexual activity, such as seminal and vaginal fluids. Some people like the taste of them, the smell of them, or how they feel on their body. Other bodily fluids are usually not associated with sexual activity or arousal, but a paraphilia specific to being sexually aroused by feces (solid waste that is expelled through the anus) is called *coprophilia* (kah-pruh-FILL-ee-uh). Sexual gratification is achieved by watching someone defecate on themselves, defecate on someone else, or having someone defecate on them (Crooks & Baur, 2011)

Urophilia

There seems to be some acceptability of urinating on a consenting sexual partner or consenting to being urinated on by a sexual partner when a couple is in the shower. Even though when someone urinates on a sexual partner in the shower, it's usually not performed to elicit sexual excitement in either partner. However, for individuals who exhibit *urophilia* (yoo-roh-FILL-ee-uh), urinating on a consenting sexual partner, or giving consent to a partner to urinate on them (and not necessarily in a shower) is sexually arousing to them (Crooks & Baur, 2011).

Vomerophilia

Another bodily fluid that has been found to sexually arouse some individuals is vomit. Vomit can be defined as the forceful involuntary expulsion of the contents of one's stomach through the mouth (*Merriam-Webster Collegiate Dictionary*, 2008). *Vomerophilia* (also known as *emetophilia*) can be defined as being sexually aroused by vomit (*Art and Popular Culture Encyclopedia*, 2009). The individual consents to be vomited on or to vomit on a consenting sexual partner for sexual arousal.

Autoerotic Asphyxiophilia

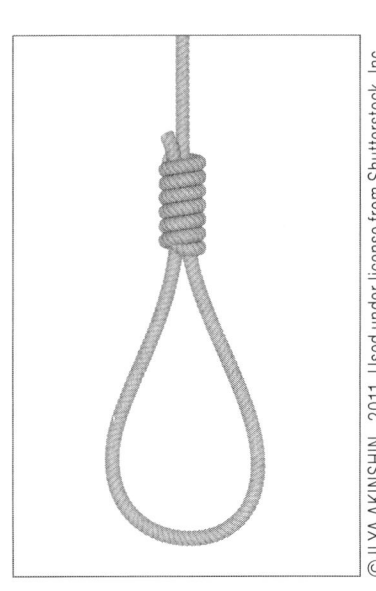

According to the *Urban Dictionary* (2011), *autoerotic asphyxiophilia* (uh-fix-uh-FILL-ee-uh) is defined as experiencing oxygen deprivation during sexual stimulation to heighten the pleasurable sensations during orgasm. Other words used to describe this behavior are *scarfing*, *breath control play*, and *terminal sex* (Jenkins, 2000). Reducing the amount of oxygen to the brain is believed to enhance masturbation sensations and orgasm intensity by producing more endorphins as the body approaches the state of asphyxia, along with light-headedness and exhilaration (Resnik, 1972).

Oxygen deprivation can be achieved by strangulation, either by hanging oneself, tying a cord, wire, or necktie around the neck, or placing a plastic bag over the head (to name a few procedures). This behavior has a high likelihood of death or serious injury. Hundreds of young adult males in the United States are believed to die from autoerotic asphyxiophilia every year (Jenkins, 2000).

COERCIVE PARAPHILIAS

Voyeurism

Voyeurism (voi-yur-IH-zum) can be defined as experiencing sexual arousal through secretly watching others in the nude or participating in sexual activity (APA, 2000). Voyeuristic behaviors are among the most common of potentially law-breaking sexual behaviors (Långström & Seto, 2006). The voyeur may go to great lengths to intrude on another's privacy, by looking through strangers' windows in different neighborhoods, or if in a high rise building, using a telescope to look through other windows in an adjoining building. Many times the voyeur may masturbate while watching an unsuspecting person or couple, especially if the risk of discovery is high (Crooks & Baur, 2011).

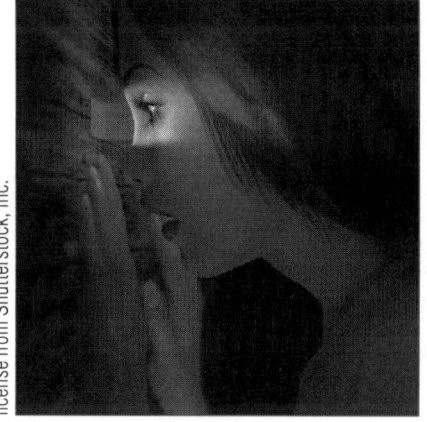

Exhibitionism

In exhibitionism, individuals expose their genitals to strangers for sexual arousal (Långström, 2010). After an encounter, they masturbate fixating on the stranger's reaction—which is usually shock or horror. Women or girls are usually the target and the event takes place in locations where there would be an easy escape for the exhibitionist. Exhibitionistic behavior is the second most common of potentially law-breaking sexual behaviors (Långström & Seto, 2006).

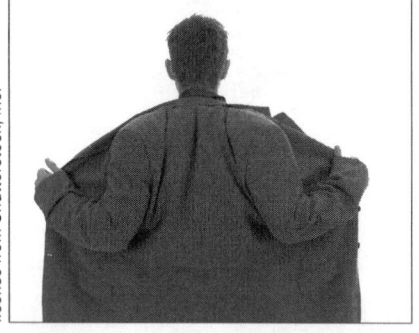

Frotteurism

The French verb *frotter* means to rub or to create friction (Långström, 2010). Thus, in *frotteurism* (frah-toor-IH-zum), individuals obtain sexual gratification by touching or rubbing their genitals against strangers, usually women or girls (APA, 2000). This can frequently occur in locations with a lot of people, like crowded subway trains or elevators.

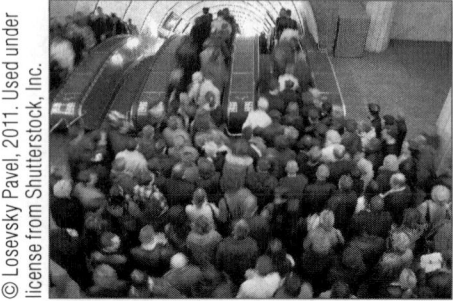

Necrophilia

Necrophilia (ne-kruh-FILL-ee-uh) is a rare paraphilia in which an individual is sexually aroused by sexual contact with a corpse (APA, 2000). Most people would consider this behavior incomprehensible and 40 of the 50 U.S. states have some type of law that defines what constitutes illegal actions with human corpses (Troyer, 2008). According to Troyer (2008), only four states (Arizona, Georgia, Hawaii, and Rhode Island) explicitly use the word necrophilia in their statutory code.

Individuals who exhibit necrophilic behaviors are believed to have a motive to attempt to gain possession of an unresisting or nonrejecting partner. They can obtain a corpse for sexual pleasure, murder someone for their body, or envision the acts but not act on them. Crooks and Baur (2011) also mention individuals procuring services of a prostitute where she or he will act like a corpse for the customer's sexual gratification.

Zoophilia

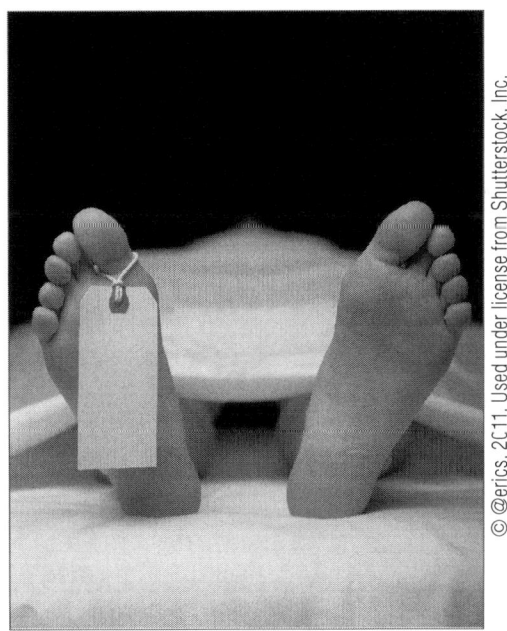

Zoophilia (zoh-oh-FILL-ee-uh), also known as *bestiality*, can be defined as having sexual contact with an animal (APA, 2000). Throughout history, sexual acts with animals have been suggested in cave drawings, ancient Egyptian artifacts, and Greek and Roman mythology (Peretti & Rowan, 1982). Even so, most religious doctrines condoned severe punishment for such indiscretions. For example, in the late 1200s, anyone convicted of engaging in bestiality was burned to death (Hensley, Tallichet, & Dutkiewicz, 2010). Individuals who exhibit zoophilic behaviors may engage in penile-vaginal/penile-anal intercourse, and/or orally stimulate the genitals of the animal, and/or have their genitals orally stimulated by the animal (Miletski, 2002). The animals most frequently involved in sexual contact with humans are cats, dogs, donkeys, ducks, geese, goats, and sheep (Crooks & Baur, 2011).

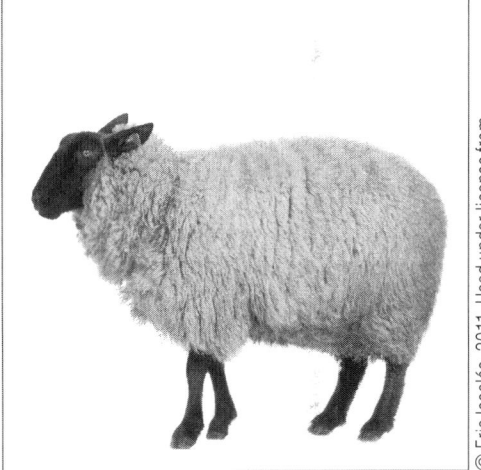

LOW TREATMENT RATE

Few individuals who engage in paraphilic behaviors voluntarily seek treatment (Garcia & Thibaut, 2011). Especially with illicit, atypical sexual behaviors, individuals may feel shame, experience social stigma, and face negative legal consequences if they disclose to family and friends or try to seek help (Långström, 2010). Rarely do people who exhibit paraphilias acknowledge the need for change, especially if they feel they are not harming anyone or they don't care if they are causing harm to others or themselves. Moreover, the behaviors can be highly reinforcing given the immediate sexual gratification some induce (Lussier & Piché, 2008), as well as the excitement that many acts can elicit, especially if there is a risk of danger to oneself or to others. Also, many individuals who exhibit paraphilias perceive that they lack control in stopping their behavior and do not believe intervention can help them.

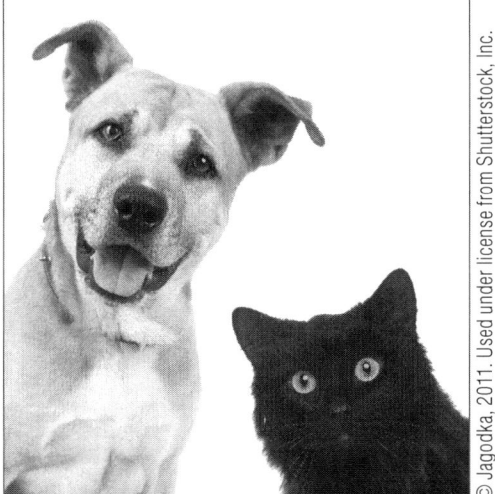

SUCCESSFUL TREATMENTS

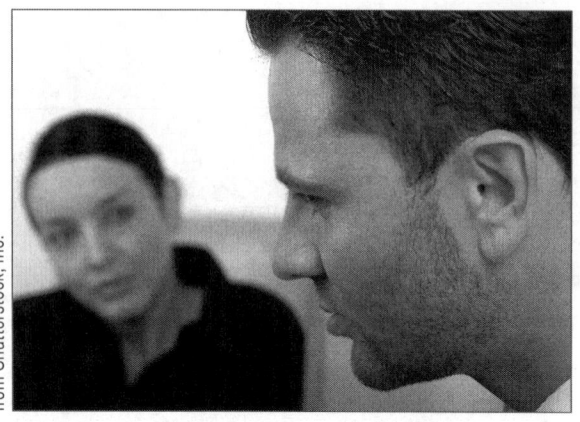

There are interventions that have been successful in treating individuals who exhibit paraphilias. Even though some individuals seek treatment on their own, most seem to be made to participate in the intervention by their family or the court system. Most research on paraphilias and ways to reduce their incidence have been conducted on males. Currently, with behavioral techniques developed to redirect what sexually arouses males (i.e., orgasmic reconditioning), exhibiting various paraphilias have been successful (Plaud & Martini, 1999). The combination of psychotherapy and medication is associated with better results when compared to either approach alone. It is also recommended that a minimal duration of treatment of three to five years be given for those exhibiting severe paraphilia with a high risk of sexual violence (Garcia & Thibaut, 2011). Social skills training is also offered to individuals who have difficulty in obtaining and maintaining interpersonal relationships and resort to paraphilic behaviors (like exhibitionism, voyeurism, or frotteurism) for "companionship."

Reflections

Few topics seem to elicit such varied emotional responses as the subject of paraphilias. Even so, certain behaviors that were once considered unacceptable (such as oral sex, same-sex sexual contact, and nonmarital sexual noncontact) no longer provoke negative reactions as much as they once did. What atypical sexual behaviors evoked strong negative emotions in you? Which ones were not bothersome at all? And which ones generated positive feelings?

Critical Thinking Questions

1. What sexual behaviors do you think your parents' and grandparents' generations did not find acceptable, but your generation does? What factors in society do you think influenced how we perceive certain sexual acts?

2. Why do you think that some states in the U.S. do not have a law against necrophilia? Why do you think some states have laws that are vague in defining what constitutes sexual contact with a corpse?

3. Do you believe the U.S. should remove certain paraphilias from its list of mental disorders like Sweden did in 2008? If so, which ones do you think should be removed and why? If not, what reasons would you give for keeping the list of paraphilias identified as mental disorders the same?

How Much Do You Remember from the Chapter?

1. Which paraphilia is considered *coercive*?
   a. partialism
   b. sexual masochist
   c. necrophilia
   d. fetishism

2. Which paraphilia is considered *noncoercive*?
   a. zoophilia
   b. vomerophilia
   c. exhibitionism
   d. voyeurism

3. Which paraphilia is considered *coercive*?
   a. urophilia
   b. autoerotic asphyxiophilia
   c. frotteurism
   d. coprophilia

4. Which paraphilia is considered *noncoercive*?
   a. necrophilia
   b. autoerotic asphyxiophilia
   c. frotteurism
   d. zoophilia

5. Which treatment option below was not discussed in the chapter as a successful treatment available for decreasing participation in atypical sexual behaviors?
   a. orgasmic reconditioning
   b. group therapy with individuals who vary in their paraphilias
   c. social skills training
   d. drug treatment with therapy

Challenge Yourself!

(1–16) • Match the paraphilia with its definition:

1. Urophilia _____
2. Voyeurism _____
3. Vomerophilia _____
4. Zoophilia _____
5. Partialism _____
6. Exhibitionism _____
7. Sexual masochist _____
8. Frotteurism _____
9. Coprophilia _____
10. Autoerotic asphyxiophilia _____
11. Necrophilia _____
12. Sexual sadist _____

a. aroused by oxygen deprivation
b. aroused by viewing or having sex with a corpse
c. aroused by inflicting pain
d. aroused by watching others nude
e. aroused by having sex with animals
f. aroused by receiving pain
g. aroused by a particular body part
h. aroused by contact with feces
i. aroused by contact with urine
j. aroused by rubbing against an nonconsenting individual
k. aroused by vomit
l. aroused by exposing genitals to strangers

Websites

www.aasect.org/
American Association of Sexuality Educators, Counselors and Therapists

www.psych.org/
American Psychiatric Association

www.sexscience.org/
Society for the Scientific Study of Sexuality

References

American Psychiatric Association. (APA). (2000). *Diagnostic and statistical manual of mental disorders—text revision* (4th ed.). Washington, DC: Author.

Art and Popular Culture Encyclopedia. (2009). *List of paraphilias*. Retrieved from www.artandpopularculture.com/List_of_paraphilias

Crooks, R., & Baur, K. (2011). *Our sexuality* (11th ed.). Belmont, CA: Wadsworth/Cengage Learning.

Garcia, F., & Thibaut, F. (2011). Current concepts in the pharmacotherapy of paraphilias. *Drugs, 71*(6), 771–790.

Hanson, R. (2010). Dimensional measurement of sexual deviance. *Archives of Sexual Behavior, 39*, 401–404.

Heil, P., & English, K. (2009). Sex offender polygraph testing in the United States: Trends and consequences. In D. Wilcox (Ed.), *The use of the polygraph in assessing, treating, and supervising sex offenders: A practitioner's guide* (pp. 181–216). Chichester, UK: Wiley.

Hensley, C., Tallichet, S., & Dutkiewicz, E. (2010). Childhood bestiality: A potential precursor to adult interpersonal violence. *Journal of Interpersonal Violence, 25*, 557–567.

Jenkins, A. (2000). When self-pleasuring becomes self-destruction: Autoerotic asphyxiation paraphilia. *International Electronic Journal of Health Education, 3*(3), 208–216.

Kinsey, A., Pomeroy, W., & Martin, C. (1948). *The sexual behavior of the human male*. Bloomington, IN: Indiana University Press.

Kinsey, A., Pomeroy, W., Martin, C., & Gebhard, P. (1953). *The sexual behavior of the human female*. Bloomington, IN: Indiana University Press.

Krueger, R. (2010). The DSM diagnostic criteria for sexual sadism. *Archives of Sexual Behavior, 39*, 325–345.

Langdridge, D., & Barker, M. (2007). *Safe, sane and consensual: Contemporary perspectives on sadomasochism*. Basingstoke, UK: Palgrave Macmillan.

Långström, N. (2010). The DSM diagnostic criteria for exhibitionism, voyeurism, and frotteurism. *Archives of Sexual Behavior, 39*, 317–324.

Långström, N., & Seto, M. (2006). Exhibitionistic and voyeuristic behavior in a Swedish national population survey. *Archives of Sexual Behavior, 35*, 427–435.

Lowenstein, L. (2002). Fetishes and their associated behavior. *Sexuality & Disability, 20*, 135–147.

Lussier, P., & Piché, L. (2008). Frotteurism: Psychopathology and theory. In D. Laws & W. O'Donohue (Eds.), *Sexual deviance: Theory, assessment, and treatment* (2nd ed., pp 131–149). New York, NY: Guilford Press.

Masters, W., & Johnson, V. (1966). *Human sexual response*. Boston, MA: Little Brown

Merriam-Webster. (2008). *Merriam-Webster's Collegiate Dictionary* (11th ed.). Springfield, MA: Merriam-Webster.

Miletski, H. (2002). *Understanding bestiality and zoophilia*. Bethesda, MD: East-West Publishing.

Peretti, P., & Rowan, M. (1982). Variables associated with male and female chronic zoophilia. *Social Behavior & Personality, 10*(1), 83–87.

Philaretou, A., Phellas, C., & Karayianni, A. (2006). *Sexual interactions: The social construction of atypical sexual behaviors*. Boca Raton, FL: Universal Publishers.

Plaud, J., & Martini, R. (1999). The respondent conditioning of male sexual arousal. *Behavior Modification, 23*, 254–268.

Resnik, H. (1972). Eroticized repetitive hangings: A form of self-destructive behavior. *American Journal of Psychotherapy, 26*, 4–21.

Richters, J., de Visser, R., Rissel, C., Grulich, A., & Smith, A. (2008). Demographic and psychosocial features of participants in bondage and discipline, 'sadomasochism' or dominance and submission (BDSM): Data from a national survey. *Journal of Sexual Medicine, 7*, 1660–1668.

Roach, M. (2008). *Bonk: The curious coupling of science and sex*. New York, NY: W. W. Norton & Company.

Stekel, W. (1930). *Sexual aberrations: The phenomenon of fetishism in relation to sex, disorders of the instincts and emotions the parapathiac disorders*. New York, NY: Liveright Publishing.

Troyer, J. (2008). Abuse of a corpse: A brief history and re-theorization of necrophilia laws in the USA. *Mortality, 13*(2), 132–152.

Urban Dictionary. (2011). *Auto erotic asphyxiation*. Retrieved from www.urbandictionary.com/define.php?term=erotic%20asphyxiation

Williams, D. (2006). Different (painful!) strokes for different folks: A general overview of sexual sadomasochism (SM) and its diversity. *Sexual Addiction & Compulsivity, 13*, 333–346.